GASTROENTEROLOGY and HEPATOLOGY
A CLINICAL HANDBOOK

EDITORS

Nicholas J Talley
MD, PhD, MMedSci (Epi), FRACP, FRCP (London), FRCP (Edin), FAFPHM, FACP, FACG, AGAF

Professor of Medicine, Mayo Clinic College of Medicine; Chair, Department of Internal Medicine, Mayo Clinic, Jacksonville, FL; Consultant Gastroenterologist, Mayo Clinic Jacksonville, FL, USA

Isidor Segal
MBBCh, PhD, FRACP, FRCP (London), AGAF

Emeritus Professor (University of Witwatersrand, Johannesburg), Gastroenterology Department, Prince of Wales Hospital, Sydney, NSW

Martin D Weltman
MBBCh, PhD, FRACP, FAChAM

Associate Professor of Medicine, University of Sydney, NSW; Senior Staff Specialist Gastroenterologist and Head of Department of Gastroenterology and Hepatology, Nepean Hospital, NSW; Clinical Director, Drug and Alcohol Services, Sydney West Area Health Service, NSW

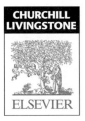

CHURCHILL LIVINGSTONE

ELSEVIER

Sydney Edinburgh London New York Philadelphia St Louis Toronto

ELSEVIER

Churchill Livingstone
is an imprint of Elsevier

Elsevier Australia
(a division of Reed International Books Australia Pty Ltd)
30–52 Smidmore Street, Marrickville, NSW 2204
ACN 001 002 357

National Library of Australia Cataloguing-in-Publication Data

---

Talley, Nicholas Joseph.
    Gastroenterology and hepatology : a clinical handbook.

    Bibliography.
    Includes index.
    ISBN 978-0-7295-3775-9 (pbk.).

    1. Gastroenterology - Handbooks, manuals, etc. I. Segal,
    Isidor. II. Weltman, Martin D. III. Title.

    616.3

Publishing Editor: Sophie Kaliniecki
Publishing Services Manager: Helena Klijn
Edited by Deborah McRitchie
Proofread by Tim Learner
Design and typesetting by DiZign
Index by Merrall-Ross International
Printed by Ligare

Printed using vegetable-based inks on paper manufactured from sustainable forests

ae, bett

GASTROENTEROLOGY
and HEPATOLOGY

A CLINICAL HANDBOOK

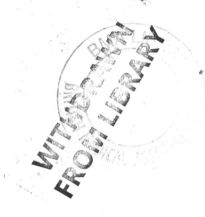

Please note that some drugs
referred to in this text may
not be available in Australia.

CONTENTS

Hepatology

FOREWORD 1

With the increasing use of internet facilities and web-based educational programs, such as www.UpToDate.com, the role of print texts is changing. Large, comprehensive and authoritative text books such as *Harrison's Principles of Internal Medicine* will continue to have a role in medical education, but smaller more specialised books will probably be less commonly used. There remains a place, however, for ready references that can be available at the bedside and in clinics.

In this 'pocket' volume, Professors Talley, Segal and Weltman have produced one such aid. This book provides the essentials of gastroenterology and hepatology in an easily accessible form, while focusing primarily on the disorders commonly encountered in wards and clinics. A notable feature that should ensure the book finds a niche in clinical practice is the sharp focus on clinical problems as they confront the internist or student.

Thus, in contrast to the usual format of clinical textbooks, we find chapters devoted specifically to common symptoms and signs that lead patients to consult their practitioner. Examples include, inter alia, sore mouth, anal pain, rectal bleeding, obesity and abnormal liver function tests, liver disorders in pregnancy and a family history of liver disease.

This novel approach to medical education at the bedside or in the clinic should prove popular with students and staff at various levels and we can anticipate regular updates. A comprehensive index adds to the practicability and appeal of this innovative book.

Lawrie W Powell AC, MD, PhD, FRCP, FRACP
Professor Emeritus of Medicine
The University of Queensland
Director of Research, Royal Brisbane and Women's Hospital
Brisbane, Australia

FOREWORD 2

What, another gastroenterology book? How can we justify the appearance of another title in this field? To provide an adequate response to these questions, one must come up with some solid evidence to indicate that this new kid on a congested block is different and differentiated from the rest. I believe that this 'pocket' text succeeds admirably in this regard. It, firstly, represents a welcome return to the *vade mecum* format that was so popular in the past and has become a favourite of our harried and harassed juniors yet again. There is a lot of information out there: gastroenterology and hepatology have witnessed tremendous change with the appearance of new diseases, a vast array of new technology and very new approaches to 'old' problems. This volume provides a precise, up-to-date, evidence-based and appropriately referenced summary of the important issues in the field. These are not the infallible utterances of the great and the good, but rather a sensible and clinically salient distillation of a mass of information by real doctors! It should answer the burning question, guide appropriate and safe therapy and lead the reader to sources of further and more detailed information. The jury is in: this new title is more than justified!

Eamonn MM Quigley MD, FRCP, FACP, FACG, FRCPI
Professor of Medicine and Human Physiology,
Head of the Medical School
National University of Ireland
Cork, Ireland
President, World Gastroenterology Organisation (WGO-OMGE),
Vice-President, American College of Gastroenterology

PREFACE

This is an exciting time in the field of gastroenterology. There have been major advances in the diagnosis and treatment of luminal gut and liver disease that have been nothing short of revolutionary. Furthermore, new challenges continue to emerge, such as the growth of complications after obesity surgery and medical problems after liver transplantation. This book aims to succinctly summarise a practical, modern approach to diagnosis and treatment in gastrointestinal and liver diseases. The text is organised around a key topic or clinical problem to help maximise learning and retention. The chapters contain a summary of key points and relevant algorithms to assist with planning care. Important topics often omitted in textbooks, such as how to prepare patients for endoscopic procedures, anaesthesia for endoscopy, colon cancer screening issues, the sore mouth, eating disorders, obesity surgery for the gastroenterologist, nutritional assessment in gastrointestinal and liver disease, family history of liver disease and food allergies, are all covered here. We hope that the book will be carried around and referred to frequently in the outpatient setting. The chapters have all been written by experts who have synthesised available material, so that it can be easily digested and utilised by the reader.

We would like to acknowledge our mentors and students who have taught us so much, and who continue to inspire us. We are particularly grateful to all the contributors who have so graciously provided their expertise for this book. Finally, we would like to thank our families for their support during the long, laborious writing and editing process.

Nicholas J Talley
Isidor Segal
Martin Weltman
June 2007

CONTRIBUTORS

Dr Minoti Apte
Liverpool Hospital, Sydney,
Australia

Professor Nadir Arber
Tel Aviv University, Tel Aviv,
Israel

Dr Simon Benstock
Sydney, Australia

Dr Simon Chew
Nepean Hospital, Sydney,
Australia

Professor Ian James Cook
St George Hospital, Sydney,
Australia

Professor Darrell Crawford
Greenslopes Private Hospital,
Brisbane, Australia

Associate Professor Paul Desmond
St Vincent's Hospital,
Melbourne, Australia

Dr John Darke
Nepean Hospital, Sydney,
Australia

Dr Katherine Ellard
Royal North Shore Hospital,
Sydney, Australia

Dr Jeffrey Engelmann
St George Private Hospital,
Sydney, Australia

Dr Arie Figer
Tel Aviv University, Tel Aviv,
Israel

Professor Jacob George
Westmead Hospital, Sydney,
Australia

Dr Martin Grehan
Nepean Hospital, Sydney,
Australia

Associate Professor Paul Haber
Royal Prince Alfred Hospital,
Sydney, Australia

Dr Hugh Harley
Royal Adelaide Hospital,
Adelaide, Australia

Professor Gerald Holtmann
Royal Adelaide Hospital,
Adelaide, Australia

Dr Brett Jones
Royal North Shore Hospital,
Sydney, Australia

Dr Jenny Kaldor
Royal Hospital for Women,
Sydney, Australia

Dr Hossam Kandil
University of Pittsburgh,
Pittsburgh, PA, USA

Dr Revital Kariv
Tel Aviv University, Tel Aviv,
Israel

Associate Professor Peter Katelaris
Concord Hospital, Sydney,
Australia

Dr Greg Keogh
Prince of Wales Hospital,
Sydney, Australia

Dr Robert Kim
Prince of Wales Hospital,
Sydney, Australia

Dr Michael Kohn
The Children's Hospital at
Westmead, Sydney, Australia

Dr Rupert Leong
Concord Hospital, Sydney, Australia

Associate Professor Christopher Liddle
Westmead Hospital, Sydney, Australia

Dr Graeme MacDonald
Royal Brisbane Hospital, Brisbane, Australia

Dr Jenny McDonald
Wollongong Hospital, Wollongong, Australia

Dr Ian D Norton
Royal North Shore Hospital, Sydney, Australia

Professor Stephen O'Keefe
University of Pittsburgh, Pittsburgh, PA, USA

Dr Paul Pavli
Canberra Hospital, Canberra, Australia

Dr Stephen Philcox
Nepean Hospital, Sydney, Australia

Dr Nghi Phung
Nepean Hospital, Sydney, Australia

Associate Professor Stephen Riordan
The Prince of Wales Hospital, Sydney, Australia

Dr Stuart Roberts
The Alfred Hospital, Melbourne, Australia

Professor Ian Roberts-Thomson
Queen Elizabeth Hospital, Adelaide, Australia

Professor Isidor Segal
Prince of Wales Hospital, Sydney, Australia

Dr Bill Sievert
Monash Medical Centre, Melbourne, Australia

Dr Simone Strasser
Royal Prince Alfred Hospital, Sydney, Australia

Professor Joseph Sung
Prince of Wales Hospital, Hong Kong

Dr Michael Talbot
St George Hospital, Sydney, Australia

Professor Nicholas Talley
Mayo Clinic College of Medicine, Jacksonville, FL, USA and University of Sydney, Nepean Hospital, Sydney, Australia

Dr Philip Truskett
Prince of Wales Hospital, Sydney, Australia

Dr Brynn Wainstein
Sydney Children's Hospital, Sydney, Australia

Emeritus Professor D Murray Walker
Westmead Dental Hospital, Sydney, Australia

Dr Katrina Watson
St Vincent's Hospital, Melbourne, Australia

Associate Professor Martin Weltman
Nepean Hospital, Sydney, Australia

Professor Jeremy Wilson
Liverpool Hospital, Sydney, Australia

Professor Shing Wong
Prince of Wales Hospital, Sydney, Australia

ABBREVIATIONS

α_1-ATD alpha$_1$-antitrypsin deficiency
AAA aromatic amino acid
AA Alcoholics Anonymous
ADPKD autosomal dominant polycystic kidney disease
ADPLD autosomal dominant polycystic liver disease
ADRAC Adverse Drug Reactions Advisory Committee
AFLP acute fatty liver of pregnancy
AFP alpha-fetoprotein
AIDS acquired immunodeficiency syndrome
AIH autoimmune hepatitis
ALD alcohol-related liver disease
ALDH aldehyde dehydrogenase
ALF acute liver failure
ALP alkaline phosphatase
ALT alanine aminotransferase
AMA antimitochondrial antibody
AN anorexia nervosa
ANCA antineutrophil cytoplasmic antibody
Anti-LKM Ab anti-liver/kidney microsomal antibody
ANUG acute necrotising ulcerative gingivitis
APC adenomatous polyposis coli
APGARS acute post-gastric reduction surgery
ARDS acute respiratory distress syndrome
ARM anorectal manometry
ASA American Society of Anesthesiologists
ASCA anti-*Saccharomyces cerevisiae* antibody
AST aspartate aminotransferase
AVMs arteriovenous malformations

BCAA branched-chain amino acid
BDv barium defecography
BEE basal energy expenditure
BET balloon expulsion test
BIE bioelectrical impedance
BMI body mass index
BPD biliopancreatic diversion
BUN blood urea nitrogen

CA 19-9 carbohydrate antigen
CABG coronary artery bypass graft
CAM complementary and alternative medicines
CBC complete bl ood count
CCD charged couple device
CCK cholecystokinin
CDT carbohydrate-deficient transferrin
CE capsule endoscopy
CEA carcinoembryonic antigen
CE-CT contrast enhanced computed tomography
CF cystic fibrosis
CFTR gene for cystic fibrosis (cystic fibrosis transmembrane regulator)
CMV cytomegalovirus
CNS central nervous system
COPD chronic obstructive pulmonary disease
COX 2 cyclo-oxygenase 2
CRC colorectal cancer
CRP C-reactive protein
CT computed tomography
CTT colonic transit time
CTZ chemoreceptor trigger zone
Cu copper
CVS cyclic vomiting syndrome

DBE double-balloon enteroscopy
DCBE double-contrast barium enema
DCC deleted in colon cancer gene

DEXA	dual energy X-ray absorptiometry	FNH	focal nodular hyperplasia
DIC	disseminated intravascular coagulation	FOBT	faecal occult blood test
		FTH	ferritin heavy chain
DLE	discoid lupus erythematosus	FTL	ferritin light chain
DNA	deoxyribonucleic acid	GAVE	gastric antral vascular ectasia
DU	duodenal ulcer		
		GGT	gamma-glutamyltransferase
EBV	Epstein-Barr virus	GI	gastrointestinal
ECF	epirubicin, cisplatin and infused fluorouracil	GIST	gastrointestinal stromal tumours
ECG	electrocardiogram	GORD	gastro-oesophageal reflux disease
EGD	oesophagogastro-duodenoscopy	GSH	glutathione
EGFR	epidermal growth factor receptor	GU	gastric ulcer
EGG	electrogastrography	H_2-RA	histamine H_2-receptor antagonist
EHEC	enterohaemolytic *Escherichia coli*	HAART	highly active antiretroviral treatment
EoG	eosinophilic gastroenteropathy	*HAMP*	hepcidin gene
EPG	electrophoresis	HAV	hepatitis A virus
EPS	epigastric pain syndrome	HBcAb	hepatitis B core antibody
ERC	endoscopic retrograde cholangiography	HBeAb	hepatitis B e antibody
		HBeAg	hepatitis B e antigen
ERCP	endoscopic retrograde cholangiopancreatography	HBsAg	hepatitis B surface antigen
		HBV	hepatitis B virus
ES	endoscopic sphincterotomy	HCC	hepatocellular carcinoma
ESR	erythrocyte sedimentation rate	β-hCG	human chorionic gonadotrophin
ETR	end-of-treatment response	HCV	hepatitis C virus
EUS	endoscopic ultrasound	HDL	high-density lipoprotein
EUS-FNA	endoscopic ultrasound guided fine needle aspiration	HDV	hepatitis D virus
		H&E	haematoxylin and eosin
		HE	hepatic encephalopathy
EVR	early virological response	HELLP	haemolysis, elevated liver enzymes and low platelets syndrome
FAP	familial adenomatous polyposis	HEV	hepatitis E virus
FDG PET	fluorodeoxyglucose position emission tomography	*HFE*	hereditary haemochromatosis gene
		HH	hereditary haemochromatosis
Fe	iron		
FFP	fresh frozen plasma	HHV-3	herpes zoster/varicella zoster
FHF	fulminant hepatic failure		
FLAGS	intervention for alcohol abuse: feedback/listen/advise/goals/strategies	HHV-5/CMV	cytomegalovirus
		HIV	human immunodeficiency virus
FNA	fine-needle aspiration	*HJV*	hemojuvelin gene

HLA	human leucocyte antigen	LOS	lower oesophageal sphincter
HNPCC	heredity non-polyposis colorectal cancer	LUS	laparoscopic ultrasound
HSV	herpes simplex virus	M	metastases
5-HT	serotonin	MAC	*Mycobacterium avium* complex
HVPG	hepatic vein-portal vein pressure gradient	MBS	modified barium swallow
		MCHC	mean corpuscular haemoglobin concentration
IBD	inflammatory bowel disease		
IBS	irritable bowel syndrome		
IBS-A	irritable bowel syndrome, alternating between diarrhoea and constipation	MCH	mean corpuscular haemoglobin
		MCNs	mucinous cystic neoplasms
IBS-C	irritable bowel syndrome with predominant constipation	MCV	mean corpuscular volume
		MDF	Maddrey Discriminant Function
IBS-D	irritable bowel syndrome with predominant diarrhoea	MELD	Model for End-stage Liver Disease
ICD	International Classification of Diseases	MPFF	micronised purified flavonoid fraction
ICP	intracranial pressure	MRCP	magnetic resonance cholangiopancreatography
IEPG	immunoelectrophoresis	MRI	magnetic resonance imaging
IgE	immunoglobulin E		
IgG	immunoglobulin G	MSI	microsatellite instability
IM	intramuscular		
INR	international normalised ratio	N	lymph node
		NAFLD	non-alcoholic fatty liver disease
IPMN	intraductal papillary mucinous neoplasms	NASH	non-alcoholic steatohepatitis
IR	insulin resistance		
IU	international unit	NBT-PABA	*N*-benzoyl-L-tryosyl-para-aminobenzoic acid
IV	intravenous		
		NG	nasogastric
K	potassium	NHMRC	National Health and Medical Research Council of Australia
KF	Kayser-Fleischer rings		
KU/L	kilounits per litre		
		NNH	number needed to harm
LAGB	laparoscopic adjustable gastric band	NNT	number needed to treat
		NSAID	non-steroidal antiinflammatory drug
LCHAD	long-chain 3-hydroxyacyl-CoA dehydrogenase	NUD	non-ulcer dyspepsia
LDH	lactate dehydrogenase		
LFLA	faecal lactoferrin latex agglutination	OLT	orthotopic liver transplantation
LFTs	liver function tests		
LKM	liver-kidney microsomal antibodies	PAS	periodic acid-Schiff
		PBC	primary biliary cirrhosis
LOH	loss of heterozygosity	PCLD	polycystic liver disease

PCM	protein–calorie malnutrition	SIM	specialised intestinal metaplasia
PCR	polymerase chain reaction	SLE	systemic lupus erythematosus
PCT	porphyria cutanea tarda		
PDS	postprandial distress syndrome	SPECT	single-photon emission computed tomography
PEG	percutaneous endoscopic gastrostomy	SPINK1	serine protease inhibitor Kazal type 1 gene
PEG	polyethylene glycol	SPT	skin prick test
PEG-J	percutaneous endoscopic gastrostomy with post-pyloric J extension	SSRI	selective serotonin reuptake inhibitor
		STD	sodium tetradecyl sulfate
PEJ	direct endoscopic jejunostomy	SVR	sustained virological response
PEM	protein–energy malnutrition	T	tumour
PET	positron emission tomography	T_3	triiodothyronine
		T_4	thyroxine
PET-CT	positron-emission tomography - computed tomography	TACE	transarterial chemoembolisation
		TB	tuberculosis
PHG	portal hypertensive gastropathy	TCA	tricyclic antidepressants
		TFR	transferrin receptor
PI	protease inhibitor	TIPS	transjugular intrahepatic porto-systemic shunt
PN	parenteral nutrition		
PNALD	parenteral nutrition-associated liver disease	TNF	tumour necrosis factor
		TPMT	thiopurine methyltransferase
PPC	polyenylphosphatidylcholine		
PPI	protein pump inhibitor	TPN	total parenteral nutrition
PRSS1	cationic trypsinogen gene	TSH	thyroid stimulating hormone
PSC	primary sclerosing cholangitis		
		TS	thymidylate synthase
PTC	percutaneous transhepatic cholangiography	U	urea
		UC	ulcerative colitis
R0	complete resection	UDCA	ursodeoxycholic acid
RBC	red blood cell	US	ultrasound
RFA	radiofrequency ablation		
RYGBP	Roux-en-Y gastric bypass	VBG	vertical banded gastroplasty
		VC	virtual colonoscopy
SAAG	serum-to-ascites albumin gradient	VEGF	vascular endothelial growth factor
SAMe	S-adenosylmethionine		
SBFT	small bowel follow-through	WCC	white cell count
SBP	spontaneous bacterial peritonitis	WD	Wilson's disease
		WHO	World Health Organization
SD	standard deviation		
SGA	subjective global assessment		

Chapter 1

SORE MOUTH

KEY POINTS

- The commonest fungal infection in the mouth is *Candida albicans*. Always look for a predisposing factor (systemic disease, drugs, diabetes or HIV infection).
- In gingivitis, a red line limited to the entire gingival margin (linear gingival erythema) can be a marker of HIV infection.
- Recurrent aphthous ulcers tend to start in childhood or adolescence, and heal spontaneously in 2–10 days. The cause is unknown. Major aphthae are more severe and can persist for months, healing by scar formation.
- Gastrointestinal causes of oral ulceration include coeliac disease, Crohn's disease and ulcerative colitis.
- The bullous eruption of pemphigus (usually pemphigus vulgaris) may be restricted to the mouth before a skin rash appears.
- Mucous membrane pemphigoid selectively involves the mucosa lining the mouth, conjunctiva, pharynx, oesophagus, larynx and vagina. Skin lesions are uncommon.
- A minority of leucoplakias are potentially malignant.
- More than 90% of oral malignancies are squamous cell carcinomas.
- Do not confuse the burning mouth syndrome with heartburn.

EXAMINATION OF THE MOUTH

Wear gloves, a mask and spectacles or goggles for oral examinations.

Extraoral

Is there any facial swelling, asymmetry or altered cutaneous sensation? Are the submandibular and other cervical lymph nodes palpable?

Intraoral

Ask the patient to open their mouth wide. Normally 2½ finger breadths can be inserted between upper and lower incisors.

Does the patient's breath have an offensive odour (halitosis) due to gum disorders (periodontitis), alcohol or tobacco, ketones in untreated or poorly managed diabetes (predominantly type 1) or due to liver failure?

A good light source is very helpful. If available, a head-light or a dentist's light are ideal rather than a battery pencil torch. A pair of dental mirrors helps to both retract the lips, cheeks and tongue and illuminate the mouth. A gauze square is essential to hold (gently) and retract the tongue to inspect the floor of the mouth and ventral surface and lateral margins of the tongue, relatively common sites for precancerous growths and cancers. Subtle changes are best detected by drying the oral mucosa with a gauze square (or air syringe, if available).

Examine each part of the mouth in turn: vermilion margin and inner mucosal surface of lips, buccal mucosa, retromolar trigone, gingivae, the lateral margins, ventral surface, dorsum and base of tongue and hard and soft palate. Note any grossly decayed, loose or discoloured teeth. This systematic approach ensures that small lesions will not be overlooked. Inflammation of the palate covered by dentures is usually due to *Candida* (denture stomatitis). Ask the patient to remove any dentures and assess their cleanliness. Note whether they are old, unstable or ill fitting.

CAUSES OF SORE MOUTH

The causes of sore mouth are listed in Table 1.1.

Infections

Fungal infections

These are usually due to *Candida*. Thrush (acute pseudomembranous candidiasis), usually due to *Candida albicans*, is a relatively common cause of sore mouth. The diagnosis can usually be made clinically from the scattered white plaques resembling clotted milk that are easily wiped off the oral mucosa, leaving a red base. If doubt remains, laboratory confirmation is available by microscopy and culture of a swab. Always look for predisposing factors. Systemic causes include pharmacotherapy with immunosuppressive drugs, steroids, cytotoxic therapy, or antibiotics, as well as human

TABLE 1.1: Causes of sore mouth

Trauma	*Gastrointestinal* Coeliac disease Crohn's disease Ulcerative colitis

Infection
Bacterial
  Dental
  Tuberculosis
  Syphilis
Fungal
  Candida
Viral
  Herpes simplex (HSV-1 & 2)
  Herpes zoster (varicella zoster, HHV-3)
  Cytomegalovirus (HHV-5)
  Hand-foot-mouth disease (coxsackievirus)
  Herpangina
	Bullous or erosive
	Pemphigus
	Cicatrising mucous membrane pemphigoid
	Erythema multiforme
	Systemic lupus erythematosus

	Potentially malignant Leucoplakia Lichen planus Lichenoid reactions – drugs graft versus host disease – amalgam fillings Discoid lupus erythematosus Oral submucous fibrosis
Idiopathic Aphthous ulceration Geographical tongue ACE inhibitors (scalded mouth sensation) Sarcoidosis	*Xerostomia* Sjögren's syndrome Drugs: antihypertensive, diuretic Radiotherapy
Haematological Anaemias: iron, vitamin B_{12}, folate deficiency Neutropenias Leukaemias	*Malignant* Squamous cell carcinoma Kaposi's sarcoma Non-Hodgkin's lymphoma

immunodeficiency virus (HIV) infection, particularly before HAART begins, and diabetes.

Management

Topical antifungals, amphotericin B 10 mg lozenges three times daily for 1 week, dissolved slowly in mouth or nystatin pastilles 100,000 units or lozenges 500,000 units, allowed to dissolve in mouth or as a suspension 100,000 units/mL four times daily for 1 week. In immunocompromised states, oral itraconazole (contraindicated in acute hepatitis) 100–200 mg daily for 1 week may be needed.

Denture stomatitis

This appears as a fiery, red inflammation of the palate under the upper dentures and is a chronic form of *Candida* infection associated with the habit of continuous day and night wearing of dentures and poor hygiene. A candidal angular stomatitis (angular cheilitis) at the corners of the mouth may result. Advise the patient to clean the dentures with a brush and to leave them out at night in a 1% sodium hypochlorite disinfectant solution (e.g. Milton), and prescribe topical amphotericin B 10 mg lozenges three times daily for 1 week.

Median rhomboid glossitis

Median rhomboid glossitis is a red area of papillary atrophy in the midline of the posterior third of the tongue. It may remain asymptomatic or cause occasional soreness. It appears to be a chronic acquired oral candidiasis and not a developmental anomaly as previously supposed. Predisposing factors include tobacco smoking, continuous night and day denture wearing and steroid sprays for asthma or HIV infection. The condition is quite harmless and management involves attending to predisposing factors and topical amphotericin B 10 mg lozenges three times daily for 1 week to alleviate soreness.

Viral infections

Herpes simplex (human herpes virus type 1, less commonly 2)

Oral herpes simplex infections usually present in young children with fever, malaise, enlarged tender submandibular lymph nodes, widespread small irregular mouth 'ulcers' and swollen inflamed gums (often dismissed as 'teething'). The diagnosis can usually be made clinically, but laboratory tests include a smear for microscopy, swab for culture or direct immunofluorescence of a saline mouth rinse and a blood sample to show an immediate rise in IgM antibody. Aqueous 0.2% chlorhexidine mouth baths or, for the immunocompromised, aciclovir 400 mg five times daily for 5 days or famciclovir for aciclovir-resistant infections. Recurrent herpes simplex infections are usually restricted to the lips (herpes labialis or 'cold sores'), and only rarely affect the oral cavity, which may be involved, however, where HSV is reactivated in immunocompromised states. Early application of 5% aciclovir or penciclovir cream is useful for treating cold sores.

Varicella zoster virus (human herpes virus 3)

Patients with varicella zoster virus infections are usually middle aged or elderly. After prodromal symptoms of facial pain and fever, vesicles appear on the face or as ulcers in the mouth in a unilateral distribution corresponding to one or more divisions of the trigeminal nerve (V2 or V3, less often V1). Chlorhexidine mouth baths and famciclovir 500 mg three times daily for 7 days speeds healing and also reduces the likelihood of post-herpetic neuralgia. Don't forget that this reactivation of human herpes virus 3 may be a marker of malignancy (e.g. lymphoma) or immunosuppression.

Cytomegalovirus (human herpes virus 5)

Infections may uncommonly present as mouth ulceration due to reactivation in immunosuppressed states or, rarely, as a parotitis.

Bacterial infections

Dental causes

Teeth which are grossly carious, heavily filled or with severe periodontal (gum) disease or partly erupted wisdom teeth can cause severe odontogenic infections with toothache and rapid, painful swelling of the mouth, jaws and face, and limited mouth opening (trismus). Refer the patient to a dentist. If delay is unavoidable, amoxycillin (exclude penicillin allergy) 500 mg three times daily or amoxycillin 500 mg and clavulanic acid 125 mg three times daily as well as paracetamol and codeine will provide some relief.

Gum disorders

Gingivitis

Chronic gingival inflammation is common and results from bacterial plaque and calculus deposits on the teeth. The gum margins are red, bleed easily while brushing teeth or eating but usually this gingivitis is painless. A red line limited to the entire gingival margin (linear gingival erythema) can be a marker of HIV infection.

Acute necrotising ulcerative gingivitis (ANUG, Vincent's stomatitis) is uncommon except in immunocompromised states, e.g. with uncontrolled HIV infection or during chemotherapy. Tobacco smoking or excessive fatigue may be contributing factors. Typically the patient is a teenager presenting with pain, gingival ulceration and halitosis. ANUG responds quickly to metronidazole 200 mg three times daily for 4 days (patients should avoid alcohol during treatment).

Haematological

Iron deficiency anaemia

In severe anaemias there may be general features such as dyspnoea on exertion, angina, or ankle swelling and pale conjunctivae, nail beds and palmar creases.

In the mouth, look for angular cheilitis (angular stomatitis) and a smooth sore tongue (glossitis). The Paterson-Kelly (Plummer-Vinson) syndrome of atrophic glossitis, angular cheilitis, koilonychia and dysphagia due to pharyngeal webs associated with iron deficiency anaemia is uncommon, but carries a significant risk of oral and pharyngeal cancer.

A hypochromic microcytic blood film and low red cell values, low serum ferritin or transferrin saturation, usually with a reduced haemoglobin level, will confirm the diagnosis. A cause should be identified before starting iron therapy.

Vitamins

The oral signs of atrophic glossitis and angular stomatitis due to vitamin B_{12} and folate deficiency are essentially similar to those for iron deficiency. Vitamin B_2 (riboflavin) deficiency can present with angular cheilitis and a magenta coloured glossitis.

Dry mouth (xerostomia)

Patients with xerostomia are mostly middle aged or elderly women and complain of difficulty in eating, swallowing, altered taste and an uncomfortably leathery dry mouth. The tongue is depapillated with a 'cobblestone' appearance, the normal pool of saliva is absent and the buccal mucosa is glazed, erythematous and adherent. Dental caries becomes a problem and oral *Candida* infections can occur.

There are many causes of dry mouth (see Table 1.2). Note that salivary flow rates do not significantly decrease with ageing, but medication is a significant cause of xerostomia in the elderly. The symptoms can be relieved by sips of tap water (usually contains fluoride), or conveniently delivered with a plastic spray bottle. Fluoride in toothpaste, plus a sodium fluoride 0.2% mouth rinse, 10 mL once a week, protects against caries. Sugar-free sweets usefully promote salivation. *Candida* infections causing thrush or a red dry sore mouth with angular cheilitis respond to nystatin or amphotericin B (as detailed above). Poor denture hygiene or a continuous day-and-night wearing habit favour candidiasis.

TABLE 1.2: Causes of dry mouth (xerostomia)

Reduced salivary flow

Medication	*Salivary gland diseases*
Antihypertensive	Irradiation
Diuretic	Sjögren's syndrome
Antihistamine	Sarcoidosis
Anti-parkinsonian	HIV
Antidepressant	Amyloidosis
Antipsychotic	Haemochromatosis
Cytotoxic	*Dehydration*
Antispasmodic	Diabetes mellitus (uncontrolled)
Anti-HIV	Diabetes insipidus
	Renal failure
	Haemorrhage

Normal salivary flow
  Psychogenic

ORAL ULCERATION

The causes of oral ulceration are listed in Table 1.3.

Traumatic

Traumatic ulcers from lip, cheek or tongue biting or due to ill fitting dentures are common. They are usually solitary and irregular. After the cause is removed, the ulcer heals spontaneously and a chlorhexidine mouth rinse speeds healing.

TABLE 1.3: Causes of mouth ulceration

Trauma	*Viral infection*
Idiopathic	Herpes simplex
Aphthous	Varicella zoster
Herpetiform	Cytomegalovirus
	Herpangina
Gastrointestinal	*Bacterial infection*
Coeliac disease	Tuberculosis
Crohn's disease	Syphilis
Ulcerative colitis	
Haematological	*Drug induced*
Neutropenia	Topical aspirin 'burn'
Anaemias: iron, vitamin B_{12} or	Non-steroidal antiinflammatory
folate deficiency	Cytotoxic
Leukaemia	
Autoimmune	
Dermatological	*Neoplastic*
Lichen planus/lichenoid reaction	Squamous cell carcinoma
Lupus erythematosus (DLE or SLE)	Minor salivary gland carcinoma
Behçet's syndrome	Kaposi's sarcoma
Bullous	
Pemphigus vulgaris	
Cicatrising mucous membrane	
pemphigoid	
Angina bullosa haemorrhagica	
(blood blisters)	

DLE = discoid lupus erythematosus; SLE = systemic lupus erythematosus.

Recurrent aphthous ulcers

These tend to start in childhood or adolescence. Minor aphthae occur in crops of 2–10 simultaneous ulcers with an erythematous halo and yellow or grey slough on the lips, cheeks, sides and ventral surface of the tongue and heal spontaneously in 7–10 days. The cause remains unknown. Any pain and discomfort is usually minor but responds to topical steroids such as triamcinolone acetonide 0.1% paste (rather messy), or fluocinonide 0.1% in Orabase or betamethasone 0.05% in Orabase if more severe or an aqueous chlorhexidine 0.2% mouthrinse. Associated folate, iron or B$_{12}$ deficiencies or anaemias should be corrected.

Major aphthae are much more severe and may last weeks or months, healing by scar formation. The treatment remains rather unsatisfactory. Topical lignocaine gel applied to ulcers before meals can help. Prednisone, azathioprine, thalidomide and possibly pentoxifylline may be occasionally used by specialists in severe cases, but preferably in short bursts only. Specialists may prescribe thalidomide (a known teratogen) or zidovudine for the major aphthae associated with HIV infection.

Haematological

Low blood levels of functional circulating neutrophils may predispose to oral ulceration. In agranulocytosis the neutropenia is profound, with general features such as fever, malaise, septicaemia and gingival, oral and pharyngeal ulceration. Bone marrow disease (e.g. leukaemia or aplastic anaemia), drugs (e.g. cytotoxic agents or sulfamethoxazole/trimethoprim) or HIV are important causes.

Coeliac disease

There may be an atrophic glossitis or angular stomatitis due to malabsorption of iron, folate or vitamin B$_{12}$. Oral ulceration resembling aphthae may occur and remit on a gluten-free diet after the diagnosis of coeliac disease has been confirmed and haematinic deficiencies corrected. The teeth may be hypoplastic, grooved or pitted beginning in childhood.

Crohn's disease

Oral manifestations include aphthous-like ulcers. There may also be a diffuse swelling of the lips and face, mouth ulcers, angular stomatitis, thickened, corrugated buccal mucosa and small polyps in the mandibular sulci of the lips and cheeks. The gingivae may be red and swollen. A mucosal biopsy is necessary and shows non-caseating granulomas. Endoscopy and other investigations for intestinal Crohn's disease will then be needed. Tuberculosis and sarcoid will need to be excluded.

A similar clinical and histological appearance is occasionally encountered in patients in whom investigations for intestinal Crohn's disease are negative. This condition has been called 'orofacial granulomatosis' and may respond to dietary elimination of ingredients such as cinnamon or monosodium glutamate or other dietary additives. Others assert that these lesions are Crohn's disease. Topical steroids applied to the ulcers may be helpful.

Ulcerative colitis

Even in uncontrolled ulcerative colitis, oral lesions are infrequent. They include aphthous-like ulcers or more chronic ulcers equivalent to pyostomatitis gangrenosum. Pyostomatitis vegetans is another oral manifestation. Topical steroids (see above) can help.

Pemphigus

The bullous eruption of pemphigus (usually pemphigus vulgaris) may be restricted to the mouth before a skin rash appears. The bullae are intraepithelial and rupture quickly to form erosions which, unrecognised, may lead to delays in diagnosing this serious condition. The oral mucosa is fragile and the epithelium easily detached. The diagnosis is confirmed by a biopsy for histology (fixed specimen) direct immunofluorescence (unfixed specimen) and blood test to detect antibodies to the intercellular attachment protein desmoglein-3. Drug-induced or paraneoplastic pemphigus should be considered in the differential diagnosis.

Mucous membrane (cicatricial) pemphigoid

Women aged between 50 and 70 years are more commonly affected by this autoimmune disorder. Cicatricial pemphigoid selectively involves the mucosa lining the mouth, conjunctiva, pharynx, oesophagus, larynx and vagina. Skin lesions are uncommon. The blisters may be haemorrhagic and remain intact before rupturing to form erosions. The gums may be red and atrophic (desquamative gingivitis). Healing is by scarring. Aqueous chlorhexidine 0.2%, 3 times daily, or topical steroids (see above) can be helpful in less severe cases, but systemic steroids or other immunomodulators may be needed. An ophthalmic opinion is essential if eye involvement is suspected, as scarring of the conjunctiva or cornea is a serious complication.

Erythema multiforme

Young men are most often affected by this bullous eruption. Target or iris-like skin lesions on the limbs and erosions in the mouth are pathognomonic. In severe cases, the conjunctiva or genital mucosa may also be involved, with fever (toxic epidermal necrosis or Stevens-Johnson syndrome). Occasionally only the mouth is involved.

Infections, particularly recurrent herpes simplex (labial herpes), drugs, pregnancy, or malignancy are known triggers. The diagnosis is usually apparent clinically and systemic steroids (e.g. prednisone) may be needed for up to 14 days in severe cases. Ophthalmic advice should be obtained as corneal involvement can lead to scarring or blindness. Hospital admission is advisable for Stevens-Johnson syndrome.

Erosive lichen planus
This can be a cause of oral ulceration (see below).

Geographic tongue (glossitis migrans)
Multiple red areas of localised atrophy of the papillae with a white margin appear for a few days on the dorsum of the tongue, forming map-like patterns moving across the tongue, causing soreness and discomfort, before healing spontaneously. Relapses may follow weeks or months later. The cause remains unknown and the treatment is symptomatic and unsatisfactory (e.g. topical triamcinolone acetonide 0.1% paste or benzydamine oral rinse).

White lesions

Keratosis
Many white mucosal patches result from friction from the teeth or tobacco smoking and are usually reversible and non-dysplastic.

Lichen planus
Middle-aged women are mostly affected by lichen planus. The characteristic itchy red violet polygonal skin papules on the forearms and shins may be absent. Typically, white interconnecting striae and papules form a lace-like pattern especially on the buccal mucosa and ventral surface of the tongue, usually in a bilaterally symmetrical distribution. The gingivae can be red and atrophic (desquamative gingivitis). Ulceration in the erosive form may be severe. The diagnosis is often obvious clinically but a biopsy should be undertaken in doubtful cases. Remember that lichenoid reactions to drugs or dental fillings or graft-versus-host reaction may mimic idiopathic lichen planus quite closely. Aqueous chlorhexidine 0.2% and topical steroids provide some relief for the soreness. Brief courses of systemic prednisone, retinoids or other immunosuppressive agents may be used by specialists in cases of severe erosive lichen planus. Oral cancer is a rare complication

of long-standing erosive lichen planus, especially in middle-aged or elderly women.

Leucoplakia and erythroplakia

Leucoplakia has been defined as a predominantly white lesion that cannot be characterised as part of any other disease (i.e. not lichen planus, thrush, aspirin necrosis, etc). A minority of leucoplakias are potentially malignant and usually appear speckled, fissured, indurated or nodular. A biopsy is essential to exclude other causes and to detect dysplasia and its severity or to rule out early invasive carcinoma. Where clinically practicable, removal of moderately or severely dysplastic leucoplakias by surgery or laser is advisable.

Erythroplakias present as velvety-red plaques in the elderly and a biopsy usually shows severe dysplasia or early cancer. Excision is required.

Oral hairy leucoplakias

These corrugated white plaques particularly on the sides of the tongue are due to Epstein-Barr virus infection and occur in immunocompromised states, particularly in HIV-AIDS, but cases in organ transplant recipients have been reported. The changes are innocuous but will respond to aciclovir.

Other causes

Other causes include chronic *Candida* infection and tertiary syphilis (rare nowadays).

Squamous cell carcinoma

Over 90% of oral malignancies are squamous cell carcinomas. Most patients are middle-aged or elderly and more men than women are affected. Tobacco smoking and alcohol ingestion and, in immigrants from Asia, betel quid or Areca nut use are the main risk factors.

The lower lip (due to sunlight) and the lateral margins, ventral surface of the tongue and floor of the mouth are the most common sites affected.

A solitary ulcer with a raised indurated margin, which persists for 3 weeks despite any treatments, *must be biopsied to exclude a carcinoma*. A swelling, a white patch or gingival swelling causing loosening of the adjacent teeth, are other presentations.

Burning mouth syndrome

Postmenopausal women may develop a diffuse burning sensation of the tongue, lips and cheeks. This tends to be present on waking and gradually worsens during the day but does not usually interfere with sleep. The mouth is clinically normal.

Dentures that are ill fitting or worn continuously day and night causing *Candida* infection and inflammation of the palate may cause soreness of the mouth. Allergy to the acrylic denture base material is very rare. Lichen planus, anaemia, untreated diabetes mellitus or 'scalded mouth' sensation, due to ACE inhibitors, should be excluded. Vitamin B, C or other micronutrient deficiencies or postmenopausal oestrogen deficiency have been proposed as causes but not confirmed.

These local or systemic causes cannot be identified in most patients with burning mouth syndrome. Depression or anxiety, obsessional traits or recent adverse life events such as the death of a close relative, or divorce, etc, seem to be significant in many patients and combined cognitive therapy and antidepressants may prove helpful.

SUMMARY

Clinical examination of the mouth: Prerequisites include gloves, goggles (or spectacles), mask, dental mirror and gauze swabs. Examine each part of the mouth systematically. Assess if halitosis is present. Then examine the head and neck.

Causes of sore mouth: Think about infections (fungal, viral, bacterial), gum disorders (gingivitis), dry mouth (xerostomia: medicines are an important cause in the elderly as is poor denture hygiene) and haematological causes (iron deficiency, vitamin B_{12} and folate deficiency) (Figure 1.1).

Oral ulceration: The differential diagnosis includes trauma, recurrent aphthous ulcers, haematological (agranulocytosis), coeliac disease, Crohn's disease and ulcerative colitis, pemphigus, and mucous membrane pemphigoid, erythema multiforme and erosive lichen planus and squamous cell carcinoma.

White lesions: Many white mucosal patches result from friction of the teeth or tobacco smoking, and are usually reversible and non-dysplastic. A biopsy is recommended.

Squamous cell carcinoma: More than 90% of oral malignancies are squamous cell cancers. Tobacco smoking, and intake of alcohol, betel quid or areca nuts are the main risk factors.

Burning mouth syndrome: This is a diffuse burning sensation of tongue, lips and cheeks typically in middle-aged or elderly patients. It is not heartburn! The mouth clinically looks normal. Antidepressants may be helpful.

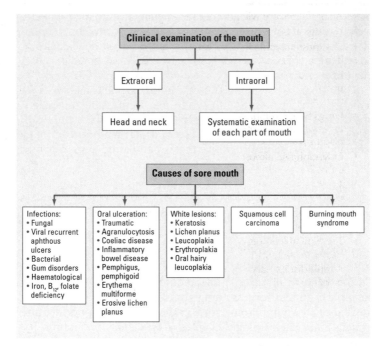

FIGURE 1.1: Sore mouth flow chart.

FURTHER READING

1. Scully C, Cawson RA. Medical problems in dentistry. 5th edn. Edinburgh: Churchill Livingstone, 2005.
2. Walker DM. Oral disease. In: Pathy MSJ, Sinclair AJ, Morley JE (Eds). Principles and practice of geriatric medicine, volume 1. 4th edn. Chichester: John Wiley and Sons, 2006:261–77.

Chapter 2

DYSPHAGIA AND ODYNOPHAGIA

KEY POINTS

- A careful history will yield the likely diagnosis in 80% of cases.
- The site of bolus hold-up is not reliable if perceived in the neck.
- The most valuable investigations for oesophageal dysphagia are a barium swallow, endoscopy and oesophageal manometry.
- Endoscopy is essential to identify and biopsy the lesion but precise diagnosis may require additional radiography and manometry.
- Drugs likely to induced oesophageal ulceration include tetracycline antibiotics, potassium, iron supplements and bisphosphonates.   .
- Odynophagia almost always has an infective, inflammatory or corrosive aetiology.
- The three cardinal features of oesophageal dysmotility are dysphagia (for solids and liquids), chest pain and regurgitation.
- If endoscopy is suggestive of dysmotility, oesophageal manometry is the best way to confirm this.
- The typical features of neurogenic pharyngeal dysphagia are highly accurate.
- A multidisciplinary approach to the management of oropharyngeal dysphagia is important.

DYSPHAGIA

Taking the dysphagia history

A good history will elucidate the site and the general pathophysiological process in 80% of cases, and is vital before embarking on a focussed and cost effective utilisation of specific diagnostic techniques. Frequently, patients will describe food sticking or holding up either retrosternally or in the neck. However, more atypical symptoms can include regurgitation, a sense of fullness retrosternally and hiccup. Dysphagia is distinguished from odynophagia (pain on swallowing) by the perception of actual bolus hold up. The aims of the history are to:

- determine whether dysphagia is actually present (i.e. distinct from globus sensation and xerostomia)
- establish whether the site of the problem is oesophageal or pharyngeal
- distinguish between a structural and a motor abnormality.

Where does the food stick?

Retrosternal hold-up suggests that the disorder lies within the oesophagus. If the site of hold-up is in the neck, the pathology can lie either in the oesophagus or in the pharynx (Figure 2.1). Due to referred sensation, the site of perceived hold-up is above the suprasternal notch in 30% of cases where the actual hold-up is within the oesophageal body. Therefore, the next batch of questions aims to distinguish pharyngeal from oesophageal dysfunction.

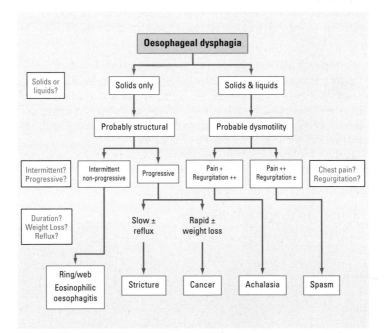

FIGURE 2.1: Differentiating oesophageal disorders.

Is one or more of the four cardinal symptoms of pharyngeal dysfunction present?

The four cardinal symptoms of pharyngeal dysfunction are:

1 Delayed or absent oropharyngeal swallow initiation
2 Deglutitive post-nasal regurgitation or egress of fluid through the nose during swallowing
3 Deglutitive cough indicative of aspiration
4 The need to swallow repetitively to achieve satisfactory clearance of swallowed material from the hypopharynx.

Supportive but less specific symptoms of oropharyngeal dysphagia include: bolus hold-up in the neck, piecemeal swallows, oral spill or drooling, dysphonia, throat clearing, garbled voice and weight loss.

If one or more of these symptoms is/are present the dysphagia is probably oropharyngeal, either structural or neuromyogenic, and further history and investigation should proceed accordingly (see below).

If oesophageal dysphagia is suspected, the next step is to establish whether it is a structural or motor disorder (Tables 2.1 and 2.2).

Is the dysphagia for solids or liquids?

Typically the patient with a motor disorder (e.g. achalasia, diffuse spasm) will describe dysphagia for liquid and solids while structural disorders will cause dysphagia for solids only. As the calibre of the oesophagus narrows, the size of the bolus required to cause obstruction becomes progressively smaller.

If the problem is likely to be a structural oesophageal disorder, the following enquiry will define the likely cause.

How long has dysphagia been present; is it intermittent, is it progressive?

Longstanding dysphagia is compatible with a benign condition. Slowly progressive, longstanding dysphagia, particularly if reflux is or has been experienced, is highly suggestive of a peptic stricture. A short history of dysphagia particularly with rapid progression (weeks or months) and associated weight loss is highly suggestive of oesophageal cancer. Longstanding, intermittent, non-progressive dysphagia purely for solids is indicative of a fixed structural lesion such as a distal oesophageal ring or proximal oesophageal mucosal web.

TABLE 2.1: Structural oesophageal disorders causing dysphagia

- Peptic stricture
- Mucosal rings
  - Lower (e.g. Schatzki's ring)
  - Multiple rings
    (e.g. eosinophilic oesophagitis)
  - Cervical webs

- Carcinoma
- Corrosive strictures
  - Caustic, pill-induced
- Oesophageal diverticula
- Benign tumours
- Extrinsic (vascular compression, tumour)

TABLE 2.2: Aetiology of pharyngeal dysphagia*

Structural	Neuromyogenic
• Tumour	• Stroke
• Stenosis	• Head trauma
– Post-surgical	• Parkinson's disease
– Radiation	• Amyotrophic lateral sclerosis
– Idiopathic	• Multiple sclerosis
• Zenker's diverticulum	• Myasthenia gravis
• Cricopharyngeal bar	• Myopathies (inflammatory,
• Web	metabolic)
• Extrinsic compression	
* Common causes. List not intended to be comprehensive.	

What does the patient do when the bolus sticks?

Sipping water will frequently relieve obstruction due to a structural lesion causing solid bolus dysphagia. However, if the patient sips water in the context of a solid bolus impaction, this will result in immediate regurgitation of the water indicative of complete bolus obstruction. If the bolus is catching very high (e.g. at the cricopharyngeus) patients learn very quickly not to sip water as it results in immediate coughing and spluttering due to laryngeal penetration.

Does the patient regurgitate?

While regurgitation can be associated with solid bolus hold-up *during* a meal, spontaneous regurgitation *between* meals (generally fluid and 'frothy' saliva) is highly suggestive of dysmotility (see below).

If the problem is likely to be an oesophageal motility disorder, the following enquiry will define the likely cause.

The three cardinal features of oesophageal dysmotility are dysphagia (for solids and liquids), chest pain and regurgitation.

Regurgitation during the meal as well as spontaneous regurgitation *between* meals or at night (generally fluid and saliva) is highly suggestive of dysmotility. The regurgitated fluid/food is generally not noxious to taste (unlike reflux-related regurgitation).

Does the patient experience chest pain or discomfort?

Oesophageal spasm and achalasia typically cause chest pain. While frequently described as heavy or crushing, it can be indistinguishable from the typical 'heartburn' of reflux. The pain frequently occurs during the meal but can be quite unpredictable and sporadic or nocturnal. Sipping antacids or even water can relieve the related dysmotility, thus further confusing distinction from reflux pain.

If oesophageal dysmotility is strongly suspected, distinction between achalasia and oesophageal spasm can be difficult at times. Achalasia is very much more common than spasm. In achalasia, chest pain is more prominent early in the disease, but over the years tends to diminish and may disappear as dysphagia and regurgitation worsen. In contrast, the chest pain of spasm is the predominant symptom and can be quite severe. Due to poor oesophageal clearance, regurgitation is frequently more impressive in achalasia than it is in the case of spasm. The oesophagus generally dilates over time in the context of achalasia, but this is less prevalent with spasm. Finally, there can be significant overlap between the two syndromes and spasm can evolve into more typical achalasia over time as they both share a similar underlying inhibitory neuropathic process. Oesophageal motility disorders can be classified as either primary (e.g. achalasia or diffuse oesophageal spasm) or secondary (e.g. scleroderma) (Table 2.3).

Examination of the patient with dysphagia

In the context of oesophageal dysphagia, the physical examination is generally unremarkable. However one should examine the skin for features compatible with connective tissue disorders particularly scleroderma and CREST syndrome. Muscle weakness or wasting might be evident if myositis is present, and this can overlap with other connective tissue disorders affecting the oesophagus. Signs

TABLE 2.3: Classification of oesophageal motility disorders	
Primary	**Secondary**

• Achalasia
• Diffuse oesophageal spasm
• Other
  – Non-specific oesophageal motor disorder
  – Overlap syndrome
  – 'Nutcracker'
  – Hypertensive lower oesophageal sphincter
	• Scleroderma
	• Other connective tissue disorders
	• 'Achalasia-like'
	  – Pseudoachalasia
	  – Chagas disease
	• Parkinson's disease
	• Diabetes
	• Myopathy/dystrophy

of malnutrition, weight loss and pulmonary complications from possible aspiration should be looked for. If pharyngeal dysphagia is suspected, careful evaluation for neuromuscular disorders is important (see below).

Diagnostic tests for oesophageal dysphagia

The most valuable investigations include a barium swallow, endoscopy and oesophageal manometry. Endoscopy will frequently obviate the need for barium radiology. However, the barium swallow, particularly with the addition of video sequences of the oesophageal body, can be very useful when the endoscopy fails to identify an abnormality and/or when oesophageal motility studies are atypical or equivocal. For example, one might identify so-called 'corkscrew' oesophagus indicative of diffuse oesophageal spasm. The hallmark of achalasia is oesophageal dilatation, a 'birdbeak' tapering at the cardio-oesophageal junction and the oesophagus typically supports a column of barium, often mixed with food and mucus. However, more subtle radiographic features in the early stages of achalasia might include loss of mid and distal oesophageal peristalsis and delayed clearance of barium from the distal oesophagus. Barium radiology will identify many structural abnormalities such as diverticula, strictures, rings and webs, tumours and ulcerative pathology.

Endoscopy is virtually always indicated in the dysphagic patient. It is necessary to identify and biopsy ulcerative pathology, malignancy and infective oesophagitis. A normal endoscopy, however, does not rule out a structural abnormality. Consider taking mid-oesophageal biopsies to rule out eosinophilic oesophagitis (abnormal mucosal eosinophilia in the oesophagus on histology [>24 eosinophils/ high power field]) in the setting of any case of unexplained dysphagia or food impaction. The ringed oesophagus is not always apparent unless adequate distension or insufflation of the oesophagus is achievable. The so-called 'multi-ringed' oesophagus, characteristic of eosinophilic oesophagitis, may have very subtle features such as longitudinal furrows, the 'feline' oesophagus with typical corrugation compatible with longitudinal shortening as well as the development of mucosal rings. Reflux oesophagitis and ulcerative oesophagitis (e.g. herpes simplex, cytomegalovirus [CMV], *Candida*) have typical appearances. Strictures can be biopsied and dilated at the time of endoscopy. The finding of food, fluid or salivary residue within the oesophagus is highly suggestive of dysmotility, particularly achalasia.

If endoscopy is normal or the history is suggestive of dysmotility, oesophageal manometry is the best way to confirm this. The characteristic features of achalasia are failure of lower oesophageal sphincter relaxation and aperistalsis. Typical although not always present is a hypertensive lower oesophageal sphincter. Oesophageal spasm is diagnosed in the context of normal sphincter relaxation, synchronous oesophageal pressure waves (>20% of wet swallows) and intermittent, normally progressive oesophageal peristalsis. Variably present, but not necessary for diagnosis, are high amplitude oesophageal pressure waves (>180 mmHg) and prolonged (>6 seconds) oesophageal pressure waves. The features of scleroderma oesophagus are complete absence of peristalsis and absence of lower oesophageal sphincter tone. Despite the virtual absence of propulsive motor activity in the scleroderma oesophagus, dysphagia in this syndrome is generally related to reflux-induced strictures. While manometry is the gold standard for diagnosis of motor disorders, in equivocal or atypical cases (approximately 5%) this must be interpreted in the context of the clinical and radiological features.

Diagnostic approach in suspected oropharyngeal dysphagia

The aetiology of pharyngeal dysphagia can be considered in 2 broad categories; structural disorders or neuromyogenic causes (Table 2.2). The range of potential neuromyogenic causes of pharyngeal dysphagia is broad but the most common is stroke. At least 50% of stroke patients experience pharyngeal dysphagia.

While considering the likely underlying cause in a patient, there are four fundamental issues to consider in the work-up of these patients as listed in Table 2.4.

TABLE 2.4: Approach to oropharyngeal dysphagia

- Identify correctable structural causes (e.g. cervical web, pharyngeal diverticulum)
- Identify treatable systemic disorders (e.g. inflammatory myopathy, myasthenia gravis)
- Establish the aspiration risk
  - Is non-oral feeding indicated?
- Establish the mechanics of dysfunction
  - Is the pattern of dysfunction amenable to therapy?

Identify correctable structural causes
The structural abnormalities are often readily diagnosed by endoscopy or radiography. These are generally managed effectively endoscopically or surgically (e.g. dilatation, resection, cricopharyngeal myotomy).

Identify treatable systemic disorders
Sometimes the cause is not obvious. In such cases, the underlying disease may have a systemic basis that warrants primary therapy in its own right. These conditions include:
- inflammatory myopathy (e.g. polymyositis, dermatomyositis)
- toxic/metabolic myopathy (e.g. thyrotoxicosis, drugs)
- myasthenia gravis
- extrapyramidal movement disorders (e.g. Parkinson's disease, drug-induced dyskinesia).

In addition to the history and physical examination targeting these four categories, a biochemical screen including creatinine phosphokinase, erythrocyte sedimentation rate, thyroid function tests and acetylcholine receptor antibodies should be done if in doubt. If clinical and biochemical indicators of muscle or neuromuscular function is evident, electromyography, perhaps followed by muscle biopsy, needs to be considered.

Establish the aspiration risk
This is achieved by a video radiographic swallow study sometimes called the modified barium swallow (MBS). This is frequently

conducted by the speech pathologist in conjunction with the radiologist. The MBS will determine the presence, the severity and the timing of aspiration. During the examination, the speech pathologist may modify the patient's swallow technique, head posture and swallowed bolus consistency to determine whether the aspiration can be eliminated by such manoeuvres. This is important in tailoring patient management and deciding whether non-oral feeding (by percutaneous endoscopic gastrostomy [PEG] or nasogastric [NG] tube) might be indicated.

Establish the mechanics of dysfunction

Again this is achieved with the aid of an MBS (with or without manometry). The purpose is to determine whether the pattern of dysfunction is amenable to swallow therapy and to establish the optimal dietary consistency to both minimise aspiration and maximise deglutitive pharyngeal clearance. A multidisciplinary approach to management is important and the speech language pathologist will, on the basis of the video radiographic findings, design a therapeutic programme involving swallow behaviour modification and dietary modification before embarking on an education programme for the patient. If, despite this, the patient continues to lose weight and/or suffers from pulmonary complications such as aspiration pneumonia, gastrostomy (PEG) feeding tube may become necessary.

PAIN ON SWALLOWING (ODYNOPHAGIA)

Odynophagia is the symptom of pain on swallowing, generally arising from irritation of an inflamed or ulcerated mucosa by the swallowed bolus during its passage through the pharynx or oesophagus. The aetiology is generally infective, inflammatory or corrosive (Table 2.5). Infective causes are most often encountered in the immunocompromised host. The symptom of odynophagia nearly always warrants endoscopic investigation.

Gastro-oesophageal reflux disease

In reflux disease, odynophagia almost always occurs in the context of oesophagitis. The patient typically describes a sensation of pain or discomfort coincident with passage of the bolus through the oesophagus, sometimes combined with a sense of transient bolus hold-up. The sense of bolus arrest can dominate the symptom complex if the oesophagitis has progressed to stricture formation, but is not infrequently perceived even in the absence of a stricture. The symptom of odynophagia always warrants endoscopic investigation. For a detailed account of investigation and management of reflux disease, refer to Chapter 3.

Oesophageal candidiasis

This infection usually occurs in patients receiving prolonged courses of antibiotics or who are immunosuppressed (e.g. as a result of human immunodeficiency virus [HIV] or chemotherapy) or who are using systemic or inhaled steroids. Conditions commonly associated with oesophageal candidiasis include diabetes, lymphoma and other malignancies particularly during chemotherapy when these patients are neutropenic. The oesophageal infection may be accompanied by oral or pharyngeal candidiasis, particularly in the context of acquired immunodeficiency syndrome (AIDS). The endoscopic features are white plaques on an erythematous mucosa which can progress to necrosis and ulceration. Diagnosis is confirmed by brushings and biopsy demonstrating hyphae and tissue invasion by the organism. The features can be similar to those of infections due to herpes simplex virus (HSV) or CMV and biopsy is necessary to distinguish between these conditions. Therapy is aimed at treating the underlying disease or conditions that predispose to the infection. Specific antifungal therapy, such as nystatin or amphotericin lozenges, are useful for oropharyngeal but not oesophageal candidiasis. Oral fluconazole is recommended for oesophageal candidiasis. Unresponsive cases may benefit from an intravenous echinocandin (e.g. caspofungin).

TABLE 2.5: Aetiology of odynophagia	
Infective	*Inflammatory or corrosive*
• Herpes simplex virus (HSV) • Cytomegalovirus (CMV) • Candidiasis	• Reflux oesophagitis • Radiation injury • Caustic ingestion • Pill-induced
Infective (pharyngeal)	*Miscellaneous*
• Tonsillitis • Pharyngitis • Paratonsillar abscess • Retropharyngeal abscess	• Spontaneous intramural haematoma • Crohn's disease • Pemphigus

Herpes simplex virus (type 1) oesophagitis

While frequently seen in the immunosuppressed patient, herpetic oesophagitis can occur spontaneously in the healthy, immunocompetent individuals. The endoscopic appearances can vary from discrete, punched out ulcers to confluent, extensive ulceration. Endoscopic biopsy, showing ground glass nuclei and typical eosinophilic (Cowdry's type A) inclusion bodies, will confirm the diagnosis. Treatment involves suspension, if possible, of drugs such as corticosteroids or cytotoxic agents. The antiviral agent aciclovir is active against this virus.

Cytomegalovirus oesophagitis

This oesophageal infection is seen most frequently in patients with AIDS, bone marrow transplantation and other immunodeficiency states. Endoscopic features are of extensive ulceration and characteristic inclusion bodies and giant cells are seen on biopsy. Effective antiviral agents include ganciclovir, foscarnet and cidofovir.

Drug-induced oesophageal ulceration

A number of medications, if allowed to dwell in the oesophagus, can cause severe local ulceration, pain and stricture. Factors predisposing to this phenomenon include: swallowing tablets without water, delayed oesophageal transit and extrinsic compression. Drugs particularly likely to cause this syndrome include: tetracycline, potassium and iron supplements and bisphosphonates.

Caustic oesophageal injury

This is frequently caused by ingestion of household substances including strong bleach, alkali or acid solutions. Interestingly, the severity of the corrosive injury doesn't always correlate with the severity of the pain and odynophagia. Hypothetically there is an increased risk of perforation during endoscopy in these patients. However, if it is done early (within 48 hours) and the scope is not pushed passed points of circumferential ulceration, the procedure is safe and important as it establishes the extent and severity of damage. A chest X-ray is also important as it can detect pulmonary infiltrates due to aspiration and possible signs of perforation. Therapy includes IV fluids and airway management as appropriate. The use of steroids is controversial and there is no high-level evidence supporting its efficacy. If steroids are used, they should be used in partial thickness burns and with concurrent antibiotics. If oral feeding cannot be resumed early, enteral or parenteral feeding is considered.

SUMMARY

A good history will elucidate the site and the general pathophysiological process in 80% of cases. The aims of the history are to:

1 determine whether dysphagia is actually present
2 establish whether the site of the problem is oesophageal or pharyngeal
3 distinguish between a structural and a motor abnormality.

The most important investigations for oesophageal dysphagia include a barium swallow, endoscopy and oesophageal manometry. The aetiology of suspected oropharyngeal dysphagia can be considered in two broad categories: structural disorders or neuromyogenic causes. A multidisciplinary approach to the management of oropharyngeal dysphagia is essential.

The aetiology of odynophagia is usually infective, inflammatory or corrosive. Odynophagia in reflux disease almost always occurs in the context of oesophagitis. Other causes of odynophagia include; oesophageal candidiasis, herpes simplex virus (type 1), cytomegalovirus, drug-induced oesophageal ulceration and caustic oesophageal injury.

FURTHER READING

Achem SR, Devault KR. Dysphagia in aging. J Clin Gastroenterol 2005; 39:357–71.

Castell DO, Richter J, eds. The esophagus. 4th edn. Philadelphia: Lippincott Williams & Wilkins; 2004.

Cook IJ, Kahrilas PJ. American Gastroenterological Association clinical practice guidelines: management of oropharyngeal dysphagia. Gastroenterology 1999; 116(2):455–78.

Ferguson DD, Foxx-Orenstein AE. Eosinophilic esophagitis: an update. Dis Esophagus 2007; 20:2–8.

Ronkainen J, Talley NJ, Aro P, et al. Prevalence of oesophageal eosinophils and eosinophilic oesophagitis in adults: the population-based Kalixanda study. Gut 2007; 56:615–20.

Chapter 3

HEARTBURN, ACID REGURGITATION AND BARRETT'S OESOPHAGUS

KEY POINTS

- Gastro-oesophageal reflux disease (GORD) is defined as a condition that develops when the reflux of stomach contents causes troublesome symptoms or complications.
- Most GORD is non-erosive. About one-third of patients have oesophagitis (erosions).
- GORD is associated with excessive oesophageal acid exposure. Some patients have symptoms triggered by weakly acidic reflux episodes.
- Dysphagia occurs with GORD but this and weight loss, anaemia or bleeding is an indication for endoscopy to exclude strictures or malignancy.
- GORD symptoms overlap with peptic ulcer disease and functional dyspepsia. In some GORD patients, epigastric pain may be the major symptom of GORD.
- A positive response to a therapeutic trial of protein pump inhibitor (PPI) therapy supports the diagnosis of GORD.
- Endoscopy is warranted if the diagnosis is unclear or when symptoms persist or are refractory or there are alarm symptoms.
- Goals of management are to relieve symptoms, reduce risk and restore quality of life.
- Proton pump inhibitors (PPIs) are the most effective pharmacotherapy for GORD providing rapid and reliable symptom resolution and healing of oesophagitis in most patients.
- Management involves an initial trial of PPI therapy then a tailored long-term treatment plan using the lowest effective PPI dose and frequency. Surgery is an option for a selected minority.
- Barrett's oesophagus confers an increased risk of oesophageal adenocarcinoma.

DEFINITIONS AND SPECTRUM

Heartburn is defined as a burning sensation in the retrosternal area and regurgitation as the perception of flow of refluxed gastric content into the mouth or hypopharynx. These are the cardinal symptoms of gastro-oesophageal reflux. Reflux is a physiological event but excessive reflux exposes the patient to the risk of physical complications or symptoms that impair quality of life. Gastro-oesophageal reflux disease (GORD) is defined as a condition which develops when the reflux of stomach contents causes troublesome symptoms or complications. Thus, in the absence of physical complications the definition depends on the impact of symptoms on an individual. Frequently, significant impairment of well-being (quality of life) occurs when symptoms occur on two or more days a week. GORD can be divided into oesophageal syndromes and extra-oesophageal syndromes (Figure 3.1). The

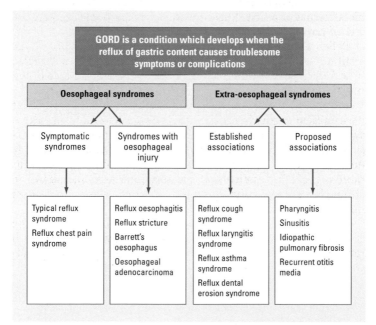

FIGURE 3.1: The definition of GORD and its constituent syndromes.*
*Reproduced with permission Am J Gastroenterol 2006; 101:1900–20.

former includes symptomatic syndromes of typical reflux symptoms and reflux induced chest pain and syndromes associated with oesophageal injury including oesophagitis (erosive GORD), strictures, Barrett's oesophagus and the small risk of oesophageal adenocarcinoma. Extra-oesophageal reflux syndromes include the established associations with cough, laryngitis and asthma as well as other putative associations.

EPIDEMIOLOGY, RISK FACTORS AND NATURAL HISTORY

Reflux symptoms are common with 15%–20% of adults experiencing heartburn at least once a week. GORD prevalence is higher in Western countries but is increasing elsewhere, particularly in Asia. This is thought to be due to an increase in Western lifestyle factors that may contribute to the development of GORD.

Obesity, alcohol consumption (>7 standard drinks a week), hiatal hernia or a first-degree relative with heartburn increase the risk of having reflux symptoms.

Patients with scleroderma, chronic respiratory disease, the institutionalised or intellectually handicapped and patients nursed in a supine position for prolonged periods are at increased risk of GORD.

In most patients, GORD is a chronic disorder and may have been present regularly for years prior to presentation. In others, symptoms may wax and wane while a minority may have transient symptoms. Milder symptoms may vary in intensity and occur only on some days. With increasing severity, symptoms tend to occur more often. Many patients will require long-term management, although in a minority symptoms do not relapse or relapse infrequently after a course of treatment.

Most patients with GORD have normal oesophageal mucosa at endoscopy (Figure 3.2). Only about one-third of patients with reflux disease have reflux oesophagitis confirmed by endoscopically visible mucosal breaks (erosions or ulceration).

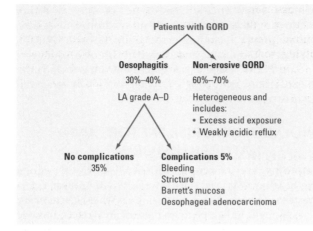

FIGURE 3.2: The spectrum of gastro-oesophageal reflux disease (GORD).

PATHOPHYSIOLOGY

GORD is usually associated with excessive exposure of the oesophagus to gastric contents, particularly acid and pepsin. This is largely the result of an increased frequency of reflux episodes, but impaired clearance of stomach contents from the oesophagus is also a factor. The degree of excess oesophageal acid exposure correlates with the likelihood and severity of oesophagitis. The pathophysiology of non-erosive GORD appears heterogeneous. Some patients have excess oesophageal acid exposure whereas, in others, symptoms appear to be triggered by weakly acidic reflux episodes. Functional heartburn is a term used to describe apparently typical GORD symptoms that have no definable relationship with acid exposure.

The tonic activity of the lower oesophageal sphincter (LOS) prevents reflux. When LOS function is impaired there is an inappropriate increase in transient LOS relaxations, which permit an increase in reflux episodes. In addition some reflux episodes occur because of defective basal LOS pressure.

Hiatal hernia is common in reflux disease. Hiatal hernia increases the likelihood that reflux will occur by impairing LOS function. However, the presence of a hiatal hernia does not necessarily mean that reflux disease is present.

Obesity is associated with an increased risk of GORD. It promotes reflux by a number of mechanisms including increased intra-abdominal pressure, reduced oesophageal clearance and gastric emptying, reduced LOS tone and the increased likelihood of hernia. Factors that may aggravate reflux include dietary components such as fat, chocolate, caffeine and alcohol as well as possibly smoking and some drugs.

DIAGNOSIS

Symptom recognition and assessment

The diagnosis of GORD is mostly based on symptom assessment. The most characteristic and common symptom is heartburn. However, it is important to use descriptive language such as 'a burning feeling rising up from the stomach or lower chest towards the neck', as the term 'heartburn' is widely interpreted and has variable meaning in different cultures. Regurgitation is also common. Excessive belching, odynophagia and waterbrash (sudden filling of the mouth with saliva) also occur in GORD. Periodic dysphagia is not infrequent, but new onset, frequent or progressive dysphagia is an indication for prompt endoscopy to exclude mechanical obstruction due to peptic strictures or malignancy. Overt bleeding occurs occasionally but is rarely severe. Occult iron deficiency may result from oesophagitis or from Cameron lesions (linear erosions caused by mechanical trauma due to the effect of the diaphragm on a hiatal hernia sac). However, iron deficiency should not be ascribed to oesophagitis or hiatal hernia without considering colonic causes for blood loss.

Accurate recognition of heartburn has reasonable sensitivity for the diagnosis of reflux. Assessment of the duration, frequency and severity of this and other symptoms and of the impact of symptoms on quality of life will determine if GORD is present and allow grading of the severity of the condition, which in turn guides the intensity of therapy.

Atypical symptoms include chest pain, which may mimic cardiac pain, and symptoms associated with extra-oesophageal manifestations of GORD including cough, sore throat, hoarseness and wheeze. GORD should be considered in patients who present with no other apparent cause for these symptoms although most patients with reflux-induced extra-oesophageal symptoms will also have typical GORD symptoms.

Symptoms of GORD may be similar to those of other upper gut disorders, especially peptic ulcer disease and functional dyspepsia. About two-thirds of patients with reflux symptoms will also complain of upper abdominal pain or discomfort (dyspepsia). In some GORD patients epigastric pain may be the major symptom of GORD and in these cases it is difficult to distinguish GORD from other conditions.

About 40% of patients with irritable bowel syndrome also complain of reflux symptoms. Such an overlap suggests both conditions may be part of the spectrum of a broader gastrointestinal disorder representing variations in the presentation of an irritable gut.

GORD symptom severity is not a reliable guide to the presence or severity of oesophagitis. In some patients, particularly the elderly or intellectually disabled patients, severe oesophagitis may be present with only mild symptoms. The presence of dysphagia, odynophagia, nocturnal choking, haematemesis or weight loss should alert the clinician to the possibility of severe or complicated GORD, or to an alternative serious diagnosis.

The therapeutic trial as a diagnostic test

A symptom-based diagnosis of GORD is often followed by a therapeutic trial of a standard dose of a proton pump inhibitor (PPI), and a response to this is inferred to support the diagnosis of GORD. When there is uncertainty about the diagnosis, particularly when there are atypical or extra-oesophageal symptoms, twice-daily PPI dosing is used. The optimal duration for this 'PPI test' is not known. Typical symptoms often respond within 2 weeks but, for extra-oesophageal symptoms, up to 8 weeks of treatment may be required. The PPI test is often assumed to have major diagnostic value for GORD but meta-analysis reveals that the sensitivity and specificity of this is moderate only, although it may be comparable to that of oesophageal pH monitoring.

INVESTIGATIONS

The role of endoscopy

It is inappropriate to investigate every patient with suspected GORD. Patients who have mild, typical reflux symptoms and no alarm symptoms may be given a trial of therapy without investigation.

Endoscopy is warranted if the diagnosis is unclear, because symptoms are either non-specific or atypical for GORD or are 'mixed' with upper gut symptoms, such as epigastric pain (Table 3.1). Endoscopy should also be undertaken for symptoms that persist or are refractory to treatment, when complications are suspected or there are alarm symptoms present (weight loss, dysphagia, odynophagia, bleeding or anaemia).

TABLE 3.1: Endoscopy recommendations

Indications for early endoscopy
- Alarm symptoms: dysphagia, odynophagia, weight loss, bleeding, anaemia
- Diagnostic problems: e.g. mixed, non-specific or atypical symptoms
- Symptoms are refractory to initial treatment
- Provision of reassurance when verbal reassurance is inadequate
- Preoperative assessment

Additional situations in which endoscopy may be appropriate
- Patients with long-standing troublesome symptoms
- To tailor drug treatment
- To detect and manage Barrett's oesophagus

Endoscopy is specific but not sensitive for the diagnosis of GORD as most patients have non-erosive GORD. However, it has an important role in the evaluation of GORD in selected patients. It allows the exclusion of alternative diagnoses, an assessment of the severity of oesophagitis (graded A–D by the LA classification), the diagnosis of complications and may allay physician and patient anxiety.

Barium swallow has a minor role in investigating GORD, except in some cases where it may be useful to plan management in patients with persistent dysphagia when a stricture is suspected or for the assessment of a large hiatal hernia.

Ancillary tests

24-hour ambulatory oesophageal pH monitoring

Only a minority of patients need ancillary testing. A pH study tests whether symptoms are temporally related to the occurrence of reflux. Measurement of the amount of reflux that occurs is of lesser diagnostic value. pH monitoring is also useful in patients in whom the diagnosis is unclear after endoscopy and a therapeutic PPI trial. It is used particularly in patients with suspected extra-oesophageal manifestations of GORD. It also has a role in assessing the adequacy of acid suppression in patients taking PPIs with presumed GORD who continue to have symptoms on therapy.

Newer diagnostic techniques include oesophageal impedance measurement. This may identify and correlate weakly acidic reflux episodes with symptoms, but is not widely available.

MANAGEMENT OF GORD

The goals of management in primary care are to recognise and treat symptoms, reduce risk and restore quality of life in patients suffering from GORD. Medical therapy is the mainstay of treatment with surgery appropriate for a select minority. The role of endoscopic therapy remains to be established.

Medical therapy

PPIs are the most effective therapy for GORD, providing rapid and reliable symptom resolution and healing of oesophagitis in most patients (80% after 8 weeks). Management involves a first phase of diagnosis, assessment of severity and initial trial of once-daily PPI therapy, usually given before breakfast, for 4–8 weeks (Figure 3.3). Patients with prominent evening or nocturnal symptoms may be dosed before the evening meal. A positive initial response to PPI therapy supports the clinical diagnosis, relieves symptoms, reassures the patient and heals oesophagitis if present. While the majority of patients with GORD will achieve good control of symptoms, a substantial minority will not. These patients are more likely to have non-erosive GORD with less acid reflux demonstrable and are less responsive to acid suppression.

The second or maintenance phase involves tailoring an individualised long-term plan using the lowest dose and frequency of drug possible. The aim is to control symptoms and minimise relapses, reduce the risk of complications of the disease or of therapy and to minimise costs. Patients with longstanding, severe symptoms or a higher grade of oesophagitis need continuous PPI therapy, as relapse is inevitable if treatment is withdrawn. A few patients need twice-daily dosing. Milder disease is treated with less intense therapy. A trial of treatment cessation is warranted in patients with short-term symptoms as not all patients relapse. An attempt can be made to 'step down' to a lower PPI dose or to an H_2-receptor antagonist (H_2-RA). Intermittent, self-directed ('on demand') therapy is effective for some patients with less frequent symptoms. Patient-directed use of antacids, antacid/ alginate combinations or 'over the counter' H_2-RAs may be helpful for the relief of mild and occasional reflux symptoms but are adjunctive treatment only for significant GORD. Prokinetic agents have little role in management.

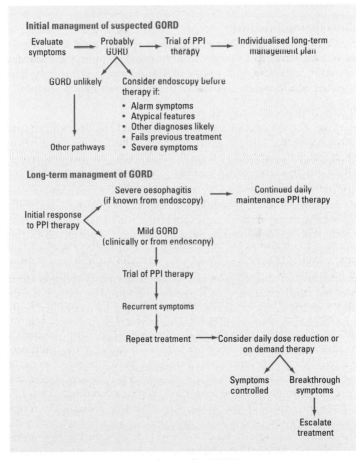

FIGURE 3.3: Management pathways for GORD.

GORD = gastro-oesophageal reflux disease; PPI = proton pump inhibitor.

PPIs are safe drugs but minor adverse effects may include headache, nausea and diarrhoea. There is a slightly increased risk of community acquired pneumonia, and bacterial gastroenteritis. Interstitial nephritis occurs rarely with PPI use. Initial concerns about potential risk of long-term acid suppression have not been realised after 20 years of PPI usage, but ongoing surveillance is required. PPIs have a very low rate of clinically important drug interactions.

Lifestyle modification

Weight loss in obese patients improves symptoms of GORD and should be advised. Lifestyle modification including dietary fat reduction, avoidance of foods that precipitate symptoms and smoking cessation are adjunctive measures that may be helpful.

Surgical therapy of GORD

Laparoscopic fundoplication may provide effective long-term control of reflux symptoms. Results are operator dependent and, as such, vary considerably. Patient selection is crucial to outcome. Patients who respond well to PPIs usually obtain good symptom control with surgery and in these patients the decision is one of informed choice. Those with atypical symptoms, who are endoscopy negative and unresponsive to acid suppression fare poorly with fundoplication. Surgery should be considered in the few patients with medically refractory GORD and in patients with problematical 'volume reflux' or symptoms derived from large and particularly para-oesophageal hernia. Fundoplication does not cause regression of Barrett's epithelium or reduce cancer risk. There is a risk of death (0.2%) and serious morbidity from fundoplication. Although the absolute risk is relatively small, it exceeds that for PPIs. Perioperative complications include surgical mishap and the need for conversion to open fundoplication. Common adverse effects are inadequate symptom control (re-operation rate 3%–6%) and a need for ongoing antisecretory medication (20%–60%) which increases over time. Troublesome new symptoms include dysphagia, 'gas bloat' syndrome and diarrhoea, and these may be difficult to manage.

Endoscopic antireflux therapy

Endoscopic procedures have been developed as alternatives to laparoscopic fundoplication. Adequate comparative short-

and long-term efficacy data are lacking and safety issues are unresolved. Although these techniques are being used, at present such techniques should be considered experimental and their use confined to clinical trials in major centres.

GORD, PPIs and *Helicobacter pylori*

Helicobacter pylori infection is present frequently in patients with GORD as both conditions are common. However, *H. pylori* does not cause GORD. Similarly, infection does not reduce the risk of developing GORD, except in the minority of patients in whom infection causes marked gastric mucosal atrophy with reduced acid secretion. These patients are somewhat less likely to develop severe oesophagitis and Barrett's mucosa but are at greatly increased risk of gastric adenocarcinoma and eradication therapy is advisable. Reflux symptoms are not better controlled with PPIs in patients who are *H. pylori*-positive and eradication of *H. pylori* does not significantly increase the risk of GORD developing.

In *H. pylori* infected patients, PPI therapy causes a worsening of the histological grade of gastritis and an accelerated risk of gastric mucosal atrophy and intestinal metaplasia. This is not seen when PPIs are used in uninfected patients or in those in whom *H. pylori* has been eradicated prior to long-term PPI use. As these changes are risk factors for gastric adenocarcinoma, eradication of *H. pylori* is recommended prior to long term PPI therapy for GORD, particularly in younger patients.

PPIs affect the accuracy of biopsies (urease test and histology) and breath tests for *H. pylori* so testing is best done prior to PPI therapy or after cessation of PPIs for at least one week and preferably two.

Barrett's oesophagus

Definitions of Barrett's oesophagus vary, but the core component is the presence of metaplastic columnar epithelium from the gastro-oesophageal junction and extending proximally. Specialised intestinal metaplasia (SIM) is often identified in this metaplastic epithelium and it is the presence of SIM that confers the risk of progression to dysplasia and adenocarcinoma. For this reason the presence of oesophageal SIM identified by histological examination of biopsy specimens is considered a prerequisite for the diagnosis of Barrett's oesophagus by some, whereas others prefer to describe Barrett's oesophagus on endoscopic appearances and then specify the presence or absence of SIM after biopsy results are available. The endoscopic description of Barrett's oesophagus should include a standardised measure of extent.

About 4%–8% of Caucasian patients with GORD who undergo endoscopy will have Barrett's oesophagus. Caucasian males aged over 50 years have the highest risk for the development of Barrett's oesophagus and progression to adenocarcinoma. Obesity and smoking are added risk factors.

The majority of people with a Barrett's oesophagus remain undiagnosed and unaware of the condition. The frequency and severity of heartburn are not useful for the prediction of the presence of Barrett's oesophagus. There is no evidence that acid control by PPIs or surgery reverses the condition. Whether PPI therapy reduces the risk of progression to dysplasia remains to be confirmed.

There is no evidence that general population screening for Barrett's oesophagus will affect mortality from oesophageal adenocarcinoma. Furthermore, there is no convincing evidence that screening all patients with GORD for Barrett's oesophagus by endoscopy would be of benefit. Targeted screening of individuals at higher risk of developing the condition has been proposed. When patients who have endoscopy to evaluate GORD are found to have Barrett's oesophagus, ongoing endoscopic surveillance is often offered, although there is no unequivocal evidence for a clinical or health economic benefit from such a strategy. When Barrett's oesophagus is found, multiple biopsies should be obtained in four quadrants at 2 cm intervals along the Barrett's mucosa to determine if SIM is present and to search for dysplasia or cancer. The highest yield for this occurs at the initial diagnosis of Barrett's oesophagus and not during subsequent surveillance. The risk of progression to cancer appears greater for those with long-segment Barrett's oesophagus (>3 cm) and has been estimated to be about 0.5% annually. Surveying patients with short-segment Barrett's oesophagus (<3 cm) or SIM occurring just at or above the gastro-oesophageal junction is controversial as the cancer risk is lower.

When Barrett's oesophagus is found or suspected in the presence of oesophagitis, epithelial atypia or dysplasia may be misdiagnosed. In this case the examination needs to be repeated after mucosal healing with PPIs. Surveillance of Barrett's oesophagus after initial diagnosis aims to identify patients who progress to high-grade dysplasia or early adenocarcinoma so that appropriate intervention can be provided to improve survival. The optimal surveillance interval is not defined. Generally, 2–3-yearly biopsies are recommended.

As the likelihood of Barrett's oesophagus increases with advancing age, many patients with Barrett's oesophagus have substantial comorbidities and increased risk for mortality from other causes. Moreover, oesophagectomy for high-grade dysplasia or cancer has significant risks in older patients. For these reasons, endoscopic techniques for treating Barrett's oesophagus and dysplasia are being trialled in specialised centres. Such techniques include endoscopic mucosal resection or ablative methods such as photodynamic therapy, laser therapy, multipolar electrocoagulation, argon plasma coagulation, radiofrequency ablation and cryotherapy. Whether ablation therapy eliminates or significantly reduces the risk of cancer or reduces the need for ongoing surveillance is not known and it is yet to be determined whether the risks associated with these therapies are less than the risk of Barrett's oesophagus progressing to cancer.

When low grade dysplasia is found, repeat endoscopy with biopsies should be done within 6 months, with the patient on PPIs, to determine if high-grade dysplasia has been missed. If low-grade dysplasia persists, re-surveillance at 6 months and then annually is recommended.

When high-grade dysplasia is found, it is mandatory to have the pathology reviewed by another pathologist and, if there is doubt, to repeat the biopsies. About one-third of patients with high-grade dysplasia have an underlying cancer and a variable number (15%–60%) will progress to cancer within 4 years especially when high-grade dysplasia is multifocal. When high-grade dysplasia is confirmed, consideration for oesophagectomy is an option in patients fit for surgery. An alternative is intensive surveillance (every 3 months) until intramucosal cancer is detected, then surgery (as not all dysplasia will progress to cancer), but such a strategy is problematical. If the patient declines or is not fit for surgery, endoscopic techniques are an option.

SUMMARY

Heartburn is defined as a burning sensation in the retrosternal area. Regurgitation is the perception of flow of reflux gastric content into the mouth or hypopharynx. GORD is defined as a condition that develops when the reflux of stomach contents causes troublesome symptoms or complications. Risk factors for GORD include hiatal hernia, obesity and increasing age. Most GORD is non-erosive (endoscopy-negative reflux disease). About one-third of patients have oesophagitis (erosions or mucosal breaks). GORD is associated with excessive oesophageal acid exposure. Some patients have symptoms triggered by weakly acidic reflux episodes. GORD encompasses oesophageal syndromes and extra-oesophageal syndromes. The diagnosis of GORD is mostly symptom based. Typical symptoms are heartburn and acid regurgitation. Other symptoms include excessive belching, odynophagia and waterbrash. Atypical symptoms include chest pain, cough and sore throat. Dysphagia occurs with GORD, but in conjunction with weight loss, anaemia or bleeding is an indication for endoscopy to exclude strictures or malignancy. Notably, GORD symptoms can overlap with peptic ulcer disease and functional (non-ulcer) dyspepsia. In some patients with GORD, epigastric pain is the major symptom. Many patients with irritable bowel syndrome (IBS) also complain of reflux symptoms, suggesting that both conditions may be part of the spectrum of a broader gastrointestinal disorder. Assessment of the duration, frequency and severity of symptoms and the impact of symptoms on quality of life allows grading of GORD severity and guides therapy. A positive response to a therapeutic trial of PPI therapy supports the diagnosis of GORD, although both false positives and false negatives occur with a PPI trial. Endoscopy is warranted if the diagnosis is unclear or when symptoms persist or are refractory, or if there are alarm symptoms. The goals of management are to relieve symptoms, reduce risk and restore quality of life. PPIs are the most effective pharmacotherapy for GORD providing rapid and reliable symptom resolution and healing of oesophagitis in most patients. Management involves an initial trial of a PPI and a tailored long-term plan using the lowest dose and frequency of drug. Antireflux surgery is an option for a selected minority or those who prefer not to take acid suppression therapy. Weight loss in obese patients may improve symptoms of GORD and should be advised. Barrett's oesophagus is a premalignant condition conferring an increased risk of oesophageal adenocarcinoma. However, there is controversy regarding optimal screening, surveillance and treatment for this condition currently.

FURTHER READING

DeVault KR, Castell DO. Updated guidelines for the diagnosis and treatment of gastroesophageal reflux disease. Am J Gastroenterol 2005; 100:190–200.

Katelaris PH. An evaluation of current GERD therapy: a summary and comparison of effectiveness, adverse effects and costs of drugs, surgery and endoscopic therapy. Best Pract Res Clin Gastroenterol 2004; 18 Suppl:39–45.

Moayyedi P, Talley NJ. Gastroesophageal reflux disease. Lancet 2006; 387:2086–100.

Sharma P, McQuaid K, Dent J, et al. A critical review of the diagnosis and management of Barrett's esophagus: the AGA Chicago Workshop. Gastroenterology 2004; 127:310–30.

Vakil N, van Zanten SV, Kahrilas P, et al. Global Consensus Group. The Montreal definition and classification of gastroesophageal reflux disease: a global evidence-based consensus. Am J Gastroenterol 2006; 101:1900–20.

van Pinxteren B, Numans ME, Bonis PA, et al. Short-term treatment with proton pump inhibitors, H2-receptor antagonists and prokinetics for gastro-oesophageal reflux disease-like symptoms and endoscopy negative reflux disease. Cochrane Database Syst Rev. 2006; 3: CD002095.

Chapter 4

DYSPEPSIA AND FUNCTIONAL DYSPEPSIA

KEY POINTS

- Dyspepsia is defined as pain or discomfort located in the central upper abdomen.
- Dyspepsia may coexist with and be difficult to differentiate from gastro-oesophageal reflux disease.
- The most common cause of organic dyspepsia is reflux oesophagitis, followed by peptic ulcer disease.
- Functional dyspepsia accounts for over 60% of all dyspepsia.
- If identified, all cases of *Helicobacter pylori* in patients with dyspepsia should be treated.

DEFINITIONS

The definition of dyspepsia is controversial, with some authorities including reflux symptoms whereas others do not. An international committee of clinical investigators that meets in Rome have routinely excluded reflux symptoms.

Dyspepsia has historically been defined as pain or discomfort located in the upper abdomen (mainly in or around the midline as opposed to the right or left hypochondrium). Discomfort may include bloating, fullness, early satiety, postprandial fullness or nausea. Dyspepsia may be either *organic*, implying an organic, systemic or metabolic disease has been identified as the cause, or *functional*, where there is no identifiable explanation for the symptoms. Functional dyspepsia is also known as idiopathic or non-ulcer dyspepsia.

The Rome III committee has redefined functional dyspepsia and limited the term to refer to the four following symptoms: bothersome post-prandial fullness, early satiation, epigastric pain, or epigastric burning. The remaining symptoms of discomfort listed above have been allocated clinical entities of their own, and together they comprise the functional gastroduodenal disorders (Table 4.1). In addition, as shown in Table 4.2, there are two new diagnostic categories within functional dyspepsia; namely postprandial distress syndrome (PDS) and epigastric pain syndrome (EPS).

There is some overlap between symptoms of gastro-oesophageal reflux disease (GORD) and dyspepsia. Heartburn is traditionally excluded from the Rome II and III criteria for dyspepsia, although in Rome III a burning sensation confined to the epigastrium is not considered to be heartburn unless it also radiates retrosternally. Despite the exclusion of heartburn, reflux oesophagitis is the most common structural finding when patients with dyspepsia are evaluated by upper endoscopy in Western nations. Heartburn more than twice weekly strongly suggests GORD in favour of dyspepsia.

TABLE 4.1: Functional gastroduodenal disorders

- Functional dyspepsia
  - Postprandial distress syndrome
  - Epigastric pain syndrome
- Belching disorders
  - Aerophagia
  - Unspecified excessive belching
- Nausea and vomiting disorders
  - Chronic idiopathic nausea
  - Functional vomiting
  - Cyclic vomiting syndrome
- Rumination syndrome in adults

TABLE 4.2: Subtypes of functional dyspepsia

Diagnostic criteria* for postprandial distress syndrome

Must include *one or both* of the following:

1. Bothersome postprandial fullness, occurring after ordinary sized meals, at least several times per week
2. Early satiation that prevents finishing a regular meal, at least several times per week

Supportive criteria

1. Upper abdominal bloating or postprandial nausea or excessive belching can be present
2. Epigastric pain syndrome may coexist

TABLE 4.2: Subtypes of functional dyspepsia *(continued)*

Diagnostic criteria* for epigastric pain syndrome

Must include *all* of the following:

1. Pain or burning localised to the epigastrium of at least moderate severity at least once per week
2. The pain is intermittent
3. Not generalised or localised to other abdominal or chest regions
4. Not relieved by defecation or passage of flatus
5. Not fulfilling criteria for gall bladder and sphincter of Oddi disorders

Supportive criteria

1. The pain may be of a burning quality but without a retrosternal component
2. The pain is commonly induced or relieved by ingestion of a meal but may occur while fasting
3. Postprandial distress syndrome may coexist

*Criteria fulfilled for the last 3 months with symptom onset at least 6 months before diagnosis

---

Uninvestigated dyspepsia refers to new onset or recurrent dyspepsia for which no diagnostic investigations have yet been performed and subsequently a specific diagnosis has not been reached. This has implications for both diagnostic and management pathways.

EPIDEMIOLOGY

The prevalence of dyspepsia in the Western society is approximately 25%, although the true prevalence depends on the population being studied. The annual incidence is cited between 1% and 10%. As similar numbers of patients experience resolution of their symptoms, fairly constant prevalence rates occur. Women suffer marginally more than men and symptoms tend to improve slightly with age.

CAUSES

Organic

Organic causes of dyspepsia are many and varied as outlined in Table 4.3, but the majority of cases are due to peptic ulcer disease, gastro-oesophageal reflux and malignancy.

TABLE 4.3: Causes of organic dyspepsia

Luminal
- Peptic ulcer disease
- Gastric or oesophageal neoplasms
- Gastro-oesophageal reflux disease
- Gastroparesis (diabetes, post-vagotomy, scleroderma, chronic intestinal pseudo-obstruction)
- Infiltrative gastric disorders (Ménétrier's syndrome, Crohn's, eosinophilic gastroenteritis, sarcoidosis, amyloidosis)
- Malabsorptive disorders (coeliac sprue, lactose intolerance)
- Gastric infections (cytomegalovirus, fungal, tuberculosis, syphilis)
- Parasites (*Giardia lamblia, Strongyloides stercoralis*)
- Chronic gastric volvulus
- Chronic intestinal ischaemia

Medications
- Ethanol
- Aspirin/NSAIDs
- Antibiotics (macrolides, sulfonamides, metronidazole)
- Theophyllyine
- Digitalis
- Glucocorticoids
- Iron, potassium chloride
- Niacin, gemfibrozil
- Narcotics
- Colchicine
- Quinidine
- Oestrogens
- Levodopa
- Nitrates
- Loop diuretics
- ACE inhibitors

Pancreaticobiliary
- Chronic pancreatitis
- Pancreatic neoplasms
- Biliary colic (cholelithiasis, choledocholithiasis, sphincter of Oddi dysfunction)

Systemic
- Diabetes mellitus
- Thyroid disease
- Hyperparathyroidism
- Adrenal insufficiency
- Collagen vascular disorders
- Renal insufficiency
- Cardiac ischaemia, chronic heart failure
- Intra-abdominal malignancy
- Pregnancy

Adapted from Feldman M, Friedman LS, Sleisenger MH. Sleisenger and Fordtran's gastrointestinal and liver disease. 7th edn. Philadelphia: WB Saunders; 2002.

Peptic ulcer disease is implicated in up to 10% of cases of dyspepsia. A chronic duodenal ulcer is most often associated with *Helicobacter pylori* infection, whereas chronic gastric ulcers are also associated commonly with aspirin or non-steroidal antiinflammatory drug (NSAID) use. There is poor correlation between symptoms and the presence of ulcers in NSAID users. COX 2 inhibitors produce fewer symptoms than traditional NSAIDs, but the risk of dyspepsia is still increased.

Endoscopic criteria for reflux oesophagitis are found in 15% of patients with dyspepsia. Non-erosive gastro-oesophageal reflux disease may be readily confused with functional dyspepsia, but it often still responds to acid suppression therapy.

Adenocarcinoma of the stomach or oesophagus is seen in fewer than 2% of patients referred for endoscopy, and the vast majority (98%) are over 45 years of age. Alarm symptoms that may suggest the possibility of malignancy include:

- unintended weight loss
- persistent vomiting
- progressive dysphagia
- odynophagia
- anaemia
- haematemesis
- palpable abdominal mass or lymphadenopathy
- unexplained iron deficiency anaemia
- family history of upper gastrointestinal cancer
- previous gastric surgery
- jaundice.

Functional gastroduodenal disorders

Functional gastroduodenal disorders account for around 60% of presentations but are a diagnosis of exclusion. Current criteria require the presence of symptoms during the last 3 months occurring at least several times per week, with symptom onset at least 6 months before diagnosis and no evidence of structural disease on endoscopy (Tables 4.1 and 4.2).

The underlying pathophysiology of functional gastroduodenal disorders is incompletely understood. Gastric motility is abnormal in around 60% of cases with observed changes including delayed (or less often accelerated) gastric emptying, impaired proximal stomach accommodation leading to antral distension, and variable myoelectric activity. None of these changes convincingly correlate with symptoms. Use of a gastric barostat balloon has demonstrated visceral hypersensitivity in over 40% of patients with dyspepsia.

In addition to its role in peptic ulcer disease and stomach cancers, *H. pylori* infection may account for some cases of functional dyspepsia. A Cochrane review of eradication therapy showed a small but statistically significant difference in favour of *H. pylori* treatment after 12 months of follow-up.

Other

No foods have been causally implicated in dyspepsia, but coffee and foods with a high fat content may aggravate symptoms.

Acid secretion is normal in functional dyspepsia, but acid sensitivity may be relevant in a subset. A minority (one-third at most) respond to acid suppression over placebo.

Anxiety and depression may aggravate symptoms and may promote healthcare seeking for dyspepsia, but a causal link with functional dyspepsia is not established.

MANAGEMENT

Figure 4.1 shows an algorithm for the approach to the patient with uninvestigated dyspepsia. Taking a thorough history with appropriate physical examination to clarify whether the symptoms are pancreatic, biliary or colonic in origin is an essential first step. Once a specific diagnosis has been made, treatment should be directed towards the specific condition. If uncomplicated dyspepsia is a consideration, discontinuing use of aspirin/NSAIDs and, if present, treatment of symptoms of GORD with a proton pump inhibitor (PPI) should be instituted. It is critical to make an assessment of the presence of alarm symptoms and signs. Older age and/or presence of alarm features indicates the need for early endoscopy, whereas the remainder may be managed with a 'test and treat' strategy (referring to establishing the presence/absence of *H. pylori*).

Non-invasive testing for *H. pylori* utilising either a urea breath test or a stool antigen immunoassay is appropriate in most patients. Serology is less accurate and is generally not recommended unless there is no alternative. Those who are already undergoing endoscopy should have a biopsy routinely obtained based on current guidelines. In these patients, rapid urease testing (e.g. CLOtest) with or without histology is usually performed.

The most accurate non-invasive test is the urease breath test with a sensitivity and specificity of 88%–95% and 95%–100%, respectively, however PPI or H_2-receptor antagonist use, recent upper gastrointestinal bleeding or antibiotics or bismuth use may induce false negative results. In these situations, alternative strategies should be considered. Similarly, endoscopic diagnosis with a biopsy urease test is highly sensitive and specific with the same caveats. Biopsies taken for histology may be examined in the event of a negative test.

First-line treatment for *H. pylori* is triple therapy with combinations of two antibiotics and one adjunctive agent over 7–14 days; a meta-analysis has demonstrated slight superiority with a two-week treatment period. The most common regimen includes a PPI (e.g. omeprazole 20 mg twice daily) with amoxicillin 1 g twice daily and clarithromycin 500 mg twice daily. Metronidazole may be substituted for amoxicillin in penicillin-sensitive patients, although the levels of metronidazole resistance are increasing significantly. Success rates of over 80% have been achieved in most trials.

Response to therapy may be assessed most effectively with a urea breath test performed at least 4 weeks after completing antibiotic therapy, and at least one week after stopping PPI therapy. Treatment failures are most commonly treated with a second-line regimen of quadruple therapy utilising bismuth, a PPI and alternative antibiotics such as metronidazole and tetracycline for a further 2 weeks. Rescue therapy for subsequent treatment failures involves changing the antibiotics to levofloxacin or rifabutin along with a PPI. If symptoms persist despite eradication of *H. pylori*, a trial of PPI should be undertaken. Alternative diagnoses should be considered if there is a continued lack of response and consideration also given to gastric emptying studies and psychological assessment (Figure 4.1).

When an organic diagnosis cannot be made and the presumptive diagnosis is a functional gastroduodenal disorder, the first step involves reassuring the patient of the benign nature of the condition. Next, despite the lack of convincing evidence, recommendations usually include smoking cessation and stopping or reducing consumption of coffee and alcohol, in addition to advice to eat several small low-fat meals per day.

PPIs and H_2-receptor antagonists are superior to placebo in the treatment of functional dyspepsia. Prokinetic agents, such

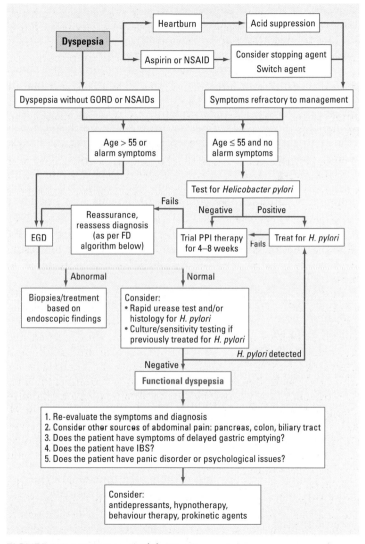

FIGURE 4.1: Management of dyspepsia.

EGD = endoscopic gastroduodenoscopy; FD = functional dyspepsia; GORD = gastro-oesophageal reflux disease; IBS = irritable bowel syndrome; NSAIDs = non-steroidal antiinflammatory drugs; PPI = proton pump inhibitor.

as metoclopramide or domperidone, also appear to be modestly effective. Domperidone has the advantage of limited crossing of the blood–brain barrier and, consequently, exhibits fewer centrally-mediated side effects compared with metoclopramide.

One small study demonstrated some symptom improvement with amitriptyline. Unfortunately, most trials evaluating antidepressants in functional gastrointestinal disorders have not investigated dyspepsia independently of other disorders such as irritable bowel syndrome, so firm conclusions specifically related to their effects in dyspepsia cannot be drawn. Finally, studies have shown that patients with functional dyspepsia have higher scores on a variety of psychological parameters including anxiety, depression and neuroticism when compared with the community controls. A recent study of patients who had failed to respond to conventional pharmacologic treatments showed that psychotherapy or hypnotherapy may have both short- and long-term beneficial effects.

SUMMARY

Dyspepsia refers to pain or discomfort in the epigastric area. Most patients with dyspepsia have functional dyspepsia but aspirin or non-steroidal antiinflammatory drugs can often cause similar symptoms. Gastro-oesophageal reflux disease can present with epigastric pain or burning rather than typical heartburn. Endoscopy is indicated to rule out serious disease for patients who are older or who have alarm symptoms or signs. In younger patients without alarm features, a trial of empiric therapy is generally appropriate. Currently, testing for *H. pylori* using the urea breath test or stool antigen test is recommended. If the patient is positive, treatment for *H. pylori* is indicated. If the patient does not have *H. pylori* infection, a trial of acid suppression with a PPI for 4–8 weeks is usual first-line empiric therapy. If the patient has a negative endoscopy and documented functional dyspepsia, treatment options include antidepressants, prokinetic agents and psychological treatments if acid suppression or *H. pylori* eradication fails.

H. pylori causes gastritis, peptic ulcer disease and gastric adenocarcinoma. A minority of patients with functional dyspepsia and *H. pylori* infection will respond to anti-*H. pylori* therapy. False negative test results for *H. pylori* can occur in the setting of recent acid suppression. Ideally, patients should be off acid suppression therapy for 1–2 weeks prior to testing to avoid false-negative results. If standard triple therapy with a PPI, amoxicillin and clarithromycin fails to eradicate the infection, then the usual next management approach is to use quadruple therapy combining a PPI, bismuth, metronidazole and tetracycline for 2 weeks.

FURTHER READING

Ford AC, Forman D, Bailey AG, et al. Initial poor quality of life and new onset of dyspepsia: results from a longitudinal follow-up study. Gut 2007; 56:321–7.

Gisbert JP. Accuracy of *Helicobacter pylori* diagnostic tests in patients with bleeding peptic ulcer: a systematic review and meta-analysis. Am J Gastroenterol 2006; 101:848–63.

Tack J, Lee KJ. Pathophysiology and treatment of functional dyspepsia. J Clin Gastroenterol 2005; 39:S211–16.

Tack J, Talley NJ, Camilleri M, et al. Functional gastroduodenal disorders. Gastroenterology 2006; 130:1466–79.

Talley NJ, Vakil NB, Moayyedi P. American Gastroenterological Association technical review on the evaluation of dyspepsia. Gastroenterology 2005; 129:1756–80.

Chapter 5

NAUSEA AND VOMITING

KEY POINTS

- Nausea and vomiting are most often secondary to extra-gastrointestinal processes.
- A systematic approach to diagnosis and management is imperative given the multitude of causes.
- Review all medications and consider their side effects.
- The metabolic consequences and complications of vomiting should be an integral part of patient assessment.
- A therapeutic trial of antiemetics and/or prokinetics is a reasonable approach if a specific cause is not found after appropriate investigations.
- Chronic unexplained nausea and vomiting may respond to tricyclic antidepressant therapy.

INTRODUCTION

Nausea and vomiting are common symptoms with a wide array of possible causes. Nausea describes the unpleasant subjective sensations that precede vomiting. During nausea, reflux of duodenal contents into the stomach is frequent, possibly due to increased tone of the duodenum and proximal jejunum, although this is not always present. Concurrently, gastric tone is reduced and gastric peristalsis is diminished or absent. It is important to distinguish between four distinct symptoms, namely retching, vomiting, regurgitation and rumination, that superficially may appear similar (Table 5.1). In particular, vomiting involves expulsion of gastric contents through the mouth via forceful, sustained contraction of the abdominal muscles and diaphragm when the pylorus is contracted. Occasionally, vomiting is associated with hypersalivation and defecation; cardiac dysrhythmias may rarely occur.

TABLE 5.1: Definitions of terminology associated with nausea and vomiting
Nausea: The unpleasant sensation of the imminent need to vomit, usually referred to the throat or epigastrium; a sensation that may or may not ultimately lead to the act of vomiting.
Retching: Spasmodic respiratory movements against a closed glottis with contractions of the abdominal musculature without expulsion of any gastric contents, referred to as 'dry heaves'.
Vomiting: Forceful oral expulsion of gastric contents associated with contraction of the abdominal and chest wall musculature.
Regurgitation: The act by which food is brought back into the mouth without the abdominal and diaphragmatic muscular activity that characterises vomiting.
Rumination: Chewing and swallowing of regurgitated food that has come back into the mouth through an unconscious voluntary increase in abdominal pressure within minutes of eating or during eating.
Anorexia: Loss of desire to eat, that is, a true loss of appetite.
Sitophobia: Fear of eating because of subsequent or associated discomfort.
Early satiety: The feeling of being full after eating an unusually small quantity of food.
Adapted from Quigley EM, Hasler WL, Parkman HP. AGA technical review on nausea and vomiting. Gastroenterology 2001; 120:263–86.

PATHOGENESIS

Emetic stimuli are recognised in the vomiting centre in the dorsal medulla, which is linked to other centres controlling respiration and salivation. This area is innervated by vagal and sympathetic afferents from the gastrointestinal tract, the pharynx, vestibular system, heart, peritoneum and higher central nervous system centres such as the thalamus, hypothalamus and cerebral cortex. A second area in the brain, the area postrema, is home to the chemoreceptor trigger zone (CTZ). The blood–brain barrier is essentially absent in this location, permitting substances in the circulation to stimulate the CTZ, which in turn induces vomiting, probably via the vomiting centre.

Neurotransmission in the vomiting centre and CTZ appears to be mediated via dopaminergic, serotonergic, muscarinic and histaminergic receptors, and pharmacological therapies have been developed targeting each of these (see later).

CLINICAL CONSIDERATIONS

The differential diagnosis of nausea and/or vomiting is extensive and is presented in Table 5.2. The major causes include infection, medications (particularly chemotherapeutic agents) and toxins, central nervous system pathology, organic gastrointestinal disorders, endocrine and metabolic disorders including pregnancy, systemic illnesses, psychiatric disease, postoperatively and functional gastrointestinal disorders including the cyclical vomiting syndrome.

Important aspects in the history that may assist in identifying the cause include:

- Duration of symptoms
  - Acute:
    - Gastroenteritis:
      - Viral most common, particularly when associated with diarrhoea, headache, and myalgias
      - Most resolve within 5 days
    - Toxin ingestion e.g. Staphylococci
    - Pancreatitis
    - Cholecystitis
    - Medication-related side effect
    - Pregnancy
    - Visceral pain related to inflammation, obstruction, or ischaemia
  - Chronic (present >1 month):
    - Intracranial pathology
    - Abnormal upper gastrointestinal motility
    - Metabolic or endocrine abnormality
    - Functional vomiting and cyclic vomiting
    - Gastro-oesophageal reflux disease—heartburn and oesophagitis may be absent.
- Timing of vomiting in relation to meals
  - Morning—prior to eating:
    - Pregnancy
    - Uraemia
    - Increased intracranial pressure (ICP)—may be 'projectile' and usually associated with neurological symptoms or signs
    - Functional vomiting

- During or soon after a meal:
  - Eating disorder e.g. bulimia, anorexia nervosa
  - Peptic ulcer near the pyloric channel (now very rare)
- Delayed >1 h after meals:
  - Gastric outlet obstruction or small bowel obstruction
  - Gastroparesis
- Continuous: conversion disorder
- Habitual postprandial or irregular vomiting: major depression.
- Contents and/or odour of the vomitus
  - Undigested food (usually regurgitation):
    - Zenker's diverticulum
    - Achalasia
    - Oesophageal stricture
    - Rumination
  - Partly digested food:
    - Gastric outlet obstruction
    - Gastroparesis
  - Bile-stained:
    - Small bowel obstruction (may also be feculent)
    - Post gastric surgery.
- Associated symptoms
  - Alarm symptoms such as weight loss, fevers or family history of cancer: suggest malignancy must be excluded
  - Abdominal pain: usually suggests an organic process such as obstruction. Subacute bowel obstruction, which can be missed on barium studies, may be secondary to adhesions from previous abdominal surgery
  - Neurological symptoms, e.g. neck stiffness, focal neurological deficit
  - Menstruation: pregnancy must *always* be considered in the differential.

Physical examination should be directed by the history obtained, however, abdominal examination is essential and should include assessing for tenderness with some emphasis on localisation, presence or absence of bowel sounds and a succussion splash, evidence of previous abdominal surgery, hernias and masses. Subsequently several additional areas may need review including, but not limited to, assessment for lymphadenopathy, central or peripheral neurological deficits, evidence of connective tissue

TABLE 5.2: Causes of nausea and/or vomiting

Medications and toxic aetiology

- Cancer chemotherapy
  - *Severe:* cisplatin, dacarbazine, nitrogen mustard
  - *Moderate:* etoposide, methotrexate, cytarabine
  - *Mild:* fluorouracil, vinblastine, tamoxifen
- Analgesics
  - Aspirin or non-steroidal antiinflammatory drugs (NSAIDs)
  - Gold
  - Antigout drugs
- Cardiovascular medications
  - Digoxin
  - Antiarrhythmics
  - Antihypertensives
  - Beta-blockers
  - Calcium channel blockers
  - Diuretics
- Hormonal preparations/therapies
  - Oral hypoglycaemic agents
  - Oral contraceptives

- Antibiotics/antivirals
  - Erythromycin
  - Tetracycline
  - Sulfonamides
  - Antituberculous drugs
  - Aciclovir
- Gastrointestinal medications
  - Sulfasalazine
  - Azathioprine
- Central nervous system (CNS) active
  - Nicotine
  - Narcotics
  - Antiparkinsonian drugs
  - Anticonvulsants
- Theophylline
- Ethanol abuse
- Marijuana toxicity

Disorders of the gut and peritoneum

- Organic gastrointestinal disorders
  - Pancreatic adenocarcinoma
  - Inflammatory intraperitoneal disease
  - Peptic ulcer disease
  - Cholecystitis
  - Pancreatitis
  - Hepatitis
  - Crohn's disease
  - Mesenteric ischaemia
  - Retroperitoneal fibrosis
  - Mucosal metastases

- Functional gastrointestinal disorders
  - Functional nausea and vomiting disorders
  - Cyclic vomiting syndrome
  - Irritable bowel syndrome
- Mechanical obstruction
  - Gastric outlet obstruction
  - Small bowel obstruction
  - Gastroparesis
  - Chronic intestinal pseudo-obstruction

TABLE 5.2: Causes of nausea and/or vomiting *(continued)*

Endocrine and metabolic causes
- Pregnancy
- Other endocrine and metabolic
  - Uraemia
  - Diabetic ketoacidosis
  - Hyperparathyroidism
  - Hypoparathyroidism
  - Hyperthyroidism
  - Addison's disease
  - Acute intermittent porphyria

Infectious causes
- Gastroenteritis
  - Viral e.g. Norwalk, rotavirus, adenoviruses
  - Bacterial e.g. *Staphylococcus aureus, Salmonella, Bacillus cereus, Clostridium perfringens*
- Non-gastrointestinal infections
  - Otitis media
  - Urinary tract infection
  - Jamaican vomiting sickness

CNS causes
- Migraine
- Increased intracranial pressure
  - Malignancy
  - Haemorrhage
  - Infarction
  - Abscess
  - Meningitis
  - Congenital malformation
  - Hydrocephalus
  - Pseudotumour cerebri
- Labyrinthine disorders
  - Motion sickness
  - Labyrinthitis
  - Tumours
  - Ménière's disease
  - Iatrogenic
  - Fluorescein angiography
- Seizure disorders
- Demyelinating disorders
- Emotional responses

Psychiatric disease
- Functional vomiting
- Anxiety disorders
- Depression
- Pain
- Anorexia nervosa
- Bulimia nervosa

Miscellaneous causes
- Postoperative nausea and vomiting
- Radiation therapy
- Cardiac disease
  - Myocardial infarction
  - Congestive heart failure
  - Radiofrequency ablation
- Hypervitaminosis

Adapted from Quigley EM, Hasler WL, Parkman HP. AGA technical review on nausea and vomiting. Gastroenterology 2001; 120:263–86.

disease or thyroid dysfunction, and review of fingernails and tooth enamel for signs of acid damage from recurrent vomiting.

Investigations

The choice of investigations will depend predominantly on the conclusions drawn from the history and physical examination.

Assessment of the consequences of vomiting must be performed, in particular looking for evidence of dehydration, electrolyte disturbances and the presence of a hypokalaemic metabolic alkalosis. Initial evaluation should include a full blood count, electrolytes and liver function tests, pH, an erythrocyte sedimentation rate or C-reactive protein and β-hCG in females of child-bearing age. More specific screening, such as thyroid function tests, should be performed as considered appropriate.

Further diagnostic evaluation may include erect and supine abdominal X-rays if the history suggests intestinal obstruction and an abdominal ultrasound if hepatobiliary, pancreatic or gall bladder pathology is suspected. Gastroscopy may also be considered if a mucosal lesion such as peptic ulcer disease or reflux oesophagitis is suspected, and is more sensitive and specific than radiographic studies. Visualisation of the small intestine is commonly obtained with a small bowel follow-through (SBFT) examination. Some centres advocate enteroclysis (or small intestine enema), which is more sensitive but may require the use of sedation as the technique requires placement of a nasoduodenal or oroduodenal tube. Computed tomography (CT) enterography is preferable with oral and intravenous contrast when intestinal obstruction is suspected and provides additional information about the pancreas and hepatobiliary system and can also identify the presence of abdominal masses or retroperitoneal pathology.

The commonest causes of gastroparesis are idiopathic (possibly post-viral) and diabetes mellitus. Systemic diseases such as scleroderma, systemic lupus erythematosus, polymyositis, dermatomyositis and amyloidosis may also cause gastroparesis, which is also seen after vagotomy and in association with pancreatic adenocarcinoma. Gastroparesis results in abnormal gastric emptying, however this also may be seen in up to 40% of patients with functional gastroduodenal disorders (Table 5.3).

Abnormal gastric emptying may be assessed using a radionuclide gastric emptying study in which serial images of the retention or disappearance of a radiolabelled meal from the stomach are captured by a γ-camera. Solid meals are more sensitive for detecting gastroparesis compared with liquid meals. Delayed gastric emptying is considered present if the gastric retention at 4 hours is greater than 40% of the radiolabelled meal (sensitivity 100%, specificity 70%).

Antroduodenal manometry, which can differentiate between neuropathy (abnormal contractile response with normal amplitude contractions) or myopathy (low amplitude contractions), is available in some specialised centres. It may also detect missed bowel obstruction.

Electrogastrography (EGG) measures the electrical activity of the stomach with surface electrodes in both the fasting and the postprandial states. The normal pacemaker rhythm of gastric

---

TABLE 5.3: Functional nausea and vomiting disorders

Diagnostic criteria* for chronic idiopathic nausea

Must include *all* of the following:

1. Bothersome nausea, occurring at least several times per week
2. Not usually associated with vomiting
3. Absence of abnormalities at upper endoscopy or metabolic disease that explains the nausea

Diagnostic criteria* for functional vomiting

Must include *all* of the following:

1. On average, one or more episodes of vomiting per week
2. Absence of criteria for an eating disorder, rumination or major psychiatric disease according to DSM-IV
3. Absence of self-induced vomiting and chronic cannabinoid use and absence of abnormalities in the central nervous system or metabolic diseases to explain the recurrent vomiting

Diagnostic criteria* for cyclic vomiting syndrome

Must include *all* of the following:

1. Stereotypical episodes of vomiting regarding onset (acute) and duration (less than 1 week)
2. Three or more discrete episodes in the prior year
3. Absence of nausea and vomiting between episodes

Supportive criterion

History or family history of migraine headaches

* Criteria fulfilled for the last 3 months with symptom onset at least 6 months before diagnosis.

myoelectrical activity is three cycles per minute. A reduction in or absence of the expected postprandial increase in the EGG amplitude correlates with delayed gastric emptying and antral hypomotility. Unfortunately, gastric dysrhythmias (both bradygastria and tachygastria) have been observed in the absence of altered gastric emptying, limiting its application to clinical practice.

Although uncommon in the absence of localising signs, intracranial lesions should be considered in those with severe, unexplained nausea and vomiting. Magnetic resonance imaging (MRI) is the investigation of choice to permit optimal imaging of the posterior fossa.

Assessment for an eating disorder (e.g. bulimia) or psychiatric illness (e.g. major depression) should be undertaken if organic causes prove elusive or when other factors indicate this may be the underlying cause.

Functional vomiting

Once common organic and psychiatric causes for chronic nausea and vomiting have been excluded, functional nausea and vomiting disorders need to be considered as a possible diagnosis. These are summarised in Table 5.3. The essential difference between functional and cyclic vomiting disorders is the pattern and frequency of vomiting; functional vomiting occurs at least weekly (on average), whereas cyclic vomiting syndrome (CVS) consists of stereotypical episodes of vomiting regarding onset (acute) and duration (less than 1 week), with the additional requirement for three or more discrete episodes in the prior year and the absence of nausea and vomiting between episodes. CVS is commonly associated with irritable bowel syndrome, motion sickness and, less frequently, migraine; family histories of these conditions are present in approximately 50% of patients.

MANAGEMENT

Initial management should include appropriate replacement of fluids either orally or intravenously as tolerated, with correction of any electrolyte (e.g. potassium, bicarbonate) or nutritional deficiencies that may have resulted from vomiting itself or the food aversion that may accompany these symptoms (Figure 5.1). Symptomatic management of the nausea and/or vomiting may be required while the underlying cause of the symptoms is identified

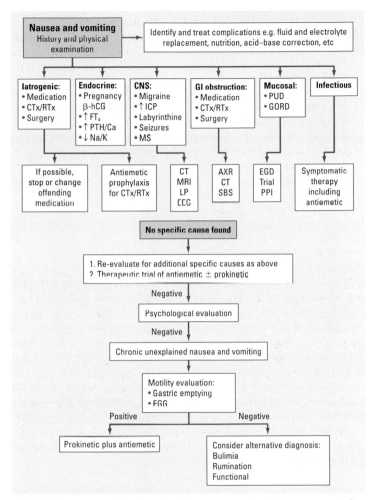

FIGURE 5.1: Suggested algorithm for assessment and management of nausea and vomiting.

Adapted from Quigley EM, Hasler WL, Parkman HP. AGA technical review on nausea and vomiting. Gastroenterology 2001; 120:263–86.

AXR = abdominal X-ray; CNS = central nervous system; CT = computed tomography; CTx = chemotherapy; EEG = electroencephalogram; EGD = endoscopic gastroduodenoscopy; EGG = electrogastrography; FT_4 = free thyroxine; GI = gastrointestinal; GORD = gastro-oesophageal reflux disease; ICP = intracranial pressure; K = potassium; LP = lumbar puncture; MRI = magnetic resonance imaging; MS = multiple sclerosis; NA = sodium; PPI = proton pump inhibitor; PTH = parathyroid hormone; PUD = peptic ulcer disease; RTx = radiotherapy; SBS = small bowel series.

and eliminated where possible. Placement of a nasogastric tube may also be required to relieve gastric distension if gastrointestinal obstruction is the cause.

Pharmacological

A variety of agents display antiemetic properties including serotonin (5-HT) antagonists, anticholinergics, H_1-receptor antagonists, phenothiazines, butyrophenones, benzamides, which also have prokinetic effects, neurokinin-1 antagonists, cannabinoids, and adjunctive agents such as benzodiazepines and corticosteroids. Examples of these agents are given in Table 5.4, which also outlines their common uses.

Prokinetic agents

Dopamine antagonists including metoclopramide and domperidone have been shown to be variably efficacious in gastro-oesophageal reflux disease, gastroparesis and functional dyspepsia. They exert both central and peripheral effects and have prokinetic effects on the oesophagus, stomach and upper small intestine. Domperidone has the advantage of fewer centrally-mediated side effects, particularly in comparison with metoclopramide. These side effects include extrapyramidal phenomena such as akathisia, dyskinesia, dystonia, opisthotonos and oculogyric crises. Both agents may induce hyperprolactinaemia, however this effect is less pronounced with domperidone.

Much less commonly used for gastroparesis is the macrolide antibiotic erythromycin, which has a dose-dependent stimulatory effect on foregut motility and inhibits isolated pyloric pressure waves and pyloric tone. Efficacy appears to be much better with intravenous administration, but gastrointestinal side effects are often dose limiting.

Treatment of functional nausea and vomiting

Treatment of unexplained nausea has not been systematically studied. Anecdotally, empiric therapy with antiemetics such as the serotonin antagonist ondansetron or low-dose tricyclic antidepressants (TCA) such as amitriptyline may be helpful.

Functional vomiting may require nutritional and electrolyte support and, once again, individual patients may respond to empiric antiemetic use and TCA therapy.

TABLE 5.4: Pharmacological agents effective in treating organic nausea and vomiting

Agent	Use	Formulation
Phenothiazines e.g. promethazine, prochlorperazine	PONV, PCNV Severe nausea and vomiting Vertigo, motion sickness, migraine	Oral, PR, IV
5-HT$_3$ antagonists e.g. ondansetron, tropisetron	PONV, PCNV	Oral, wafers, IV
Prokinetics e.g. metoclopramide, domperidone	Gastroparesis PONV, PCNV	Oral, IV (not domperidone)
Butyrophenones e.g. droperidol, haloperidol	Anticipatory and acute chemotherapy related nausea and vomiting PONV	Oral, IM, IV
Benzodiazepines e.g. lorazepam	Adjunctive in treatment of chemotherapy related nausea and vomiting	Oral, S/L, IV
Neurokinin-1 antagonists	Acute and delayed PCNV, adjunct in combination with 5-HT$_3$ antagonist and dexamethasone	Oral
Corticosteroids e.g. dexamethasone	Adjunctive in treatment of chemotherapy related nausea and vomiting	Oral, IV

5-HT = 5-hydroxytryptamine or serotonin; IM = intramuscular; IV = intravenous; PCNV = post-chemotherapy nausea and vomiting; PONV = post-operative nausea and vomiting; PR = per rectum; S/L = sublingual.

Severe episodes of cyclic vomiting may require hospitalisation for sedation and intravenous fluid and electrolyte support. If episodes are frequent or severe enough, particularly if a history of migraine is present, consideration should be given to daily treatment with agents including amitriptyline, pizotifen, cyproheptadine, phenobarbitone or propranolol; these may reduce the frequency of or eliminate episodes. Any identifiable factors known to trigger episodes, such as specific foods, emotional factors or physical stressors, should be avoided. If there is a recognisable prodrome, the episodes may potentially be aborted with early administration of ondansetron or a long-acting benzodiazepine such as lorazepam, which is beneficial for its anxiolytic, sedative and antiemetic effects. Deep sleep for several hours may prevent the episode. Early acid suppression may protect oesophageal mucosa and dental enamel from damage from acidic gastric contents.

SUMMARY

There are many causes of nausea and vomiting and therefore a careful history and physical examination is always required. A diagnosis of functional vomiting requires exclusion of eating disorders, rumination, major psychiatric disease, structural diseases such as small bowel obstruction and motility disorders such as gastroparesis. Cyclic vomiting can be diagnosed by the typical episodic nature of the symptoms with clear symptom-free intervals. Management depends on the underlying cause. In motility disorders, a combination of a prokinetic with another anti-nausea drug is often required to adequately control symptoms. Tricyclic antidepressants appear to be useful in the treatment of functional nausea and vomiting if avoidance of trigger factors is unsuccessful.

FURTHER READING

Hyman PE, Milla PJ, Benninga MA, et al. Childhood functional gastrointestinal disorders: neonate/toddler. Gastroenterology 2006; 130:1519–26.

Li BU, Misiewicz L. Cyclic vomiting syndrome: a brain–gut disorder. Gastroenterol Clin North Am 2003; 32:997–1019.

Prakash C, Clouse RE. Cyclic vomiting syndrome in adults: clinical features and response to tricyclic antidepressants. Am J Gastroenterol 1999; 94:2855–60.

Quigley EM, Hasler WL, Parkman HP. AGA technical review on nausea and vomiting. Gastroenterology 2001; 120:263–86.

Tack J, Talley NJ, Camilleri M, et al. Functional gastroduodenal disorders. Gastroenterology 2006; 130:1466–79.

CHAPTER 6

MALIGNANT CONDITIONS INVOLVING THE OESOPHAGUS, STOMACH, SMALL INTESTINE, GALL BLADDER AND BILE DUCT

KEYPOINTS

- In upper gastrointestinal tumours, accurate preoperative staging is important in determining appropriate management.
- Accurate staging includes clinical assessment and investigation of tumour and patient factors.
- Stage of disease directly correlates with outcome.
- Newer modalities of investigation include capsule endoscopy, endoscopic and laparoscopic ultrasound.
- Multidisciplinary care is now standard.
- Multimodality therapies are now common.

OESOPHAGOGASTRIC CANCERS

Gastric cancer incidence and mortality has fallen dramatically over the last 50 years in many regions, but probably remains the second most common cancer worldwide. The likely cause for this reduction is the disappearance of *Helicobacter pylori* and possibly greater consumption of fruit and vegetables, the reduced intake of salted, pickled and preserved foods, and improvements in refrigeration.

The incidence of gastric cancer varies worldwide, with the highest incidence being in Japan. Low rates can be expected in North America, India, Australia and New Zealand and northern Europe. The rates are also higher generally in lower socioeconomic groups and in males (male to female ratio 2:1). Gastric cancer is largely a disease of older age groups in most countries.

Despite a marked decline in fundal and distal tumours, there is a rising incidence of adenocarcinomas of the gastro-oesophageal junction and gastric cardia, particularly in Western nations, and predominantly in males. Comparatively high rates of this tumour are evident for the United Kingdom/Ireland, northern Europe, Australia and New Zealand, China and North America. The increase in incidence of cardia lesions has been associated with parallel increases for adenocarcinomas of the lower oesophagus, where hyperacidity, reflux oesophagitis, Barrett's oesophagus and obesity have been proposed as likely risk factors. This may imply that there are, in fact, two diseases differing from each other in epidemiology, aetiology, pathology and clinical expression. It is important to distinguish cardia and lower-third oesophageal adenocarcinoma from gastric cancer invading the lower third of the oesophagus, as treatment options may vary.

Clinical

Common presenting symptoms include weight loss, abdominal pain, nausea, anorexia and dysphagia. Easy satiety, reflux symptoms and symptoms of anaemia may be present. Background history may include previous peptic ulcer, previous history of polyps (gastric or colonic) and should include assessment of risk factors. A careful history of factors that may increase operative morbidity and mortality should also be sought (cardiac, respiratory, other systemic illness, anticoagulants, etc).

Risk factors

Oesophageal: there is a strong association between smoking and alcohol consumption and oesophageal squamous cell cancer. Human papilloma virus may be an important causative agent for oesophageal (squamous cell) cancer. Other risk factors include achalasia, chemical strictures, diverticula, previous radiation therapy and post-cricoid webs. Barrett's mucosa predisposes to oesophageal adenocarcinoma, as does smoking and obesity, while aspirin use may be protective.

Gastric: precursors of gastric cancer include chronic gastritis (autoimmune and acquired), intestinal metaplasia/dysplasia, gastric polyps (adenomatous polyps, rare in hyperplastic polyps) previous gastrectomy (>15 y post resection), pernicious anaemia and, most importantly, *Helicobacter pylori* infection. Infection with *H. pylori* induces chronic gastritis. Whether treatment of *H. pylori* infection will diminish the risk of gastric cancer is currently under investigation.

Dietary factors are important. A high consumption of fruit and vegetables is negatively correlated with risk of gastric cancer. These food items are thought to have a protective antioxidant effect. A high intake of salted foods, and potentially of smoked, cured and pickled foods, is thought to be a risk factor. These foods may include elevated levels of N-nitroso compounds, which have been shown to be potent carcinogens in animal experiments. There is also additional preliminary evidence that high-nitrate and high-starch diets may be risk factors, whereas garlic, onions and green tea may have protective effects. Ionising radiation is an established cause, based on exposure to radiation from atomic bombs and radiation therapy in certain patient groups (ankylosing spondylitis). Consumption of alcohol is weakly associated with gastric cancer, and smokers have an increased risk generally. There is a small group of patients in whom hereditary factors are important.

Examination

General physical examination may be unremarkable. However, nutritional assessment is important. Advanced disease may be identified by the presence of an epigastric mass, nodes in the left supraclavicular fossa, the presence of ascites, or a pelvic mass palpable on rectal examination as a result of peritoneal spread of tumour.

Investigations

Contrast studies: seldom used in the diagnosis and investigation of oesophageal tumours, but barium swallow may be used in the investigation of a patient with dysphagia.

Computed tomography (CT) scanning: of value in oesophageal cancer for the detection of distant metastases, particularly liver and pulmonary metastases. It can detect tracheal or bronchial invasion in up to 90% of cases, and the identification of pleural and pericardial involvement is similar. It is less accurate in the detection of nodal metastases (70% accuracy) and assessment of the cardio-oesophageal area, and the presence of diaphragmatic involvement is less secure with CT scanning. In gastric cancer, overall detection rates of the primary tumour approach 90%, but requires a high-resolution scanner, and distension of the stomach with water and contrast. CT has an accuracy of 70% in detection of nodal metastases, and the detection of distant metastases is similar to oesophageal cancer.

Magnetic resonance imaging (MRI): provides similar results to CT scanning.

Endoscopy: along with accompanying biopsy, endoscopy is an important part of the investigation of a patient with suspected oesophageal or gastric cancer.

For oesophageal cancer, 100% of early cancers can be diagnosed. The number of biopsies increases diagnostic accuracy. Advanced cancers can appear polypoidal, ulcerative or diffusely infiltrative. Barrett's mucosa can also be identified, and multiple biopsies should be performed to identify areas of high-grade dysplasia.

For gastric cancer, endoscopy can identify the site, the nature and the degree of involvement and the dimensions of the tumour. Biopsy can identify the tumour type, as the diffuse type of tumour (secreting mucin, and with no gland formation) has a worse prognosis than the intestinal tumour (which forms glandular structures). Chronic gastritis can also be identified.

Bronchoscopy: an important additional investigation in upper and middle-third oesophageal cancer to assess for evidence of invasion. Endoscopic ultrasound may be able to assess this.

Endoscopic ultrasound (EUS): a useful tool in the preoperative staging of both oesophageal and gastric cancers, and its use provides superior results to CT in the local staging of these tumours. EUS can identify involved lymph nodes in up to 90% of cases, but is less accurate in early stage disease. EUS has a central role in the initial anatomic staging of oesophageal cancer because of its high accuracy in determining the extent of locoregional disease. EUS is inaccurate for staging after radiation therapy and chemotherapy, but can be useful in assessing treatment response. For initial anatomic staging, EUS results have consistently shown more than 80% accuracy compared with surgical pathology for depth of tumour invasion. Accuracy increases with higher stage, and is >90% for T3 cancer. EUS results have shown accuracy in the range of 75% for initial staging of regional lymph nodes. EUS has been invariably more accurate than computed tomography for tumour (T) and lymph node (N) staging. EUS is limited for staging distant metastases (M), and therefore EUS is usually performed after assessment for distant metastases by CT scanning or positron emission tomography. Pathologic staging can be achieved at EUS using fine-needle aspiration (FNA) to obtain cytology from suspect lymph nodes. FNA has had greatest efficacy in confirming coeliac axis lymph node metastases with more than 90% accuracy. EUS is inaccurate for staging after radiation and chemotherapy because of its inability to distinguish inflammation and fibrosis from residual cancer, but a decrease in tumour cross-sectional area or diameter of more than 50% has been found to correlate with treatment response. Stricture due to tumour precludes full assessment of tumour size and nodal status, and dilatation to allow passage of the probe results in a high perforation rate. EUS offers the best preoperative local gastric cancer staging, with accuracies in T and N staging of approximately 78% and 70%, respectively. Although EUS is not suitable for diagnosing distant metastases, it may be more useful in detecting ascites due to the close proximity to the peritoneum.

Laparoscopy: can be performed as a separate procedure prior to final choice of therapy. Laparoscopy can identify occult peritoneal and hepatic disease in up to 25% of potentially resectable gastric cancers, thus allowing informed decision making in relation to a more significant abdominal operation. It also allows consideration of other palliative modalities.

Laparoscopic ultrasound: may combine the benefits of detection of occult metastases (laparoscopy) and nodal status (EUS). Resectability (up to 100%), TNM staging (82% accurate), nodal status (92%), T stage (96%), M stage (89%) are all significantly improved over laparoscopy alone for oesophagogastric tumours, and is as accurate as EUS. Laparoscopic ultrasound may be the optimal preoperative staging tool, and may have a complementary role to EUS in oesophageal cancer.

Management

Oesophageal cancer

The majority of cancers arising in the oesophagus are epithelial in origin (squamous or adenocarcinoma in the lower third).

Once preoperative staging has been completed, selection of primary treatment will depend on the results of staging, and the fitness of the individual patient. Radical treatment is not indicated in an infirm patient. Survival is directly correlated to stage of disease, and therefore accurate preoperative staging is important to determine whether radical treatment is indicated.

The management of oesophageal squamous cell cancer has evolved from surgery alone to definitive chemoradiation or preoperative chemotherapy or chemoradiation followed by surgery. Preoperative chemoradiation can result in a higher rate of complete resection (R0), but may result in a higher postoperative morbidity and mortality. Definitive chemoradiation has resulted in overall survival and local control rates that are comparable with those achieved with surgery alone and has been proven to be superior to radiation alone. Surgery remains the standard to which all other modalities are compared and is an acceptable option for patients with early-stage disease. For patients with locally advanced disease who are not surgical candidates, definitive chemoradiation with concurrent and adjuvant cisplatin/fluorouracil is the present standard of care.

Management of adenocarcinoma in this area is more difficult. Surgical management depends on the primary site. Oesophageal resection of lower-third adenosarcomas is the recommended surgical treatment. Radical gastric surgery is the recommended option for cardia tumours and proximal gastric cancers, with or without left thoraco-abdominal exposure. The use of neoadjuvant treatment of these tumours is evolving. Epirubicin, cisplatin and infused fluorouracil (ECF) shows significant benefit in advanced oesophagogastric cancer, particularly locally advanced disease.

Perioperative chemotherapy (pre- and postoperatively) significantly improves resectability, progression-free survival and overall survival in operable gastric and lower oesophageal cancer. Postoperative chemoradiation may be as beneficial as perioperative chemotherapy for cardia tumours.

Gastric cancer

While surgical resection remains the cornerstone of gastric cancer treatment, the optimum extent of nodal resection remains controversial, with randomised studies failing to show that the D2 (more extensive) procedure improves survival when compared with D1 dissection. This is despite data from Japan showing a survival advantage in Japanese patients. The use of neoadjuvant therapy may benefit selected patients, but may only be relevant to those patients who have a favourable response to treatment. The high rate of recurrence and poor survival following surgery provides a rationale for the early use of adjuvant treatment. Adjuvant chemotherapy or adjuvant radiotherapy used alone, do not improve survival following resection. In advanced gastric cancer, chemotherapy enhances quality of life and prolongs survival when compared with best supportive care.

Radiation can be employed for palliative treatment of bleeding gastric cancers with relief of symptoms in an acceptable number of patients.

GASTROINTESTINAL STROMAL TUMOURS (GIST)

These tumours, formerly known as leiomyomas and leiomyosarcomas, are now thought to be derived from undifferentiated stromal fibroblasts. Behaviour of these tumours correlates with the number of cells undergoing mitosis per high power field (<5 versus >5). They may be found on endoscopy, may present as a mass lesion, and can present as a result of upper gastrointestinal bleeding. Larger tumours tend to be at the malignant end of the spectrum. Recent addition of tyrosine kinase inhibitors has changed the management of these tumours. If resection is possible, gastric resection is performed. If resection is not possible, the addition of preoperative medical therapy can downstage these tumours to a resectable size. The addition of medical therapy post operatively is currently under investigation.

CARCINOMA OF GALL BLADDER

This tumour represents a small percentage (<2%) of all cancers but is the most common site of cancer in the biliary tract (80%–95% of cancers of the biliary tree). The incidence varies worldwide and the highest incidence occurs in the Andean area, in North American Indians and Mexican Americans. It is three times more common in women than in men in all populations. The highest rates in Europe are in Poland, the Czech Republic and Slovakia, and in Asia in northern and north-eastern India.

Aetiology and risk factors

Up to 85% of patients with gall bladder cancer have gallstones. This appears to be relevant if the stones are symptomatic over a long period of time. Other risk factors include obesity, chronic infections of the gall bladder (*Salmonella typhi*) and environmental exposure to chemicals (occupations in oil, paper, chemical, shoe, textile and cellulose acetate fibre manufacturing industries). The incidence is increased 14-fold 20 years after surgery for gastric ulcer. There is an association with porcelain gall bladder (calcification of the gall bladder wall), familial adenomatous polyposis (FAP)/ Gardner's syndrome. There is a high incidence of anomalous bile duct–pancreatic duct junction (pancreatic duct joins bile duct) in patients with gall bladder cancer.

Clinical presentation

The peak age incidence is over 70 years. Gall bladder cancer may be asymptomatic and is identified either on ultrasound before laparoscopic cholecystectomy, or histologically after resection for symptomatic gallstones. Less than 30% of patients are diagnosed preoperatively, and usually only those with advanced disease. The majority of these patients will present with jaundice, due to direct invasion of the hilum by the cancer.

Presentation of more advanced cancers include biliary obstruction (biochemically or clinical jaundice), acute cholecystitis or empyema.

Investigation

Biochemistry may confirm cholestasis and jaundice. Coagulation profile is important in jaundiced patients. Plain abdominal X-ray may show gall bladder calcification. Ultrasound may show a mass. CT can confirm this, and may show contrast enhancement of the suspected cancer. EUS can be helpful in preoperative staging.

Management

Surgical therapy is appropriate for disease that is localised and resectable. Laparotomy should be considered if gall bladder cancer is suspected preoperatively. Laparoscopy may be helpful in staging these patients, and may avoid laparotomy if disease is advanced. If gall bladder cancer is not suspected preoperatively, but is suspected intraoperatively, operative management ranges from completion of laparoscopic cholecystectomy, with removal of the gall bladder in a bag to avoid contamination of the port site, to laparotomy and extended resection of the gall bladder bed and regional hepato-duodenal lymph nodes. The choice will depend on operative findings and the comorbidities of the individual patient. Postoperative chemoradiotherapy may benefit selected patients. There is evidence that implantation of tumour cells may occur in port sites after laparoscopic cholecystectomy, and the biological aggressiveness of the tumour is the most likely explanation for this phenomenon as opposed to poor operative technique.

Prognosis

Most large studies of gall bladder cancer demonstrate 5%–15% overall 5-year survival. Pathologic stage remains the best prognostic factor. Most gall bladder cancers are adenocarcinomas, with a small percentage represented by adenosquamous cancer and other rare types. Early stage disease has a better prognosis, and resected disease has a better prognosis than non-resected disease (52% versus 19% for stage IV disease, respectively).

CHOLANGIOCARCINOMA

Carcinoma of the bile duct is an uncommon tumour. The overall number of cases curable by surgery is approximately 10%. Prognosis is related to anatomical location, which, in turn, determines the resectability.

Pathogenesis

There is a strong association with primary sclerosing cholangitis (PSC) and with inflammatory bowel disease. Chemical carcinogens implicated in aetiology include aflatoxin, methylene chloride and vinyl chloride monomer, with industrial exposure in factory workers. There is an increase in risk for choledochal cysts, which probably relates to an anomaly of the pancreaticobiliary junction, resulting in a common channel of variable length (bile duct joins pancreatic duct).

Pathology

The tumours are usually mucus-secreting adenocarcinomas, arising from the epithelium of any part of the biliary tract. These tumours can be multifocal. Tumours in the middle third of the bile duct are usually nodular in appearance. Lower-third tumours are generally papillary, and hilar tumours tend to be stenosing and sclerotic. Perineural invasion is a negative prognostic factor. The tumour can invade adjacent structures, including the liver, and adjacent blood vessels, including the hepatic artery and the portal vein.

Clinical

Cholestatic jaundice is the usual presentation, with or without preexisting cholestasis without jaundice. The disease may be extensive by the time jaundice develops. Systemic features of malignancy may be present, including weight loss and anorexia. Fever may be present owing to coexistent cholangitis. A history of inflammatory bowel disease should be looked for. Nutritional assessment is important, as is the assessment of medical comorbidities in relation to operative risk.

Investigations

Liver function tests will confirm the cholestatic nature of the jaundice and the level of bilirubin. Coagulation studies should be performed especially international normalised ratio (INR), particularly if endoscopic or surgical intervention is contemplated. Carcinoembryonic antigen (CEA) is expressed in the cells of cholangiocarcinomas and may be elevated in the serum. Cancer antigen 19-9 (CA 19-9) may also be elevated, but modest levels of this marker can also be found in inflammatory and infective bile duct pathology. Chronic anaemia may also be present, and a raised white cell count may suggest associated biliary sepsis. Nutritional assessment is also important.

Imaging

Ultrasound: can identify the level of obstruction in most cases, and can identify gallstones in the gall bladder. Ultrasound may identify a tumour mass and suggestion of vascular invasion may be raised. Liver secondaries may also be identified.

CT scanning: using three phase scanning, may show a mass lesion with or without local extension or lymphadenopathy. Lobar or segmental atrophy may also be identified (due to gradual, progressive bile duct obstruction, especially in tumours arising primarily in left or right main bile ducts in the hilum).

Cholangiography: is important to develop a road map of duct obstruction, especially if surgery is contemplated. Endoscopic retrograde cholangiography (ERC) can outline the level of obstruction from below, and cytology may be positive with brushings. Placement of a stent (either temporary or permanent) can also be accomplished. Percutaneous transhepatic cholangiography (PTC) can delineate the proximal ducts, and is especially important in more proximal-based tumours. Communication between the right and left bile ducts can also be outlined, and this may be important in the planning of surgical decompression.

Endoscopic ultrasound (EUS): may also be used to delineate bile duct anatomy, presence or absence of nodal metastases, and cytological diagnosis may be possible. This may be useful if surgical resection is not contemplated by virtue of stage of disease or because of patient comorbidity. With respect to accuracy of EUS, the sensitivity, specificity, positive predictive value, negative predictive value and accuracy can be as high as 86%, 100%, 100%, 57% and 88%, respectively. EUS-FNA can have a positive impact on patient management in up to 84% of patients: preventing surgery for tissue diagnosis in patients with inoperable disease, facilitating surgery in patients with unidentifiable cancer by other modalities and avoiding surgery in benign disease. Given the apparent accuracy and safety of EUS with FNA for imaging bile duct mass lesions and for obtaining a tissue diagnosis in patients with suspected cholangiocarcinoma, EUS may represent a new approach to diagnosis, especially when CT and endoscopic retrograde cholangiopancreatography (ERCP) fail. The ability to obtain a definite diagnosis has a significant impact on patient management in a significant proportion of patients.

Selective angiography: may identify hepatic arterial and portal venous involvement prior to surgery. If the main portal vein is involved, resection may be difficult or impossible. If a left bile duct hilar cholangiocarcinoma involves the right portal vein or hepatic artery, curative resection is not possible as preservation of the opposite lobe blood supply is required (and similarly for a right hilar cholangiocarcinoma).

Management

The aims of treatment are to:
• resect the primary tumour, if possible
• relieve jaundice
• treat and/or prevent cholangitis.

As a minority have surgically resectable disease, the majority of patients require biliary drainage. The options for drainage include operative drainage, endoscopic drainage and stenting, percutaneous drainage, or combined percutaneous and endoscopic approaches.

Other modalities of treatment include radiation therapy using iridium-192 with additional external beam radiation. There is some evidence that this regimen can increase 2-year and median survival for combined doses >55 Gy. Photodynamic therapy has also been used to delay biliary occlusion in unresectable cases. The place of chemotherapy for this group of patients is in evolution, with newer agents (gemcitabine, capecitabine and platin-based regimens) showing some promise in phase II trials.

The survival of patients with bile duct cancer will depend on how advanced it is. Statistically, overall only about 21% of patients with extrahepatic bile duct cancer survive 5 years, because most patients are diagnosed late.

Both stage III and stage IV are considered unresectable, indicating that the cancer cannot be completely removed surgically.

SMALL INTESTINAL TUMOURS

The small intestine, which is about 3 m in length and comprises over 60% of the mucosal area of the gastrointestinal tract, is the major site for nutritional absorption, and is relatively resistant to carcinogenesis. Small intestine carcinoma is rare compared with other parts of the gastrointestinal tract and accounts for approximately 2% of gastrointestinal malignancies, compared with 10% oesophageal, 10% stomach, and 70% from the colon and rectum. Adenocarcinoma accounts for 40%–60% of small intestine malignancies. The remainder include carcinoid tumours, lymphomas, gastrointestinal stromal tumours (GIST), sarcomas and metastases from breast, melanoma, lung and renal cell cancers.

Small intestine cancers occur most frequently in the sixth and seventh decades, and are slightly more common in men. Adenocarcinomas occur in decreasing frequency from duodenum to ileum. Other primary tumours occur in increasing frequency from proximal to distal small intestine. There is an association with coeliac disease and small intestinal lymphoma, and adenocarcinoma is associated with hereditary colorectal cancer syndromes, particularly duodenal tumours in familial adenomatous polyposis (FAP), hereditary non-polyposis colorectal cancer and Peutz-Jeghers syndrome. Small intestine adenocarcinomas are also more common in patients with Crohn's disease affecting the small intestine.

The 5-year relative survival is low for adenocarcinomas (20%–40%). Reasons for this are not clear, but these outcomes may relate to the relatively uncommon nature of the tumour, and diagnostic delays which occur as a result of the anatomical site.

Clinical

Clinically, most patients with small bowel adenocarcinoma have nonspecific signs and symptoms. The more frequent symptoms include abdominal pain and postprandial fullness (experienced by 50% of patients). Anaemia (up to 70%) and signs and symptoms of intestinal obstruction (50%) are common presentations. Up to 20% of patients may present acutely with either bleeding or obstruction, and require more urgent intervention. Other symptoms include weight loss, anorexia and fatigue. Perforation with accompanying peritonitis is an uncommon presentation.

Investigations

Endoscopy is useful for the diagnosis of duodenal adenocarcinoma, but has limited application in the investigation of more distal lesions. Push enteroscopy and double-balloon enteroscopy may be useful, usually in concert with capsule endoscopy, which employs wireless technology. These latter techniques may provide preoperative confirmation of tumours, but are not yet widely available.

CT is important in the assessment of the abdominal cavity and staging, but has variable detection rates—50% rising to 80% for detection of metastatic disease in some series.

The barium contrast study is another useful diagnostic tool, but has limited sensitivity. Small intestine enema is more sensitive than a small bowel follow-through series.

If all investigations are negative, and the index of suspicion is high, surgical intervention, either laparoscopic or open, may be indicated.

Management

Surgical resection is the gold standard of care for adenocarcinoma. Earlier stage tumours tend to occur more proximally, and this may relate to the earlier development of symptoms, and earlier detection.

Early tumour stage (stage 1 and 2) and curative resection are the only independent factors for better prognosis and long overall survival time. Lymph node metastasis is an independent predictor of disease-free survival, and probably accounts for the differences in outcome by stage. Patterns of failure post resection include peritoneal recurrence, wound recurrence, liver metastases and metastases in more distant sites, including the lungs. The role of adjuvant systemic therapy in higher risk patients is unknown.

Other tumours of the small intestine include carcinoid tumours, lymphomas, and GIST. Most small intestine carcinoids are clinically silent, and may present with local complications requiring emergent surgery, or present as metastatic disease. The rate of lymph node involvement and the prognosis of carcinoid tumours depend on their site and size. Lymph node metastases are most commonly found with small bowel carcinoids (20%–45%), providing the rationale for extended resection including the adjacent lymph node drainage area. More aggressive treatment is reserved for younger and fitter patients.

Management of GIST is similar to gastric GIST. Lymphoma may require resection if perforation, obstruction or bleeding occur. Chemotherapeutic regimens will depend on haematological advice.

FURTHER READING

American Society of Clinical Oncology website: www.asco.org. This site provides access to journal articles related to cancer topics.

Garden OJ. A companion to specialist surgical practice. Hepatobiliary and pancreatic surgery. Edinburgh: Elsevier; 2005.

Griffin SM, Raimes SA. A companion to specialist surgical practice. Upper gastrointestinal surgery. Edinburgh: Elsevier; 1997.

National Cancer Institute website: www.cancer.gov. The US National Institute of Health provides a good overview of current treatment of various cancers, including supporting level of evidence where available.

Pearson FG, Cooper JD, Deslauriers J, et al. Esophageal surgery. Philadelphia: Elsevier; 2002.

Chapter 7

ACUTE ABDOMINAL PAIN

KEY POINTS

- Acute abdominal pain is usually a surgical condition.
- Most conditions can be diagnosed by bedside assessment.
- Clinical peritonitis will usually require a laparotomy to clean the peritoneal cavity and stop continuing contamination from a perforated or ischaemic viscus.
- Peritonitis not caused by gut ischaemia or perforation of a viscus does not require a laparotomy, e.g. acute pancreatitis, salpingitis and spontaneous bacterial peritonitis.
- Surgery for localised peritoneal inflammation will not always be required and will be dictated by the presumed diagnosis and its natural history.
- Management of a patient with an acute abdomen should consist of:
  - Initial assessment and resuscitation
  - Focused assessment and investigation
  - Decision and planning of management.
- Management should not be delayed by unnecessary investigations.
- Patients who require urgent surgery for intraperitoneal bleeding or peritonitis should be resuscitated in the operating theatre while surgery is being performed.
- Contact a surgeon quickly if the patient is unstable or the diagnosis is unclear.

INTRODUCTION

Acute abdominal pain should always be considered a surgical condition. The management of the patient with acute abdominal pain can be simplified by considering appropriate clinical management pathways and not focusing on the final diagnosis. The key to this is the use of clinical symptoms and signs in combination with limited special tests to decide if the patient is best treated by urgent or planned operation or conservative management. Many of these immediate decisions can be made by the bedside with a good history and examination.

DEFINITION

Acute abdominal pain is defined as the sudden onset of severe abdominal pain. The rapidity of onset may be over minutes to hours. The pain may be localised to a specific site of the abdomen or generalised.

CAUSES OF ACUTE ABDOMINAL PAIN

Generalised abdominal pain

Constant abdominal pain

In a patient with generalised constant abdominal pain and abdominal rigidity, the working diagnosis is peritonitis. This is always secondary to some other process. Often, but not always, this is due to a perforated viscus. The role of surgery is to provide peritoneal toilet and to prevent ongoing contamination by removing or repairing the perforated viscus. There are a number of conditions that fulfill this criterion. There are other conditions, however, that may demonstrate the signs of peritonitis but not require intervention (see Figure 7.1). Typically acute pancreatitis with generalised inflammation may have tenderness and guarding but does not require a laparotomy. A diagnostic elevated lipase may be very useful in this setting. In females, pelvic inflammatory disease may show generalised signs and does not benefit from laparotomy as there is no ongoing contamination. This should be considered in appropriate clinical contexts. Spontaneous bacterial peritonitis in portal hypertension should also be considered in patients presenting with generalised abdominal pain and portal hypertension with ascites.

Beware of the patient complaining of severe constant generalised abdominal pain who appears to have a relatively soft 'doughy' abdomen to palpation. This patient may have ischaemic bowel. Suspicion may be raised if they have bloody diarrhoea and atrial fibrillation. Investigations may reveal an elevated white cell count and a metabolic acidosis. Venous obstruction is often more subtle and slowly progressive.

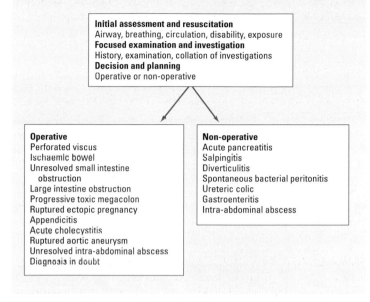

Initial assessment and resuscitation
Airway, breathing, circulation, disability, exposure
Focused examination and investigation
History, examination, collation of investigations
Decision and planning
Operative or non-operative

Operative
Perforated viscus
Ischaemic bowel
Unresolved small intestine
   obstruction
Large intestine obstruction
Progressive toxic megacolon
Ruptured ectopic pregnancy
Appendicitis
Acute cholecystitis
Ruptured aortic aneurysm
Unresolved intra-abdominal abscess
Diagnosis in doubt

Non-operative
Acute pancreatitis
Salpingitis
Diverticulitis
Spontaneous bacterial peritonitis
Ureteric colic
Gastroenteritis
Intra-abdominal abscess

FIGURE 7.1: Management of acute abdomen.

Colicky abdominal pain

Colicky abdominal pain is episodic pain that comes in waves every 4–5 minutes. It is crescendo decrescendo in nature. When it is generalised the diagnosis is usually between gastroenteritis or a bowel obstruction. Gastroenteritis will often be associated with early vomiting and diarrhoea and abdominal distension will not be a feature. Some infective forms of gastroenteritis may not produce diarrhoea.

In contrast, a bowel obstruction will usually be associated with vomiting and constipation with progressive abdominal distension. The higher the obstruction is anatomically in the intestine, the earlier the vomiting and the later the constipation. The more distal the obstructing lesion, the greater the distension. A supine and erect plain abdominal film will usually confirm the diagnosis. An erect chest X-ray should always be ordered to look for free peritoneal gas. The supine abdominal film is the most useful. With the patient lying flat it will not show the fluid levels of the erect film but it will show gaseous distended bowel down to the level of obstruction. The ileum or small intestine can be distinguished by its central position and valvulae conniventes extending across the intestinal lumen. The jejunum or large intestine is distinguished by its incomplete valves and more peripheral position.

Be very wary of the diagnosis of constipation causing abdominal pain if the rectum is empty or if abdominal tenderness is present.

Surgery is indicated for an obstructed bowel when the cause for the obstruction is unlikely to resolve. The timing is a balance between appropriate resuscitation of the patient and avoiding the development of gut ischaemia.

Small intestine obstruction is more difficult to manage than colonic obstruction as there are no objective diagnostic indicators of early bowel ischaemia. Colonic ischaemia can be predicted if the bowel lumen is distended above a 10 cm diameter, as venous drainage in the bowel wall will be impaired at this level. The caecum is the part of the large intestine usually most susceptible to distension and can be monitored clinically and radiologically.

If constant abdominal pain, worsening tenderness, fever, leucocytosis and acidosis are present, gut ischaemia should be suspected and urgent surgery is indicted.

All these signs and symptoms can be absent or late.

Localised abdominal pain

The management of focal abdominal pain relates very much to the presumed or proven diagnosis, the natural history of the condition and the morbidity if treated conservatively or operatively. Typically, appendicitis is usually treated operatively as it is known that the natural history may lead to perforation and generalised peritonitis. Appendicectomy is straightforward and is associated with low morbidity. Acute diverticulitis of the colon is usually treated conservatively with antibiotics. Diverticulitis may sometimes perforate but operative resection of the affected bowel will usually lead to a temporary colostomy and will not prevent further recurrence. Surgery is therefore reserved for the patient whose condition does not resolve with conservative management.

It is best to consider these conditions in relation to the position in the abdomen in which the signs occur.

Right upper quadrant

Pain in this region may be due to pathology in the liver, gall bladder, bile duct, hepatic flexure of the colon, appendicitis in the high-riding caecum or the duodenum. The conditions that might require early intervention include the subhepatic appendix or a perforated viscus such as the duodenum or the hepatic flexure. Pain and jaundice in this region suggests a biliary cause.

Cholecystitis may be treated conservatively but is best treated by early laparoscopic cholecystectomy. Cholangitis may respond to antibiotics but may need biliary drainage by endoscopic retrograde cholangiopancreatography (ERCP) if this fails.

Right upper quadrant pain of a sudden onset with minimal signs will frequently be due to biliary colic. Characteristically, the pain is sudden in onset, epigastric or right upper quadrant in site with radiation around or through to the back. Biliary colic is due to a stone obstructing either the gall bladder or the bile duct. The latter may be associated with jaundice.

Left upper quadrant

The diagnosis of acute pain in this area can often be the most challenging. Peptic ulcer disease and colonic pathology should be considered as well as, rarely, pancreatitis. A splenic infarct should also be considered which might be due to an embolic event in a normal spleen or a spontaneous infarct if the spleen is palpable. It should also be remembered that both upper quadrant and epigastric pain can be caused by some pathology above the diaphragm such as basal pneumonia, pleurisy, ischaemic heart disease or pericarditis.

Right iliac fossa

Any patient who complains of periumbilical pain that radiates to the right iliac fossa should be considered to have appendicitis until proven otherwise. The patient will usually have a low-grade fever and anorexia with an elevated white cell count and significant tenderness in the right iliac fossa. Abdominal imaging is usually not required in such a patient although a pelvic ultrasound may be considered in a female if a ruptured ovarian cyst is considered. Initial periumbilical pain does not usually occur in primary pelvic pathology.

Remember that the sigmoid colon can sometimes lie in the right iliac fossa and may mimic appendicitis clinically in the older patient.

In females of child-bearing age, ruptured ovarian cysts, pelvic inflammatory disease and ectopic pregnancy must always be considered. Estimation of β-hCG and pelvic ultrasound are valuable investigations here for lower abdominal and pelvic pain.

Left iliac fossa

Left iliac pain and tenderness is usually due to diverticulitis. There is often associated fever. Occasionally a palpable mass may be present, which may be an inflammatory mass or an abscess.

Loins

Loin pain is usually due to renal tract disease. The typical 'loin to groin pain' is characteristic of ureteric colic and may be associated with sepsis if the ureter is blocked. Other retroperitoneal structures such as the pancreas and the aorta may present with back or loin pain. Occasionally ureteric colic may focus with predominant pain in the iliac fossa. Local tenderness is usually not a feature. Remember both appendicitis and ureteric colic may cause microscopic haematuria.

ASSESSMENT

History and physical examination is the cornerstone of diagnosis in the acute abdomen. Most decisions concerning acute abdominal pain can be made by the bedside.

History

Taking a history of pain must begin with inquiring about the rapidity of onset. A true sudden onset of significant pain without prodromal symptoms usually indicates a perforated, obstructed or an acutely ischaemic viscus. This would include perforated peptic ulcer, biliary colic, foreign body perforation of bowel, mesenteric embolus, ureteric colic or a ruptured aneurysm. A sudden exacerbation of pain with preceding symptoms of malaise and fever may suggest perforated diverticulitis or appendicitis. If the pain is generalised, a perforated viscus is most likely.

The presence of colic and duration of symptoms will differentiate between viscus obstruction and inflammation. The presence of vomiting, diarrhoea or constipation and a previous history suggests bowel obstruction.

Physical examination

Examination should begin with a global look at the patient to assess toxicity, discomfort and distress and overall nutritional status. The presence of jaundice and anaemia and the overall hydration of the patient can also be assessed.

The vital signs—temperature pulse and blood pressure—should also be recorded.

Examination of the abdomen should be gentle. If there is significant tenderness, there is no need to make the patient unnecessarily uncomfortable. If hurt, the patient will voluntarily guard their abdominal wall, making palpation difficult. Rebound tenderness is not necessarily useful and can be more humanely replaced by eliciting percussion or cough tenderness.

As a routine, it is always important to palpate for an aortic aneurysm. The hands must be placed in the epigastrium for at least 10 seconds to feel for an expansile mass of greater than 2 cm to make the diagnosis. All hernial orifices must be palpated for a mass. A hernia causing a bowel obstruction will not always be locally painful to the patient. It will be palpable and irreducible.

Auscultation is of limited benefit. The presence or absence of bowel sounds has little diagnostic significance, even in the context of a bowel obstruction.

A rectal examination should always be performed in acute abdominal pain as an inflammatory or malignant intraluminal or peritoneal mass may be palpated. The presence and consistency of the stool and the presence of blood can be useful signs.

MANAGEMENT

The approach to managing the patient should be performed in three steps:

1 Immediate assessment and management
2 Focused assessment and investigation
3 Decision and plan of management.

Immediate assessment and management

This is really the initial resuscitation phase and should stabilise the patient's airway, breathing and circulation. This phase should only take a few minutes. If the patient can speak then the airway is clear, if not the airway will need to be secured and oxygen applied. Breathing is the mechanical act of ventilation and may be compromised by altered consciousness or a splinted diaphragm due to severe abdominal pain. Circulation may be compromised by sepsis or dehydration. Venous access should be achieved by a large bore peripheral cannula, bloods drawn for assessment and a crystalloid fluid administered. A bolus of 10 mL/kg should be administered initially. If the patient is hypoperfused, the bolus should be increased to 20 mL/kg. Next the level of consciousness and mental state of the patient should be documented. The patient should be exposed for any obvious finding, such as distension, and then covered to keep them comfortable.

Focused assessment and investigation

Once the initial resuscitation phase is initiated then a more focused assessment can be made. A history is initially taken to include a description of the presenting illness as well as past medical and surgical history, medications, allergies and fasting state. A focused abdominal examination is then performed and all findings recorded.

Decision and plan of management

A plan of action now needs to be formulated. The management decision can be enhanced by the use of appropriate blood tests, plain X-ray, abdominal ultrasound, computed tomography (CT) scan, angiography and endoscopy. The use of plain X-ray and ultrasound can be very useful in the assessment of patients with acute abdominal pain. CT may be useful if the diagnosis is unclear. It must be stressed that overinvestigation can lead to unnecessary delay and must be avoided. An investigation should only be ordered if its outcome is likely to have a significant impact on management.

Initially it must be decided if the patient requires immediate surgery, delayed surgery or observation with conservative management and further investigations. If immediate surgery is required, it should be established whether there is time or the need for preoperative stabilisation. The patient with a bleeding condition, such as a ruptured aortic aneurysm or ruptured ectopic pregnancy or a perforated viscus, is often best managed by urgent surgical intervention with no delay. Further resuscitation can occur while surgery is performed. A delay in intervention in these conditions is associated with increased morbidity and mortality.

A bowel obstruction will benefit from fluid resuscitation prior to surgery as long as bowel viability is not compromised.

The management of focal abdominal sepsis is dependent on specific factors that depend, in turn, on potential complications of the intervention. As a general rule, a focal acute inflammation of the colon is usually treated conservatively with antibiotics. If there is a large associated abscess, this will usually be treated by imaging guided percutaneous drainage or open surgery.

Appendicitis and acute cholecystitis are usually be treated surgically. In the event of a delay of more than 72 hours, both conditions are often treated conservatively with antibiotics. This is because resection of these organs at this time may lead to damage of the surrounding organs due to the attempts by these structures to wall off the inflammation. The bile duct with the gall bladder and surrounding small intestine and caecum with the appendix could be placed in jeopardy.

If a plan of management cannot be decided upon, then the role of further observation or an intervention must be considered. It is also important to decide whether the patient needs to be placed in a high dependency area based on their condition or comorbidity.

A patient should never be left in pain. Appropriate analgesia should be administered early in small frequent doses. Analgesia will not mask signs but will reduce the patient's awareness of pain. There is a duty of care to ensure frequent pain reassessment.

It is essential that communication with the treating clinician is both timely and accurate. If the patient is unstable or the diagnosis unclear, early communication with the consultant is mandatory.

SUMMARY

History and clinical examination are the cornerstones of diagnosis in the acute abdomen. Most decisions can be made at the bedside. A rectal examination should always be carried out.

The management centres on three core issues:

1 Initial assessment and management
2 Focused assessment and investigations
3 Decision and plan of management including appropriate laboratory investigations and imaging.

FURTHER READING

Abu-Yousef MM, Bleicher JJ, Maher JW. High resolution sonography of acute appendicitis. Am J Roentgenol 1987; 149:53–8.

Anderson ID. Care of the critically ill surgical patient. 2nd edn. London: Arnold; 2003.

Dang C, Aguilera P, Dang A. Acute abdominal pain. Geriatrics 2002; 57:30–42.

Davidson SJ, Murphy DG, Barbaro G. Missed diagnosis of acute cardiac ischemia. N Engl J Med 2000; 343:1492–4.

Oria A, Cimmino D, Ocampo C, et al. Early endoscopic intervention versus early conservative management in patients with acute gallstone pancreatitis and biliopancreatic obstruction: a randomized clinical trial. Ann Surg 2007; 245:10–17.

Thomas SH, William S, Cheema F. Effect of morphine analgesia on diagnostic accuracy in emergency department patients with abdominal pain. J Am Coll Surg 2003; 196:18–31.

Chapter 8

HAEMATEMESIS AND MELAENA

KEY POINTS

- Resuscitation should be instituted irrespective of the underlying cause of gastrointestinal bleeding.
- A multidisciplinary approach to management is key.
- Patients over 60 years of age and patients with comorbid conditions have a higher risk of mortality.
- Endoscopic examination should be made available to the patient within 24 hours or when the patient is stabilised.
- A combination of adrenaline injection with either thermal coagulation or haemoclips reduces the risk of recurrent bleeding.
- Proton pump inhibitors are recommended as an adjuvant to endoscopic therapy in peptic ulcer patients with a high risk of bleeding.
- Somatostatin or octreotide are effective therapy for acute variceal bleeding.
- Angiography may help identify bleeding from an unknown source.
- Indications for surgery include arterial bleeding that cannot be controlled by endoscopic haemostasis, and patients requiring massive transfusions.

INTRODUCTION

Acute gastrointestinal (GI) bleeding is one of the most common emergency conditions and is associated with significant morbidity and mortality. *Haematemesis* is the vomiting of fresh blood. Haematemesis indicates that bleeding originates from a site proximal to the ligament of Treitz. A history of fresh haematemesis usually implies a significant bleed. Vomiting altered blood that appears like coffee grounds arises from the breakdown of haemoglobin by gastric acid, and often indicates that active bleeding may have ceased. *Melaena* is the passage of black, tarry stool. It occurs when haemoglobin is converted to haematin by bacterial degradation. Ingestion of as little as 200 mL of blood can produce melaenic stool. Although melaena generally connotes bleeding proximal to the ligament of Treitz, bleeding from the small intestine or proximal colon may also cause melaena, especially when colonic transit is slow. *Haematochezia* is the passage of pure red blood or blood admixed with stool. It usually occurs as a result of bleeding in the lower GI tract. It can also be present in massive upper GI bleeding (in 10%–15% of cases).

RESUSCITATION

Irrespective of the underlying cause of GI bleeding, a patient should be resuscitated. Vital signs (blood pressure, pulse, oxygenation) should be carefully monitored. A large bore peripheral drip should be inserted for fluid replacement and, if the patient is in shock, a central line inserted. Blood transfusion should not be delayed if there is evidence of substantial volume loss. Patients with chronic liver diseases might also benefit from fresh frozen plasma and platelet transfusion. A patient with GI bleeding is best cared for by a joint team with gastroenterologists, GI surgeons and intervention radiologists. Patients with severe acute bleeding require admission to a high dependency or intensive care unit.

AETIOLOGY

The most common cause of upper GI bleeding is peptic ulcer. This is followed by mucosal erosions, Mallory-Weiss tear, oesophagitis and oesophageal/gastric varices. In the lower GI tract, the most common causes of bleeding are diverticular disease, vascular malformation, inflammatory bowel disease and colorectal neoplasia (Table 8.1). In general, bleeding from the upper GI tract is more common than lower GI tract bleeding.

High-risk patients

Significant GI bleeding is indicated by syncope, haematemesis, tachycardia (pulse rate >100 beats per minute), systolic blood pressure below 100 mmHg (13.3 kPa), postural hypotension and requiring more than 4 units of blood to be transfused within 12 hours to maintain blood pressure. Patients over 60 years of age with multiple underlying diseases (comorbidities) are at higher risk of mortality. Those admitted for comorbid medical problems (e.g. heart or respiratory failure, or a cerebrovascular bleed) who

TABLE 8.1: Causes of acute upper and lower gastrointestinal (GI) bleeding

	Upper GI bleeding	Lower GI bleeding
Common	• Gastric/duodenal ulcer • Oesophageal/gastric varices	• Diverticular disease • Angiodysplasia • Haemorrhoids
Less common	• Gastroduodenal erosions • Oesophagitis • Mallory-Weiss tear	• Colonic neoplasms • Inflammatory bowel disease • Ischaemic colitis • Radiation colitis • Upper GI bleeding • Small intestine diseases
Rare	• Upper GI malignancy • Vascular malformation	• Colonic ulcers • Rectal varices

develop GI bleeding during hospitalisation also have a higher mortality risk.

In about 80% of patients, bleeding stops spontaneously before presentation. In the remaining 20% of patients, bleeding continues or recurs during hospitalisation. The mortality in this latter group increases as much as eight-fold compared with patients without further bleeding. Peptic ulcers are a very common cause of GI bleeding and haematemesis. High-risk peptic ulcers, those actively bleeding or that have bled recently, may show stigmata of haemorrhage on endoscopy. These stigmata of recent haemorrhage include active localised bleeding (i.e. pulsatile, arterial spurting or simple oozing), an adherent blood clot, a protuberant vessel or a flat pigmented spot on the ulcer base. Stigmata of haemorrhage are important predictors of recurrent bleeding.

INVESTIGATIONS

Endoscopy

Endoscopic examination offers three functions. It:

1 Gives the most accurate diagnosis of the source of bleeding
2 Assesses the risk of recurrent bleeding (from an ulcer or varices)
3 Offers endoscopic therapy when a source of bleeding is found.

Endoscopic examination should be made available to the patient within 24 hours or when the patient has been stabilised haemodynamically. For triage, it is the best tool to determine whether a patient should be treated at home or admitted.

The following should be done during endoscopy.

- Emptying of blood and blood clot. A single dose of erythromycin (3 mg/kg) can assist visualisation by increasing gastric emptying in a massive bleed.
- Lavage of potential bleeding source (e.g. ulcer, varices, tumour) to assess the risk of recurrent bleeding.
- Endoscopic haemostasis:
  - For peptic ulcers (either actively bleeding or showing protuberant vessel or fresh clot):
    - Injection therapy using adrenaline
    - Thermocoagulation using heater probe or electrocoagulation
    - Haemostatic clips.
  - For gastric or oesophageal varices:
    - Banding ligation using single or multiple band ligators
    - Injection of sclerosant (e.g. ethanolamine, sodium tetradecyl sulfate [STD]) if banding is not possible
    - Injection of cyanoacrylate for gastric varices is an option. Balloon tamponade can buy time to provide other definitive therapy (e.g. TIPS—see below).
  - For vascular malformation:
    - Argon plasma coagulation
    - Haemostatic clips.

MANAGEMENT

Pharmacological therapy

In patients with a high risk of recurrent bleeding, pharmacologic control without endoscopic haemostasis is inadequate. Thus a combination of endoscopic and pharmacologic therapy is best practice for patients with bleeding ulcers.

Acid suppressing drugs

Acid suppressing drugs such as H_2-receptor antagonists and proton pump inhibitors (PPIs) are effective drugs to promote ulcer healing, however H_2-receptor antagonists do not control acute bleeding. As an acidic environment impairs platelet function and haemostasis, reducing the secretion of gastric acid should reduce bleeding. Potent acid suppression using intravenous PPIs (e.g. esomeprazole, lansoprazole, omeprazole, pantoprazole or rabeprazole) reduces recurrent bleeding after endoscopic therapy. PPIs should be recommended as an adjuvant to endoscopic therapy in patients with peptic ulcers with a high risk of bleeding.

Vasoactive agents

Previously, vasopressin (0.2–0.4 U/min) was the most widely used agent to reduce portal blood pressure and control variceal bleeding. Adverse effects of vasopressin such as cardiac ischaemia (in about 10% of patients) and worsening coagulopathy (by release of plasminogen activator) have discouraged the use of this drug in recent years. Terlipressin, a triglycyl synthetic analogue of vasopressin, has a longer half-life and fewer cardiac side effects and appears more effective and safe when used in combination with glyceryl trinitrate. Infusion of somatostatin and its analogue (octreotide, vapreotide) reduces portal blood pressure and azygous blood flow. They are safe and effective vasoactive agents for acute variceal bleeding. The benefit is more prominent if these vasoactive agents are given early, even before endoscopy. Octreotide has also been shown to be effective when used as an adjuvant therapy in combination with endoscopic therapy. Recurrent bleeding episodes and, hence, transfusion requirements are significantly reduced.

Antifibrinolytic agents

Antifibrinolytic agents such as tranexamic acid have not reduced the operative rate and mortality of acute GI haemorrhage. Recombinant activated factor VII (rFVIIa, eptacog alfa) may be useful in difficult cases of bleeding from oesophageal varices.

Antibiotics

Antibiotics have been recommended in management of variceal bleeding. Bacteraemia is a common occurrence after endoscopic therapy. Prophylactic antibiotics (e.g. cephalosporin or quinolone) can prevent the development of infected ascites in these patients.

Radiological therapy

Angiography is an important tool for diagnosing GI bleeding when endoscopy fails to identify the source. The advantages of angiography include accurate localisation of rapidly bleeding lesions and the potential to achieve immediate control with several treatment modalities:

- Highly-selective coil embolisation for bleeding ulcer and vascular malformation using:
  - Gelatin sponge pledgets
  - Microcoils
  - Polyvinyl alcohol particles
- Transjugular intrahepatic porto-systemic shunt (TIPS) for gastric or oesophageal varices.

Surgery

Surgery remains the most definitive method of stopping haemorrhage. However, there is little agreement on the exact indications and best timing for surgical intervention. These issues are even less clear now that endoscopic and radiological intervention are so effective. Accordingly, good cooperation among intensivists, gastroenterologists, intervention radiologists and surgeons is essential. Indications for surgery include:

- arterial bleeding that cannot be controlled by endoscopic haemostasis
- massive transfusion (i.e. total of 6–8 units of blood) required to maintain blood pressure
- recurrent clinical bleeding after initial success in endoscopic and/or angiographic haemostasis
- evidence suggestive of GI perforation.

A multidisciplinary approach to the management of upper GI bleeding is shown in Figure 8.1.

BLEEDING OF OBSCURE ORIGIN

The source of bleeding remains unidentified after gastroscopy and colonoscopy in about 5% of patients. The most common causes include angiodysplasia, small intestine neoplasms, Meckel's diverticulum, ectopic varices and conditions causing haemobilia. Bleeding as a result of these conditions is often difficult to manage. In the past, red blood cell scintigraphy and angiography were the two commonly used diagnostic tools, but the yields were very low. With the advent of capsule endoscopy and double balloon enteroscopy, the diagnosis and treatment success of these conditions is much improved. While capsule endoscopy is much more comfortable and, hence, better tolerated by patients, double balloon enteroscopy offers an opportunity to control the bleeding when a source is found.

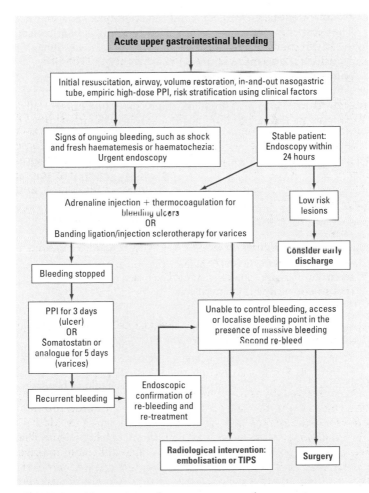

FIGURE 8.1: Management of common causes of acute upper gastrointestinal bleeding.

PPI = proton pump inhibitor; TIPS = transjugular intrahepatic portosystemic shunt.

SUMMARY

Acute GI bleeding is one of the common emergencies encountered and is associated with significant morbidity and mortality. It is important that a team approach is adopted comprising gastroenterologists, GI surgeons and interventional radiologists.

The most common cause of upper GI bleeding is peptic ulcer, followed by mucosal erosions, Mallory-Weiss tear, oesophagitis and oesophageal/gastric varices.

High-risk patients with peptic ulcers are those actively bleeding or which have bled recently and show stigmata of haemorrhage at endoscopy. There is a high mortality in approximately 20% of patients in whom bleeding has not stopped spontaneously or recurs during hospitalisation.

Endoscopic examination should be done within 24 hours or when the patient is stabilised. A combination of endoscopic and adjuvant pharmacologic therapy (PPIs and octreotide) is optimal therapy for patients with bleeding ulcers. Surgery is indicated when arterial bleeding cannot be controlled by endoscopic haemostasis and when massive transfusion is required.

FURTHER READING

Chung SS, Lau JY, Sung JJ, et al. Randomized comparison between adrenaline injection alone and adrenaline injection plus heat probe treatment for actively bleeding ulcers. Brit Med J 1997; 314:1307–11.

Gross M, Schiemann U, Muhlhofer A, et al. Meta-analysis: efficacy of therapeutic regimens in ongoing variceal bleeding. Endoscopy 2001; 33:737–46.

Leontiadis GI, Sharma VK, Howden CW. Proton pump inhibitors for acute peptic ulcer bleeding. Cochrane Database Syst Rev 2006;(1): CD002094.

Rollhauser C, Fleischer DE. Nonvariceal upper gastrointestinal bleeding. Endoscopy 2004; 36:52–8.

Chapter 9

IRRITABLE BOWEL SYNDROME

KEY POINTS

- Irritable bowel syndrome (IBS) is a highly prevalent condition affecting 15% of the population.
- IBS is defined by chronic or relapsing abdominal symptoms (pain and/or discomfort) associated with an abnormality of bowel movements (loose or hard, or more or less frequent stools at pain onset) in the absence of structural lesions.
- In the absence of alarm features (e.g. weight loss, vomiting, rectal bleeding) or advanced age, a diagnosis of IBS usually can be made with no additional testing.
- Communicating the diagnosis and explaining the prognosis is key for further treatment
- A proportion of patients with IBS suffer from concomitant anxiety or depressive disorders.
- Proper dietary assessment and advice may help identify triggers for symptoms.
- Target the dominant symptoms (i.e. abdominal pain, constipation or diarrhoea) when planning symptomatic treatment.
- Low-dose tricyclic antidepressants, psychological interventions or hypnotherapy can be considered in patients with severe symptoms not responding to the conventional therapies.

DEFINITIONS AND CATEGORIES

In less than 50% of patients with chronic or relapsing symptoms such as abdominal pain or discomfort, structural or biochemical abnormalities can be found that explain these symptoms. On the other hand, even if there are structural abnormalities, such as diverticula in the sigmoid colon, these abnormalities may not explain the symptoms in patients presenting for assessment. If there are no abnormalities explaining symptoms, a functional gastrointestinal disorder can be diagnosed.

If there is no structural abnormality to explain the symptoms, and symptoms such as pain or discomfort are associated with changes in bowel habit, irritable bowel syndrome (IBS) can be diagnosed. The most stringent definitions for functional gastrointestinal disorders have been provided by the Rome Committee, an international working party. The Rome III criteria for IBS are summarised in Table 9.1. Essentially, IBS can be diagnosed when structural lesions are absent (or unlikely based upon the clinical presentation) and the patient suffers from chronic or relapsing abdominal discomfort or pain associated with an abnormality of bowel movements (constipation, diarrhoea or alternating diarrhoea and constipation). Bloating is also common.

TABLE 9.1: Diagnostic criteria for irritable bowel syndrome (Rome III)
Recurrent abdominal pain or discomfort for at least 3 months, and symptoms at least 3 days/month associated with two or more of the following:
1. Relief of pain or discomfort with defecation
2. Onset of pain or discomfort associated with a change in bowel frequency
3. Onset of pain or discomfort associated with a change in form (appearance) of stool (loose or hard stools)

Based upon the symptoms, patients with IBS are usually categorised into one of three groups: IBS with predominant diarrhoea (IBS-D) or predominant constipation (IBS-C) or a mixed pattern of diarrhoea and constipation. Alternating refers to changing from diarrhoea to a constipation pattern (IBS-A). There is a group of patients who develop IBS symptoms after an episode of acute infectious diarrhoea, sometimes accompanied by fever, nausea and vomiting. This syndrome is now labelled post-infectious or PI-IBS. Interestingly, post-infectious IBS is usually associated with diarrhoea predominant IBS. Chronic abdominal pain or discomfort in the absence of abnormalities in stool pattern is not IBS, but is called chronic functional abdominal pain.

EPIDEMIOLOGY

The prevalence of IBS ranges from 10% to 20% in Western countries, and it is just as common in India, Japan and China. Only one out of three people who have symptoms of IBS seek medical attention. Generally, those who have more severe symptoms seek medical help. IBS is more prevalent in females. While IBS is not life-threatening, it is remarkable that affected patients have a substantial number of days off work, and thus society has to cope with the burden of IBS too.

PATHOPHYSIOLOGY OF IBS

A number of mechanisms are believed to be involved in the manifestation of IBS. Indeed, there is evidence accumulating that IBS is not one disease, but most likely represents a group of disorders with different pathophysiologies.

Genetic and environment

IBS runs in families. It is reasonable to speculate that specific genetic factors in combination with the exposure to specific environmental factors cause IBS. The environmental influences (e.g. infections or stress) most likely have different effects based upon an array of factors that include genetic predisposition.

Sensorimotor dysfunction

There is sufficient evidence from numerous studies that, at least in a proportion of patients, abnormal gut sensory function is present (increased sensitivity to innocuous stimuli in the gut).

Food intolerance

A proportion of patients report intolerance of specific foods. There is evidence for hypersensitivity but usually not food allergy. However, diets that carefully exclude these nutrients rarely succeed in providing long-lasting relief.

Gastrointestinal flora and bacterial overgrowth

Emerging evidence suggests that, at least in a subgroup of patients, small intestinal bacterial overgrowth may be present. Antibiotic therapy has improved symptoms, especially bloating, more than the placebo, but more data are needed.

Psychological factors

Up to two-thirds of patients with IBS referred to a tertiary centre suffer from depression or anxiety disorders. In addition, it is striking that IBS patients are more likely to report a history of physical or sexual abuse. However, IBS is not simply a psychological disorder.

MANAGEMENT

Even though IBS does not carry any risk for excess mortality, effective management of and treatment for these patients is important since this disorder can cause severe and sometimes disabling symptoms, impairment of quality of life and, if inappropriately treated, may trigger unnecessary costs for diagnostic and therapeutic measures. Establishing the diagnosis is the first step and, for further management, the most important step. IBS can be diagnosed in the majority of patients without any tests, simply based upon the clinical presentation. While a colonoscopy may not find structural lesions that explain the chronic symptoms in the majority of patients, it may still be helpful to reassure the patient or, if the patients are 50 years of age or older, may be a preventive measure with regard to the early detection of colonic polyps and cancer.

Diagnostic tests

For many years, IBS was considered a diagnosis of exclusion. Patients with alarm symptoms or signs (red flags) such as weight loss, fever, rectal bleeding, malnutrition (or laboratory abnormalities such as anaemia, a low albumin level or an elevated white blood count) need to undergo a diagnostic work-up before the diagnosis of IBS can be made. However, current best evidence does not support the routine use of tests in order to exclude organic gastrointestinal disease in patients with typical IBS symptoms without alarm features. Serological testing for coeliac sprue only might be useful (5% with IBS-type symptoms may have coeliac disease). However, alarm features or persistent non-responsive symptoms should prompt a more detailed diagnostic evaluation.

The diagnosis of IBS is based on patient descriptions of common symptoms and, in particular, abdominal pain or discomfort accompanied by changes in stool form or frequency, often associated symptoms such as bloating and distension. A review of the literature shows that, in patients with no alarm symptoms, the Rome criteria have a positive predictive value of approximately 98%, and that additional diagnostic tests have a yield of 2% or less. The diagnostic evaluation ideally should also include a psychosocial assessment specifically addressing any history of sexual or physical abuse because these issues significantly influence management strategies and treatment success.

While the evidence for a comprehensive diagnostic work-up to establish the diagnosis of IBS is poor, it needs to be acknowledged that the response to treatment is frequently disappointing. Even treatments that are considered to be effective only yield a gain over placebo that does not exceed 10%–20%. Thus, a large proportion of patients that are diagnosed on clinical grounds as having IBS ultimately will have further diagnostic measures simply because the symptoms do not respond to therapy or symptoms relapse after a while.

If tests are being considered, a complete blood count, erythrocyte sedimentation rate (or C-reactive protein), serum chemistry and albumin, and stool examination for ova and parasites can be ordered. However, the cost-benefit of these tests is not established. Coeliac disease serological testing (e.g. transglutaminase) should be ruled out by appropriate serological testing and appears to be cost effective. While not necessary from the perspective of establishing the diagnosis of IBS, in patients over 50 years of age, a colonoscopy is recommended due to the increased probability of colon cancer. In younger patients, colonoscopy or sigmoidoscopy with biopsies can be performed, based upon relevant clinical features (e.g. diarrhoea to exclude microscopic colitis).

The need for additional diagnostic tests such as thyroid stimulating hormone (TSH) may depend on the symptom subtype. For example, for constipation-predominant symptoms, a therapeutic trial of fibre supplementation may be sufficient. The American Gastroenterological Association guidelines recommend that in patients who do not respond to fibre, confirmation of slow colonic transit with a whole gut transit test, or evaluation for obstructed defecation with anorectal motility and balloon expulsion test, might be indicated. In patients with diarrhoea-predominant symptoms, clinical judgment will determine the further diagnostic work-up. In patients with relapsing or chronic loose/watery stools, a lactose/dextrose H_2 breath test for bacterial overgrowth, serology for coeliac sprue or biopsies of the small intestine (for *Giardia*, small bowel malabsorption) or colon (for microscopic colitis) might be necessary. Small intestine imaging might be required to rule out Crohn's disease. Other imaging procedures such as computed tomography (CT) or magnetic resonance imaging (MRI) scan may be justified in very selected patients with severe symptoms not responding to therapy, and patients whose symptoms appear to worsen over time. However, none of these can be considered routine diagnostic measures. If clinically indicated, lactose intolerance should be excluded by breath test or an exclusion diet.

Treatment

General measures

The management approach in patients with IBS is summarised in Figure 9.1. It is most important to address the patient's needs and to match their individual requirements with the management strategy. Ultimately, it must be recognised that a proper clinical assessment and carefully selected diagnostic measures are important to reassure the patient. Thus, theoretically while the decision to use a specific diagnostic test can be based simply upon the clinical presentation (symptoms, age, family history), this decision making should also address the patient's needs in order to avoid over- or under-treatment.

For a large proportion of patients, explanation of the causes of symptoms, the underlying mechanism and reassurance are probably the most important elements of treatment. Patients with mild or infrequent symptoms that do not affect quality of life may not need any further measures. On the other hand, patients who are anxious, depressed and suffer from the fear that an incurable malignancy is causing the symptoms, require, as an important 'therapeutic step', diagnostic work-up to address this concern. In fact, in these patients a colonoscopy might be considered, even if they are below the age of 50 and the risk of malignancy is excessively low, in order to provide reassurance.

General advice to patients should also include dietary recommendations. Foods that trigger symptoms should be identified and systematically avoided. A logbook to document meals and symptoms might be helpful for this purpose. Alternatively, a systematic elimination diet can be attempted. In patients with diarrhoea and bloating, artificial sweeteners sometimes contribute to the manifestation of symptoms. Thus, advice should be given to avoid (at least temporarily) nutrients and sweets with large amounts of artificial sweeteners (including soft drinks, and chewing gum, if used extensively). However, there is currently no diet that has been proven to cure IBS. Removal of foods that have high IgG responses may improve symptoms in a sub-group of patients but remains to be better tested.

IBS is a chronic or relapsing condition. Probably with the exception of fibre, medication should be only used temporarily and doses reduced or drugs discontinued as soon as possible. However, it needs to be acknowledged that a proportion of patients requires long-term maintenance therapy.

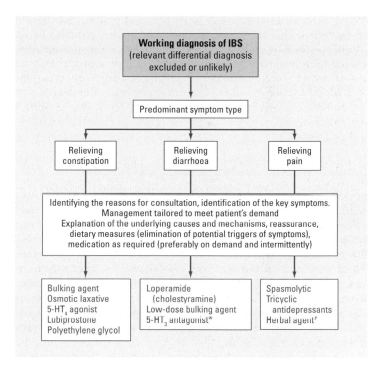

FIGURE 9.1: Management of patients with irritable bowel syndrome (IBS). After establishing the working diagnosis, the predominant symptom is used to guide therapy. It is of crucial importance to determine and tailor the management approach based upon the primary reason for consultation (i.e. a patient concerned about symptoms may require a different management approach compared with a patient with severe symptoms dramatically impairing quality of life).

5-HT = serotonin; IBS = irritable bowel syndrome.

* e.g. Alosetron, currently available in the USA with strict restrictions due to the risk of ischaemic colitis

Only if clinical trial data on efficacy and safety are available for the respective plant extract or the combinations available

Fibre (bulking agent)

Soluble fibre has been shown to affect bowel transit time but trials in IBS have provided conflicting evidence. However, in clinical practice small amounts of fibre or a fibre supplement (e.g. psyllium) are added to the diet. Exposure of these patients to large amounts of fibre should be avoided since excess fibre can cause bloating. However, it needs to be emphasised that it is a common clinical experience that many patients consuming 'standard doses' of fibre improve if doses are reduced. Thus, as a general rule fibre should be introduced in very small doses.

Antispasmodics

Use of antispasmodics (e.g. hyoscine, mebeverine) or peppermint oil may help some patients suffering from cramps or diarrhoea.

Anti-constipation agents

In patients with constipation (not responding to fibre), osmotic laxatives can be helpful. Polyethylene glycol (PEG) can be helpful for constipation. Lubiprostone is a chloride channel activator that also improves constipation. The $5-HT_4$ agonist, tegaserod, has demonstrated modest superiority over placebo.

Antidiarrhoeals

From randomised trials, it can be concluded that loperamide improves diarrhoea but not pain. Cholestyramine may help some cases. Alosetron, a $5-HT_3$ receptor antagonist, is not available in many countries and its use has been restricted because of the potential risk of ischaemic colitis. However, in clinical trials its superiority was clearly demonstrated over placebo and the antispasmodic mebeverine.

Alternative therapies

In IBS, acupuncture is no better than placebo. Psychological interventions are controversial and there are many issues in relation to study design. However, psychological interventions are probably efficacious. Traditional Chinese herbal remedies/treatments have been found in one controlled trial to be superior to placebo, but further trials are needed to confirm this finding and it cannot be concluded that all traditional Chinese medicines are efficacious.

Alterations of enteric flora may play a role in irritable bowel syndrome. There is emerging evidence that bacterial overgrowth exists in a subgroup of patients. These patients are usually characterised by bloating and abdominal distension. While antibiotic treatment or probiotics appear to improve symptoms, little is known about the long-term outcome.

In patients with pain that does not respond to the above-mentioned measures, low-dose tricyclic antidepressants can be recommended, which appear to be beneficial in a subset of patients.

Long-term prognosis

The life expectancy of patients with IBS is normal. Many patients improve over time and will become asymptomatic. However, it needs to be acknowledged that, in a proportion of patients, all the above-mentioned measures fail. Multimodal therapeutic approaches involving pain specialists and clinical psychologists can sometime improve the situation in these patients.

Perspective

IBS is a syndrome most likely due to various underlying pathophysiologies. There is no treatment that cures this condition. The high prevalence of this condition and the resulting implications for the healthcare system are significant. Better understanding of the pathophysiology will hopefully provide the opportunity to develop more effective treatments that ultimately will lead to cure.

SUMMARY

Irritable bowel syndrome (IBS) is a highly prevalent condition affecting 15% of the population. IBS is defined by chronic or relapsing abdominal symptoms (abdominal pain and/or discomfort) associated with an abnormality of bowel movements (diarrhoea and/or constipation) in the absence of structural lesions. In younger patients (<50 y), if there are no alarm symptoms (e.g. weight loss, per anal blood loss), the diagnosis can usually be made with no additional testing. Communicating the diagnosis and explaining the implications for the prognosis and future management is key for optimal treatment. Based upon the severity of symptoms and the severity of impairment of quality of life, no further therapeutic measures may be required in a subgroup of patients once the diagnosis has been established. A large proportion of patients with IBS suffer from concomitant anxiety or depression. Thus there is frequently the fear of an underlying catastrophic disease as the cause of the symptoms. In this context, further diagnostic measures may need to be done to reassure the patient. Proper dietary assessment and advice can sometimes help identify triggers for symptoms. Pharmacotherapy targets the dominant symptoms but is not disease modifying. Low doses of tricyclic antidepressants may be used in subjects not responding to standard therapy.

FURTHER READING

American Gastroenterological Association. Medical position statement: irritable bowel syndrome. Gastroenterology 2002; 123:2105–7.

Bueno L, de Ponti F, Fried M, et al. Serotonergic and non-serotonergic targets in the pharmacotherapy of visceral hypersensitivity. Neurogastroenterol Motil 2007; 19(1 Suppl):89–119.

Halvorson HA, Schlett CD, Riddle MS. Postinfectious irritable bowel syndrome—a meta-analysis. Am J Gastroenterol 2006; 101:1894–9; quiz 942.

Heading R, Bardhan K, Hollerbach S, et al. Systematic review: the safety and tolerability of pharmacological agents for treatment of irritable bowel syndrome—a European perspective. Aliment Pharmacol Ther 2006; 24:207–36.

Longstreth GF, Thompson WG, Chey WD, et al. Functional bowel disorders. Gastroenterology 2006; 130:1480–91.

Mayer EA, Tillisch K, Bradesi S. Review article: modulation of the brain–gut axis as a therapeutic approach in gastrointestinal disease. Aliment Pharmacol Ther 2006; 24:919–33.

Monsbakken KW, Vandvik PO, Farup PG. Perceived food intolerance in subjects with irritable bowel syndrome—etiology, prevalence and consequences. Eur J Clin Nutr 2006; 60:667–72.

Park JM, Choi MG, Park JA, et al. Serotonin transporter gene polymorphism and irritable bowel syndrome. Neurogastroenterol Motil 2006; 18:995–1000.

Riordan SM, Kim R. Bacterial overgrowth as a cause of irritable bowel syndrome. Curr Opin Gastroenterol 2006; 22:669–73.

Chapter 10

FOOD ALLERGIES AND INTOLERANCES

KEY POINTS

- Food allergies may affect up to 6% of the population.
- Food allergies are adverse reactions to foods mediated by the immune system. Food allergies may be mediated by antibodies e.g. IgE (immediate hypersensitivity) or they may be cell mediated (delayed hypersensitivity).
- Intolerances are adverse reactions to foods that are not mediated by the immune system.
- A thorough history is the most important aspect in the evaluation of a patient with a suspected food adverse reaction
- Allergy tests may aid in the diagnosis of a food allergy but should never be exclusively relied upon in the absence of a supportive history.
- Exclusion diets and re-challenge remain the 'gold standard' for the diagnosis of many clinical food allergy-related syndromes.
- Appropriate education regarding both the risk of a severe reaction and food avoidance is the most important aspect in the management of patients with food adverse reactions.

DEFINITIONS

Food adverse reaction: any abnormal reaction that is related to the ingestion of a food.

Food allergy: an adverse reaction to food resulting from an immune-mediated response to a food protein. Food allergic reactions are usually either IgE mediated (immediate hypersensitivity e.g. urticaria) or non-IgE (cell) mediated (delayed hypersensitivity e.g. food protein enteropathy). Some allergic diseases are associated with demonstrable IgE to foods and other allergens but a causative link has not been firmly established (e.g. eosinophilic gastroenteropathy). Isolated gastrointestinal food allergies are usually either delayed or IgE-associated.

Food intolerance: any non-immune-mediated adverse reaction to food. Intolerances are usually caused by an inherent characteristic of the patient e.g. a disaccharidase deficiency causing lactose intolerance. Intolerances may require a much larger amount of the food to cause clinical symptoms and are usually delayed in onset.

Toxic reactions: adverse reactions to foods mediated by a toxin contained in the food e.g. food poisoning or histamine in scombroid fish. These reactions occur in all people who ingest the food and are not dependent on either immune- or non-immune-mediated susceptibility.

EPIDEMIOLOGY

Food allergy of all types may affect up to 6% of children and 4% of adults. Estimates from the USA suggest that around 4% of the general population have IgE-mediated food allergy while IgE-mediated allergy to specific foods varies from between 0.5% to around 2% of the general population, especially in children. The incidence of IgE-mediated food allergy is much higher in individuals with other atopic diseases e.g. up to one-third of children with atopic dermatitis have been reported to have concomitant food allergy. IgE-mediated food allergy is also found more frequently among asthmatic patients, but is rarely the cause of wheeze in the absence of other symptoms.

CLINICAL SYNDROMES

IgE-mediated immediate hypersensitivity

A relatively small number of foods, including cow's milk, hen's egg, wheat, peanut and shellfish cause the majority of IgE-mediated immediate hypersensitivity reactions. Symptoms usually occur within minutes of ingestion of the food and very rarely occur more than 2 hours following the ingestion. Symptoms involving the gastrointestinal system include abdominal pain, nausea, vomiting and diarrhoea. Immediate hypersensitivity reactions rarely involve the gastrointestinal system in the absence of other systems. The most severe form of IgE-mediated allergy is called anaphylaxis and is defined as the involvement of any two organ systems and the respiratory or cardiovascular system. Anaphylaxis is a medical emergency and can be fatal in some cases.

Food protein-induced proctocolitis

Cell-mediated (eosinophilic) hypersensitivity, usually to cow's milk or soy, is characterised by macroscopic blood and mucus in the stool of an otherwise healthy, usually breastfed, infant. Onset is at around 2 months on average. Usually no special investigations are needed to make the diagnosis. Treatment is avoidance of the causative protein by breastfeeding mothers or, if symptoms persist or the infant is not breastfed, a hydrolysed formula may be used. This usually resolves between 1 and 2 years of age.

Food protein enteropathy

Cell-mediated (T cell) hypersensitivity, usually to cow's milk but occasionally also grains, egg and shellfish, is characterised by chronic vomiting, diarrhoea and malabsorption. The onset is usually in infancy in formula-fed infants and failure to thrive is common. Protein loss may lead to oedema and iron deficiency may follow. Diagnosis is made through a combination of endoscopy (biopsy), allergen avoidance and re-challenge. This condition generally resolves between 1 and 2 years of age.

Food protein enterocolitis

Cell-mediated (T cell) hypersensitivity is similar to, but more severe than, food protein enteropathy. It usually begins in infancy and is most often caused by cow's milk, but between 30% and 50% are also sensitive to soy. Chronic ingestion of the causative protein causes vomiting, bloody diarrhoea and lethargy that may lead to dehydration and acidosis. The clinical picture may mimic sepsis including an elevated blood neutrophil count. Re-exposure to the causative protein leads to a dramatic, but delayed ($\pm$ 2 hours) recurrence of symptoms that may lead to shock in up to 20% of cases. The diagnosis is made through an elimination diet, re-challenge with the suspected food under medical supervision and examination of the stool for blood, white cells and eosinophils (colitis). A rise in the blood neutrophil count over 3500 cells/mL may be observed. Biopsy is usually not necessary for the diagnosis. Treatment is by avoidance of the causative food and the use of hydrolysed formula. This condition usually resolves between 2 and 3 years of age.

Eosinophilic gastroenteropathy (EoG)

A group of disorders characterised by infiltration of the gut wall by eosinophils. In contrast to food protein enteropathy and enterocolitis, eosinophilic gastroenteropathy (EoG) may affect people of any age. EoG is thought to be mediated by a combination of both IgE-mediated and non-IgE-mediated allergy to food proteins. Common symptoms include vomiting, diarrhoea, dysphagia, abdominal pain and bloating. Up to 50% of patients have a personal or family history of atopy and 75% may have eosinophilia or an elevated total IgE. The diagnosis depends on demonstrating elevated numbers of eosinophils on biopsy. Adjunctive tests such as skin prick tests and atopy patch tests (discussed below) may be useful to identify causative foods in some cases. Treatment is by a combination of restrictive diet, elemental diet and, if needed, systemic corticosteroids.

ASSESSMENT

As there are no specific diagnostic tests available for many food allergens, delayed allergic reactions and food intolerances, the reproducibility of the symptoms after ingestion of a common food is often important in establishing a causal relationship. There are a number of bedside and laboratory based investigations which, when used in conjunction with a thorough history, may help to make the diagnosis of food allergy or intolerance. The sensitivity and specificity of the tests vary significantly and one should be careful about making a diagnosis of food allergy or intolerance based exclusively on a diagnostic test in the absence of a supportive history.

History

The clinical history remains the most important diagnostic tool in the assessment of a patient with a suspected adverse reaction to a food. Information relating to the temporal relationship of the symptoms with ingestion of the food may help to differentiate immediate from delayed hypersensitivity reactions. Most IgE-mediated adverse reactions to foods occur within 2 hours following the ingestion of a food, although a very small proportion of IgE-mediated reactions may be delayed for up to 6 hours. Non-IgE mediated adverse reactions occur much later, even up to 72 hours after the ingestion of a food. Other important factors in the history include previous exposure to the suspected food, with or without a reaction, the reproducibility of the adverse reaction on re-exposure to the food, the amount of food ingested and the severity of the adverse reaction. The severity of the reaction on history may help to determine further management, e.g. anaphylaxis may require the prescription of self-injectable adrenaline (EpiPen® and EpiPen Jr®). In some cases it may be recommended that the patient keep a diet diary. This may be particularly useful in cases of suspected delayed adverse reactions where the causative food, or the definite relationship between a food and the onset of symptoms, is difficult to determine.

Tests for immediate hypersensitivity

An important aspect of the diagnosis of IgE-mediated immediate food hypersensitivity is the demonstration of IgE antibody to the offending food in the presence of a supportive history.

Skin prick tests

The most commonly performed test for food specific IgE is the skin prick test (SPT). Various commercial food allergen extracts are available, or in some cases fresh foods, especially fruits, are used. A positive skin prick test results in a wheal 3 mm by 3 mm larger than a saline negative control. A histamine or codeine positive control is usually applied simultaneously. The sensitivity of a negative skin prick test is >95%. A positive skin prick test indicates the presence of IgE but has poor specificity. Diagnostic cut-offs of the skin prick test wheal size have been proposed for various foods, but it is prudent not to consider any skin prick test wheal size diagnostic of IgE-mediated food allergy in the absence of a supportive history. Furthermore, the size of the skin prick test wheal has not been shown to correlate with the severity of the reaction.

Specific IgE levels

Food-specific IgE is measured in kilounits per litre (kU/L) of serum. Most commercial assays have a range of 0.35–100 kU/L. The sensitivity of a negative food-specific IgE assay (<0.35 kU/L) is >95%, but the specificity of a positive test (>0.35 kU/L) is poor. Various diagnostic cut-off levels of food-specific IgE have been proposed but, like skin prick testing, one should be cautious about diagnosing immediate hypersensitivity to food based only on a specific IgE cut-off in the absence of a supportive history and when specific IgE levels have also not been shown to correlate with the severity of a reaction.

Atopy patch tests

Atopy patch testing, in which a food extract is applied to the patient's skin for up to 72 hours, may be helpful in the diagnosis of delayed hypersensitivity reactions e.g. food protein enterocolitis. Induration occurring at the site of the patch is considered a positive result. The sensitivity of the atopy patch test is poor but the specificity is reasonable together with a supportive history. However, nonspecific irritation of the skin is common and as such these tests should be interpreted cautiously. A lack of standardised extracts has hampered the widespread use of this testing; however, commercial atopy patch tests are being developed that may improve the usefulness of this test.

Food challenges

The 'gold standard' for the diagnosis of food adverse reactions, immediate or delayed, is the oral food challenge. This can be done either open, single blinded or double blinded. Patients ingest incremental amounts of the suspected food and are then observed for a reaction. Food challenges are potentially risky and should be performed under medical supervision with facilities for resuscitation of the patient. Food challenges are especially important in the absence of a convincing history of a causative link between an adverse reaction and a food. They are also important to confirm that a patient has become tolerant of a food to which they were previously allergic. Protocols for the performance of food challenges often vary from clinic to clinic and are usually not standardised, however, various protocols for determining minimal reactive doses of various foods etc have been proposed.

MANAGEMENT

Treatments for the specific disorders are mentioned above. In general the management of food adverse reactions involves the avoidance of the causative food. A very important aspect of the management of food adverse reactions is the appropriate education of the patient or, in the case of children, their parents or carers. Patients should be told the estimated risk of a severe, life-threatening reaction, especially in the case of IgE-mediated food allergy. They should know how to administer emergency medications (e.g. an EpiPen®), if needed, and how to access medical care urgently. Most importantly, patients need to understand that avoidance is the mainstay of treatment. They should be educated to check for the presence of the causative food in all new foods, which may often involve thorough reading of food labels. Additional support, such as liaising with schools or child care in the case of children, is often necessary. Finally, all patients with food adverse reactions should receive regular medical review to ensure that management strategies, such as restricted diets, are still necessary and appropriate.

SUMMARY

Food allergy of all types may affect up to 6% of children and 4% of adults (Figure 10.1). The clinical syndromes induced are:

1 IgE-mediated immediate hypersensitivity. Peanut and shellfish are included in this category and may cause an anaphylactic reaction
2 Food protein-induced proctocolitis. This is a cell-mediated (eosinophilic) hypersensitivity, usually to cow's milk or soy
3 Food protein enterocolitis is a cell-mediated (T cell) hypersensitivity similar to, but more severe than, food protein enteropathy. It is often caused by cow's milk but between 30% and 50% of hypersensitive individuals are also sensitive to soy
4 Eosinophilic gastroenteropathy is a group of disorders characterised by infiltration of the gut wall by eosinophils. The diagnosis depends on demonstrating elevated numbers of eosinophils on biopsy.

Critical to management is a detailed clinical history. Information relating to the temporal relationship of the symptoms with ingestion of the food may help to differentiate immediate from delayed hypersensitivity reactions.

Diagnostic tests for immediate hypersensitivity include the skin prick test for food-specific IgE, specific IgE levels and the atopy patch test. However, the gold standard for the diagnosis of food adverse reactions, immediate or delayed, is the oral food challenge.

In general, management involves avoidance of the causative food. Appropriate education of the patient or, in the case of children, their parents is pivotal.

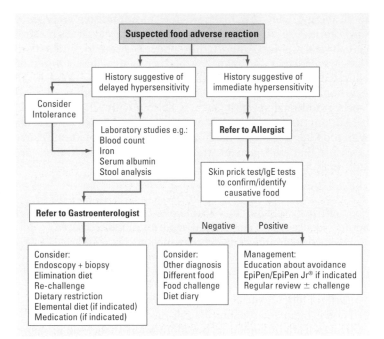

FIGURE 10.1: Approach to suspected food adverse reaction.

FURTHER READING

Bock SA, Sampson HA. Evaluation of food allergy. In: Leung DYM, Sampson HA, Geha RS, et al, eds. Pediatric allergy principles and practice. St Louis: Mosby; 2003:478–87.

Moneret-Vautrin AD. Gastrointestinal allergy in adults. Eur J Gastroenterol Hepatol 2005; 17:1293–7.

Sampson HA. Update on food allergy. J Allergy Clin Immunol 2004; 113(5):805–19.

Sampson HA, Sicherer SH, Birnbaum AH. AGA technical review on the evaluation of food allergy in gastrointestinal disorders. Gastroenterology 2001; 120:1026–40.

Chapter 11

MALABSORPTIVE DISORDERS AND COELIAC DISEASE

KEY POINTS

- Malabsorption may present with weight loss, bloating, diarrhoea and specific vitamin and nutrient deficiencies.
- Identification of the underlying cause and replacement of any nutrient deficiencies are the cornerstones of management.
- Coeliac disease, bacterial overgrowth, food-cobalamin malabsorption, pancreatic insufficiency and malabsorption after gastric surgery are commonly seen in clinical practice.
- Coeliac disease affects 1% of the population and is often undiagnosed as many patients are asymptomatic.
- IgA antibodies to tissue transglutaminase and endomysium have a high sensitivity and specificity for coeliac disease. The diagnosis is confirmed by endoscopic small intestine biopsy.
- Serological testing for coeliac disease is appropriate in cases of weight loss, iron or folate deficiency, osteoporosis, irritable bowel syndrome and in at-risk groups including first-degree relatives of diagnosed cases, type 1 diabetes, autoimmune thyroid disease and Down syndrome.
- A lifelong gluten-free diet is the only effective treatment and ameliorates the malabsorptive and neoplastic risks of coeliac disease.

INTRODUCTION

The body obtains nutrients from food by the absorption of food components that have been broken down by digestion. Malabsorption is the failure of the processes of digestion and absorption, and may present with weight loss, bloating, diarrhoea and a myriad of specific vitamin and nutrient deficiencies. Identification of the underlying cause and replacement of vitamin and nutrient deficiencies are the cornerstones of management (see Figure 11.1). An aetiologic classification of malabsorption is listed in Table 11.1 with the types commonly seen in clinical practice summarised in Table 11.2.

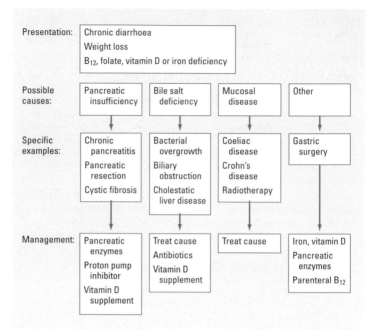

FIGURE 11.1: Management of malabsorption.

TABLE 11.1: Classification of malabsorption	
Pancreatic insufficiency	*Mucosal disease*
Chronic pancreatitis	Coeliac disease
Cystic fibrosis	Crohn's disease
Pancreatic carcinoma	Tropical sprue
	Short bowel syndrome
Bile salt deficiency	Post radiotherapy
Bacterial overgrowth	IgA deficiency and common variable
Biliary obstruction	immunodeficiency
Chronic cholestatic liver disease	Amyloidosis
Other	
Post gastric surgery	
Intestinal lymphangiectasia	

TABLE 11.2: Common types of malabsorption in clinical practice

Disorder	Clinical features	Diagnosis	Management
Coeliac disease	Often asymptomatic IBS symptoms Iron or folate deficiency Osteoporosis	1. Screening with IgA antibodies to tTG or endomysium 2. Small bowel biopsy	Lifelong gluten-free diet Monitor compliance with serology or small bowel biopsy Replace iron, folate and vitamin D deficiencies Check bone density in high-risk cases
Lactase deficiency	Bloating, abdominal cramps and flatulence	1. Disaccharidases assessed by small bowel biopsy 2. Lactose/hydrogen breath test	Reduce dietary lactose to ameliorate symptoms
Food-cobalamin malabsorption	B_{12} deficiency Fatigue, macrocytosis, neurological symptoms and signs	Low vitamin B_{12} in the absence of antiparietal cell or intrinsic factor antibodies	Parenteral B_{12} replacement
Pancreatic insufficiency	Diarrhoea, steatorrhoea or weight loss in the context of cystic fibrosis, chronic pancreatitis or pancreatic surgery	Elevated stool fat as assessed by 72 hour faecal fat	Pancreatic enzyme supplements Acid suppression with a proton pump inhibitor to reduce inactivation of enzyme activity Vitamin D supplement
Malabsorption after gastric surgery	Iron deficiency B_{12} deficiency Steatorrhoea Osteoporosis Osteomalacia	Low ferritin, B_{12} and vitamin D levels Elevated stool fat	Supplementation with iron, B_{12} and vitamin D as required Pancreatic enzyme supplements may be required

IBS = irritable bowel syndrome; tTG = tissue transglutaminase.

PANCREATIC INSUFFICIENCY

Pancreatic disease resulting in pancreatic lipase activity to less than 10% of normal will cause steatorrhoea and weight loss as a result of fat malabsorption. Common causes of pancreatic insufficiency include cystic fibrosis, chronic pancreatitis, pancreatic resection and, occasionally, pancreatic carcinoma.

Steatorrhoea is characterised by offensive pale floating stools that are difficult to flush and although often most marked in pancreatic disease, steatorrhoea can also be a feature of biliary or diffuse intestinal mucosal disease.

Testing for pancreatic insufficiency

The measurement of stool fat in a 72 hour stool collection while consuming 80–100 g of fat per day is the best validated test for pancreatic insufficiency. Excretion of more than 7 g of fat per day suggests steatorrhoea. Of note, severe diarrhoea of any cause can result in up to 14 g of stool fat daily, while a low-fat diet can result in less than 7 g of fat per day in patients with fat malabsorption.

Treatment

Treatment is with pancreatic enzyme supplements. At least 30,000 units of pancreatic lipase are given with each meal with some experts suggesting 90,000 units. The addition of a proton pump inhibitor reduces enzyme denaturation by gastric acidity.

BILE SALT DEFICIENCY

A deficiency of the detergent-like activity of bile salts in the absorption of fat is commonly found in bacterial overgrowth, Crohn's disease of the terminal ileum, surgical resection of the terminal ileum, bile salt transporter defects at the terminal ileum, chronic biliary obstruction and chronic cholestatic liver disease such as primary biliary cirrhosis and primary sclerosing cholangitis.

Bacterial overgrowth

In health, the bacteria that are cultured from the small intestinal lumen are transiently present in counts of less than 10^4 per mL of jejunal content. Stasis of luminal contents due to impaired motility or structural abnormalities can result in bacterial overgrowth.

Excess bacteria can produce malabsorption by deconjugating bile salts, rendering them inadequate for micelle formation and fat digestion. Bacterial-induced B_{12} deficiency may also occur.

Aetiology

Diabetes, scleroderma and chronic intestinal pseudo-obstruction impair small bowel motility while surgery, Crohn's disease, radiation, non-steroidal antiinflammatory drug (NSAID)-related strictures and multiple small intestine diverticula cause structural changes that promote stasis.

Diagnosis

Breath tests for carbohydrate and bile acid malabsorption have poor sensitivity and specificity and the gold standard of quantitative jejunal culture is not routinely available. In practice, a clinical diagnosis is usually made when there is a response to antibiotic therapy in the context of one of the predisposing conditions noted earlier.

Treatment

Options include nutritional supplementation, correction of structural abnormalities or antibiotic therapy on an intermittent, cyclic or regular basis with tetracycline, doxycycline, metronidazole, cephalexin or amoxycillin with clavulanic acid.

MUCOSAL DISEASE

Diseases that damage the mucosa of the small intestine will directly impair absorption. Examples include coeliac disease, Crohn's disease, tropical sprue, short bowel syndrome, post radiotherapy, IgA deficiency and amyloidosis. Coeliac disease is the most common cause of malabsorption due to mucosal disease.

Coeliac disease

In patients with coeliac disease, wheat proteins known as gluten and their equivalents in rye and barley trigger an immune response in the mucosa of the small intestine. These proline-rich proteins resist digestion and are deamidated by an enzyme known as tissue transglutaminase in the intestinal mucosa. Antigen presenting cells with specific HLA heterodimers on their surface (HLA-DQ2 in 95% and HLA-DQ8 in 5% of cases) present the antigen to CD4+ T cells resulting in an immune response that leads to mucosal damage characterised by intraepithelial lymphocytosis, villous atrophy and crypt hyperplasia. This mucosal damage or enteropathy is most marked in the proximal small intestine and impairs absorption.

Prevalence

In Caucasian populations, around 1% of individuals have coeliac disease. The prevalence is higher in certain at-risk groups including individuals with Down syndrome, type 1 diabetes, IgA deficiency, autoimmune thyroid disease and in first-degree relatives of patients with coeliac disease who have a 5% risk.

Clinical presentation

The classical presentation with weight loss, abdominal distension, lethargy and steatorrhoea is uncommon. In fact, 30% of patients are overweight at diagnosis. Many patients have no symptoms at all, termed silent coeliac disease.

Coeliac disease should be considered as a possible underlying cause in cases presenting with irritable bowel syndrome (up to 5% are affected), osteopenia or osteoporosis, infertility, iron or folate deficiency, recurrent oral aphthous ulcers and unexplained weight loss.

Diagnosis

A flow diagram summarising the diagnosis and management of coeliac disease is shown in Figure 11.1.

Testing for coeliac disease is only reliable in individuals consuming a gluten-containing diet.

In studies comparing controls with coeliac cases known to have villous atrophy on small intestine biopsy, antibodies to endomysium (IgA-EMA) and tissue transglutaminase (IgA-tTG) have been shown to have a 90%–100% sensitivity and specificity and are the recommended tests for serological screening. The IgA antigliadin antibody has approximately an 80%–90% sensitivity and specificity. The sensitivity of all of these assays is lower in cases with lesser degrees of histologic abnormality (e.g. intraepithelial lymphocytosis or crypt hyperplasia only). In IgA-deficient individuals serologic testing with IgG antibodies to the same antigens is known to have a much lower sensitivity for coeliac disease (around 30%).

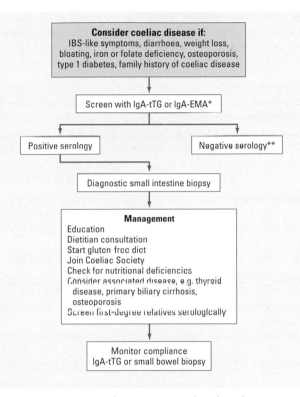

FIGURE 11.2: Diagnosis and management of coeliac disease.
*IgA deficient individuals will have negative results. **If strong clinical suspicion remains, check HLA haplotype.
IBS = irritable bowel syndrome; IgA-EMA = endomysium antibody;
IgA-tTG = tissue transglutaminase antibody.

A small intestine biopsy on a gluten-containing diet is essential to confirm a diagnosis of coeliac disease. An increased number of lymphocytes in the small intestine epithelium (intraepithelial lymphocytosis) is the earliest abnormality on routine histology, but only a minority of patients (10%) with this finding will have coeliac disease, as assessed by positive serology. Crypt hyperplasia and partial or complete villous atrophy are typical findings that are diagnostic in the presence of positive serology.

The HLA-DQ2 and DQ8 alleles that predispose to coeliac disease are present in 30% of Caucasians, and their absence effectively excludes the diagnosis of coeliac disease in cases of doubt.

Management

Management focuses on the replacement of any nutritional deficiencies and commencement of a gluten-free diet with support and monitoring.

Assessment of nutritional deficiencies. Iron, folate and vitamin D deficiencies are common at diagnosis and replaced with oral supplements. Around 12% will have associated B_{12} deficiency related to food-cobalamin malabsorption requiring parenteral replacement.

Instituting a gluten-free diet. Newly diagnosed patients must consult with a dietician for expert advice regarding a gluten-free diet and the interpretation of food labels. Joining a local support group (e.g. their state Coeliac Society in Australia) is strongly recommended for educational meetings and local contacts.

Consider associated diseases. Autoimmune thyroid disease and primary biliary cirrhosis are more common in individuals with coeliac disease.

Assessment for osteoporosis. Significant remineralisation occurs in the first 12 months on a gluten-free diet so bone density is usually assessed 12 months after diagnosis in patients at risk.

Monitoring compliance. Titres of IgA antigliadin and tTG antibodies usually fall to normal levels after 6 and 12 months of compliance with a gluten-free diet respectively. A small intestine biopsy after 6–12 months on a gluten-free diet can be useful to document histologic improvement and dietary compliance. Long-term follow-up is required.

Screen first-degree relatives serologically, as 5% will have coeliac disease.

MALABSORPTION AFTER GASTRIC SURGERY

Partial or total gastrectomy is commonly associated with malabsorption of fat, iron, vitamin B_{12} and vitamin D. Gastric atrophy with loss of acidity, rapid transit, impaired pancreatic stimulation and asynchronous pancreatic and biliary secretions contribute. Monitoring after surgery facilitates early replacement of any deficiencies.

LACTASE DEFICIENCY

A genetically determined deficiency of the brush border enzyme lactase commonly develops in adulthood, affecting 80%–100% of African and Asian individuals and 25% of Caucasians. Lactose (milk sugar) that is not digested and absorbed is metabolised by colonic bacteria resulting in diarrhoea, abdominal cramps and bloating after meals. A small intestine biopsy for measurement of disaccharidase activity or a lactose-hydrogen breath test can confirm the diagnosis. Reducing dietary lactose ameliorates the symptoms.

FOOD-COBALAMIN MALABSORPTION

Vitamin B_{12} deficiency commonly presents with fatigue or macrocytic anaemia. When severe and prolonged, neurological manifestations such as sensory neuropathy or spastic ataxia may occur. Levels of plasma homocysteine and methylmalonic acid are elevated by B_{12} deficiency and can be useful to confirm the diagnosis where serum B_{12} levels are only borderline low without clinical features of deficiency.

The most common cause of B_{12} deficiency is food-cobalamin malabsorption, where vitamin B_{12} (also known as cobalamin) cannot be liberated from food or intestinal transport proteins (70% of cases). Age-related gastric atrophy, metformin use, acid suppression with proton pump inhibitors, gastrectomy and alcohol abuse can contribute to food-cobalamin malabsorption. Less common causes of B_{12} deficiency include a dietary deficiency of B_{12} in strict vegetarians (5% of cases) and pernicious anaemia (20% of cases). Testing for antibodies to intrinsic factor and parietal cells will identify pernicious anaemia, which causes an autoimmune gastritis of the gastric body and fundus with impaired acid and intrinsic factor secretion. Antibodies to intrinsic factor have 50% sensitivity and 90% specificity for the diagnosis of pernicious anaemia, respectively, while antiparietal cell antibodies have a 90% sensitivity and 50% specificity. Currently B_{12} deficiency is treated by parenteral vitamin B_{12} replacement but there is increasing evidence that oral replacement may be satisfactory in many cases provided large doses of 0.5–1 mg are taken daily.

SUMMARY

Malabsorption occurs when there is failure of the processes of digestion and absorption. The cardinal clinical features include weight loss, bloating, diarrhoea and a myriad of specific vitamin and nutrient deficiencies. Identification of the underlying cause and replacement of vitamin and nutrient deficiencies are the cornerstones of management.

The causes of malabsorption are: mucosal disease (coeliac disease, Crohn's disease, short bowel syndrome, post-radiation therapy, IgA deficiency, amyloidosis and tropical sprue); pancreatic insufficiency, bile salt deficiency and bacterial overgrowth. The common types of malabsorption seen in clinical practice are coeliac disease, lactase deficiency, food-cobalamin malabsorption, pancreatic insufficiency and malabsorption after gastric surgery.

In patients with coeliac disease, wheat proteins known as gluten and their equivalents in rye and barley trigger an immune response in the mucosa of the small intestine. The enteropathy is most marked in the proximal small intestine and impairs absorption. The classical presentation is weight loss, abdominal distension, lethargy and steatorrhoea. However, this presentation has become uncommon and most patients are asymptomatic. Diagnostic tests for coeliac disease detect antibodies to endomysium and tissue transglutaminase. A small intestine biopsy on a gluten-containing diet is essential to confirm a diagnosis of coeliac disease. Management focuses on the replacement of any nutritional deficiencies and the commencement of a gluten-free diet with support and monitoring.

FURTHER READING

Andres E, Loukili NH, Noel E, et al. Vitamin B12 (cobalamin) deficiency in elderly patients. CMAJ 2004; 171(3):251–9.

Dewar DH, Ciclitira PJ. Clinical features and diagnosis of celiac disease. Gastroenterology 2005; 128(4 Supplement 1):S19–24.

DiMagno EP. Gastric acid suppression and treatment of severe exocrine pancreatic insufficiency. Best Pract Res Clin Gastroenterol 2001; 15(3):477–86.

Riley SA, Marsh MN. Maldigestion and malabsorption. In: Feldman M, Freidman LS, Brandt LJ, eds. Sleisenger and Fordtran's gastrointestinal and liver disease: pathophysiology, diagnosis, management. 8th edn. Philadelphia: WB Saunders; 2006.

Chapter 12

CHRONIC PANCREATITIS

KEY POINTS

- Chronic pancreatitis, chronic inflammation of the pancreas, is characterised by progressive irreversible loss of pancreatic exocrine and endocrine function.
- Chronic pancreatits manifests with chronic abdominal pain, maldigestion and secondary diabetes mellitus.
- The most common cause in Western nations is alcohol abuse.
- Autoimmune pancreatitis can present as a mass masquerading as a pancreatic malignancy.

AETIOLOGY AND PATHOGENESIS

The most common cause of chronic pancreatitis in Western nations is alcohol abuse (Table 12.1).

TABLE 12.1: Causes of chronic pancreatitis

• Chronic alcohol abuse	• Cystic fibrosis
• Idiopathic	• Tropical pancreatitis
• Hypercalcaemia	• Autoimmune
• Hypertriglyceridaemia	• Obstruction, e.g. pancreas
• Trauma	divisum, tumour, calculi
• Hereditary	

Alcohol

Alcohol accounts for 70%–90% of all cases of chronic pancreatitis in Western societies. The onset of alcoholic pancreatitis usually occurs in the fourth decade, and the majority of patients are males consuming alcohol in the order of 100–150 g/day (i.e. 10–15 standard drinks/day) in the 5–15 years prior to initial presentation. Typically, the initial clinical presentation of alcohol-mediated pancreatic injury is acute pancreatitis. However, the characteristic histological and radiological features of chronicity (atrophy, fibrosis and calcification) are already evident in a large proportion of these patients on initial presentation.

Idiopathic chronic pancreatitis

This condition has a bimodal distribution with an earlier median peak at 19 years and a late median peak at 56 years of age. This condition also presents initially as clinical recurrent acute pancreatitis manifesting chronic features over time. Several genetic defects have been linked to the development of idiopathic chronic pancreatitis. A less severe phenotype of idiopathic chronic pancreatitis in the absence of the classic full cystic fibrosis syndrome can be caused by mutations of the cystic fibrosis transmembrane conductance regulator (*CFTR*) gene on chromosome 7q31.2. Inappropriate activation of the cationic trypsinogen gene (*PRSS1*), and mutations of the serine protease inhibitor Kazal type 1 (*SPINK1*), a potent natural inhibitor of pancreatic trypsin activity, may also result in chronic pancreatitis.

Hereditary pancreatitis

This inherited form of pancreatitis caused by mutations of the cationic trypsinogen gene (*PRSS1*) on chromosome 7q35 is autosomal dominant with 80% penetrance. Trypsin activation is central to the activation of the other digestive pancreatic proenzymes. The onset of this condition is in childhood, with progression to chronic pancreatitis as early as the late teens. There is an increased risk of pancreatic cancer: 40% of patients will have cancer by age 70. Mutation of the *SPINK1* gene has been implicated in hereditary pancreatitis. Other inherited disorders that may cause pancreatitis are cystic fibrosis (see below), familial hyperparathyroidism with hypercalcaemia, familial hyperlipidaemia due to lipoprotein lipase deficiency and apolipoprotein C-II deficiency.

Cystic fibrosis

There is a correlation between the degree of abnormal *CFTR* function and severity of cystic fibrosis. Exocrine pancreatic insufficiency occurs in approximately 85% of patients with cystic fibrosis due to defective secretory capacity of bicarbonate and digestive enzymes. Chronic pancreatitis and pancreatic atrophy arises from inspissated protein-rich acinar secretions that obstruct the ducts resulting in cellular destruction and fibrosis.

Tropical pancreatitis

This form of pancreatitis is restricted to areas within 30 degrees of latitude from the equator and is associated with protein–calorie malnutrition. The pathogenesis of this condition has not been clarified.

Autoimmune pancreatitis

Autoimmune pancreatitis is characterised by the presence of autoantibodies and elevated immunoglobulins (elevated IgG4) in the serum, and lymphocytic infiltration of the pancreas. It may masquerade as pancreatitis or as a pancreatic mass mistaken for cancer. Corticosteroids are the mainstay of therapy for this condition.

Obstructive pancreatitis

Obstruction of the pancreatic duct by tumours, papillary stenosis, cysts and strictures may cause pancreatitis. In pancreas divisum, the dorsal pancreatic duct is drained by the minor papilla. Inadequacy of drainage may, in a small minority of cases of pancreas divisum, result in acute or chronic pancreatitis.

ASSESSMENT

The diagnosis of chronic pancreatitis is clinical, based on symptomatology, known risk factors and investigatory evidence.

History and examination

Abdominal pain

Abdominal pain can be variable with this condition and can range from mild discomfort to intractable severe pain associated with narcotic dependence. The pain is localised to the upper abdomen and radiates to the back. The pain may occur postprandially and may be relieved by leaning forwards. Chronic constant abdominal pain eventually develops in up to 80% of patients. A proportion of patients with chronic pancreatitis do achieve pain relief on entering a 'burnout phase' coinciding with the onset of pancreatic insufficiency and pancreatic calcification.

Steatorrhoea and diarrhoea

Pancreatic exocrine insufficiency may occur as early as 5–6 years after disease onset. Maldigestion may occasionally occur in the absence of abdominal pain. Steatorrhoea occurs in approximately

30% of patients with chronic pancreatitis, and a history of the passage of 'oil' at defecation is virtually pathognomonic of pancreatic steatorrhoea. The degree of steatorrhoea depends on the amount of fat ingested.

Weight loss

Weight loss may be marked and can be related to a number of factors (e.g. malabsorption, inadequate diet). Protein–calorie malnutrition is common.

Diabetes mellitus

Impaired glucose tolerance and secondary diabetes mellitus occur in up to 50% of patients with chronic pancreatitis.

Social sequelae

Social sequelae of chronic alcohol abuse often associated with chronic pancreatitis include unemployment and narcotic addiction.

Investigations

Serum pancreatic enzymes

The diagnosis of acute pancreatitis is made clinically and confirmed by an elevated serum amylase and/or lipase greater than three times the upper limit of normal. However, in chronic pancreatitis, the levels of these enzymes may be normal or below the normal range.

Pancreatic imaging

Abdominal X-ray, ultrasonography

Plain abdominal X-ray and ultrasound may detect the pancreatic calcification of chronic pancreatitis.

Computed tomography, magnetic resonance imaging

Computed tomography (CT) with intravenous contrast is useful for diagnosing pancreatitis, pancreatic necrosis (non-contrast enhancing segments of pancreas) and the development of fluid collections. Magnetic resonance imaging (MRI) can provide images of the pancreatic parenchyma.

Endoscopic retrograde cholangiopancreatography and magnetic resonance cholangiopancreatography

Endoscopic retrograde cholangiopancreatography (ERCP) defines abnormalities of pancreatic ducts in chronic pancreatitis. However, ERCP is invasive and can cause complications including inducing acute pancreatitis, duodenal perforation, sepsis and haemorrhage. Magnetic resonance cholangiopancreatography (MRCP) is non-invasive and can demonstrate ductal anatomy with accuracy comparable to that of ERCP.

Endoscopic ultrasonography

Endoscopic ultrasonography (EUS) of the pancreas produces high-resolution imaging of both duct and parenchyma and can aid biopsy of areas of interest. Although it shows promise, the full role of EUS in the diagnosis of chronic pancreatitis is yet to be defined.

Pancreatic function tests

Secretin/CCK/meal stimulation tests (tube tests of pancreatic function)

These tests involve the collection of pancreatic juice to measure enzyme, volume or bicarbonate output via duodenal intubation and are performed following stimulation of the pancreas by a secretagogue such as secretin or cholecystokinin (CCK) or a test meal (Lundh test). Pancreatic insufficiency is diagnosed by a low flow rate of pancreatic juice and/or decreased enzyme and bicarbonate levels in the juice. These tests are available in only a few specialised units worldwide.

Indirect tests of pancreatic function

These tests are of limited value because they miss less severe cases of chronic pancreatitis. Indirect tests of exocrine pancreatic function include the ^{13}C-/^{14}C-triolein breath test, measurement of faecal chymotrypsin and elastase, the N-benzoyl-L-tyrosyl-para-aminobenzoic acid (bentiromide; NBT-PABA) test, the pancreolauryl test and the fluorescein dilaurate test.

Faecal fat analysis

Quantitative fat analysis

The van de Kamer method is considered the gold standard test of steatorrhoea and measures the grams of faecal fat output per day. Faecal fat excretion of <7 g/day on a 100 g/day fat diet is considered normal. However the test is cumbersome and unpleasant, and requires laboratory handling of 72-hour stool collection.

Qualitative faecal fat analysis

A microscopic examination of random stool using glacial acetic acid and Sudan III stain for orange fat globules is a simple test for steatorrhoea. However, the test has only 78% sensitivity and 70% specificity.

Differential diagnosis of chronic upper abdominal pain

Peptic ulcer disease

Peptic ulcer pain is typically central epigastric, intermittent and burning in quality. Classical teaching distinguishes duodenal ulcer (DU) pain from the gastric ulcer (GU) pain by its relation to food. The pain of DU occurs in the evening and early morning and wakes the patient up from sleep between 12 am and 3 am, corresponding to times of high duodenal acid load. Hunger pains and pain relieved by food and weight gain are other features. In contrast, GU pain is aggravated rather than relieved by food and is more associated with nausea or anorexia. Patients who suffer from GU tend to be older than patients with DU and are more likely to be consuming aspirin or NSAIDs. Importantly, patients taking NSAIDs presenting with complicated ulcers often do not have antecedent abdominal pain, possibly due to the analgesic effect from the drug. Conversely, many patients who have typical ulcer-like pain turn out to have non-ulcer dyspepsia. Thus the sensitivity and specificity of typical dyspepsia for the diagnosis of peptic ulcers are low.

Less common causes of ulcers in the upper gastrointestinal tract that can present with pain are Crohn's disease, viral infections, Behçet's disease and Zollinger-Ellison syndrome.

Non-ulcer (functional) dyspepsia

Dyspepsia refers to recurrent chronic epigastric pain or meal-related discomfort. The pain of non-ulcer dyspepsia (NUD) is caused by a combination of visceral hypersensitivity and dysmotility, with possible psychosocial influences.

Malignancy

Cancers of the stomach, pancreas, colon and lymphomas may localise pain to the upper abdomen. New-onset pain in the elderly is particularly suspicious and warrants further investigation.

Biliary causes

Biliary colic is typically visceral, sudden in onset and localised in the epigastrium. Movement does not aggravate pain. Common bile duct stones may also cause jaundice, cholestasis (pale stools with dark urine) and cholangitis (fever, rigors). Cholecystitis causes a peritoneal type of pain and tenderness localised at the right upper quadrant. Sphincter of Oddi dysfunction also presents with recurrent biliary pain.

Neuropathic causes
Neuropathic pain may arise from intercostal nerve neuralgia such as from herpes zoster.

Other causes
Mesenteric ischaemia may cause epigastric or periumbilical pain made worse by eating, leading to sitophobia and weight loss. Uncommon causes of abdominal pain include poorly controlled or new onset diabetes mellitus, hypercalcaemia, porphyria and lead poisoning.

MANAGEMENT OF CHRONIC PANCREATITIS

Diet, nutrition and antioxidants
A low to moderate fat diet (30%–40% of total calories) helps reduce steatorrhoea and stimulation of pancreatic secretion. Supplementation of fat-soluble and other vitamins are indicated in deficient states. Medium-chain triglycerides, which are directly absorbed into the portal vein and do not require digestion, are rarely required. Protein intake should average 1.0–1.5 g/kg/day. Abstinence from alcohol is absolutely essential in alcoholic pancreatitis. Oxidative stress has been proposed as a mechanism in chronic pancreatitis. Whether antioxidants are useful in the treatment of chronic pancreatitis is unclear.

Treatment of pain
Appropriate and adequate treatment of the abdominal pain of chronic pancreatitis can be a challenge. In some situations, a team effort involving a gastroenterologist, surgeon, pain specialist, psychiatrist/psychologist and social worker may be required. Drug and alcohol dependence requires treatment by specialists in this field.

Analgesics
Analgesics, including non-steroidal antiinflammatory agents, paracetamol and tramadol, should be tried initially. Non-opioid analgesics, however, are often insufficient in managing pain and

patients frequently require preparations that include codeine, dextropropoxyphene, oxycodone or morphine. Long-acting agents are more effective (e.g. transdermal fentanyl). A common dilemma is differentiating between narcotic addiction and pancreatic pain as the major driving force behind the patient's presentation.

Pancreatic enzymes

Exogenous pancreatic enzymes, when administered in sufficient quantities with meals, reduce the secretion of endogenous enzymes from the pancreas through a negative feedback mechanism. This, in turn, may reduce pancreatic intraductal and interstitial pressure and provide pain relief.

Octreotide

Octreotide (300 µg/day by subcutaneous injection) can significantly reduce pancreatic secretion as measured by faecal chymotrypsin. However, pain scores and consumption of analgesics were not reduced compared to controls in a short-term trial.

Treatment of pancreatic exocrine insufficiency

For treating exocrine insufficiency, adequate amounts of pancreatic enzymes need to be taken; the treatment aims are weight stabilisation, improvement of diarrhoea and reduction in faecal fat excretion. Refractory steatorrhoea is treated with dose increase of pancreatic enzymes, use of an enteric coated formulation and introduction of acid suppression with a proton pump inhibitor (to reduce enzyme degradation in the stomach).

Treating diabetes mellitus

Achieving glucose homeostasis can be difficult in patients with secondary diabetes because of the increased potential for hypoglycaemia due to malabsorption, irregular caloric intake and impaired glucagon secretion ('brittle diabetes'). Insulin therapy should be avoided in those who continue to abuse alcohol.

Endoscopic interventional therapies

These procedures have been designed to clear the ducts of calculi (often with the aid of extracorporeal shock wave lithotripsy), relieve duct obstruction due to strictures (by stenting) or divide the pancreatic duct sphincter, with the rationale that pain from chronic pancreatitis partly originates from raised intraductal and/

or interstitial pressure. As yet these procedures have not been subjected to high-quality randomised controlled trials.

Surgery

The rationale for surgical treatment of chronic pancreatitis is to decompress the pancreatic duct and interstitium or to resect diseased tissue causing pain. Surgical treatments comprise pancreatic drainage procedures or pancreatic resection. Currently, surgery is considered for intractable pain that substantially interferes with the patient's quality of life and that cannot be controlled by medical therapy.

Pancreatic duct drainage

The Puestow procedure (lateral pancreaticojejunostomy) is performed when the main pancreatic duct in the head and body of the pancreas dilates to at least 7 mm. The rationale for this operation is to reduce intraductal pressure. This procedure has the advantage of preserving pancreatic tissue with low morbidity and mortality. In terms of pain reduction, surgery is superior to endoscopic treatment in those with a dilated pancreatic duct.

Pancreatic resection

Pancreatic resection is considered when the main duct is not dilated. Distal pancreatectomy is undertaken for disease confined to the body and tail of the gland. A pylorus-preserving Whipple procedure or duodenal-preserving resection of the pancreatic head is performed for more diffuse disease.

Coeliac plexus neurolysis

Percutaneous or EUS-guided coeliac plexus neurolysis using alcohol may provide temporary relief.

COMPLICATIONS OF CHRONIC PANCREATITIS

Pancreatic pseudocyst

Pseudocysts can occur in approximately 25% of patients with chronic pancreatitis. They present with pain, local pressure symptoms caused by mass effect, bleeding or sepsis. Symptomatic longstanding pseudocysts that are greater than 6 cm and with mature walls are usually treated. Drainage of the cyst can be percutaneous, EUS-guided, or surgical (cystogastrostomy, cystoenterostomy).

Bleeding

Gastrointestinal haemorrhage associated with pancreatitis may be from several causes. Isolated gastric varices may develop as a result of portal hypertension due to splenic vein thrombosis. Pseudoaneurysms may develop as a result of enzymatic or pressure erosion of an artery by a pseudocyst and may subsequently rupture into the peritoneal cavity or gastrointestinal tract.

Pancreatic fistula

Fistulae develop when pancreatic juice leaks from disrupted pancreatic ducts. An external fistula results from tracking of the pancreatic juice along a surgical or percutaneous tract. Internal fistulae develop following rupture of a pseudocyst (communicating with the pancreatic duct) into the peritoneal cavity, pleural cavity and other spaces. Treatment includes octreotide to reduce pancreatic secretion, endoscopic stenting of pancreatic duct obstruction downstream from the site of the leak and possibly surgery.

Pancreatic cancer

Chronic pancreatitis is associated with an increased risk of pancreatic cancer, with a cumulative risk of 1.8% (95% confidence interval [CI]: 1.0 to 2.6) for subjects followed for 10 years and 4% (95% CI: 2.0 to 5.9) for those followed for 20 years. Imaging techniques often cannot distinguish between cancer and focal pancreatitis. Screening may be appropriate in patients with hereditary pancreatitis who have a very high risk of developing cancer.

SUMMARY

Up to 50% of patients with chronic pancreatitis develop diabetes mellitus. Pancreatic imaging is a vital part of the investigation of chronic pancreatitis (see Figure 12.1). Tests include abdominal X-ray and ultrasonography to detect calcification. CT scan and MRI can detect pancreatic necrosis and fluid collections. MRCP can demonstrate ductal anatomy. EUS assesses parenchyma and duct and can biopsy suspicious lesions.

Quantitative or qualitative faecal fat analysis may assist in the diagnosis of chronic pancreatitis.

Management focuses on alcohol abstinence, improving nutrition and treatment of pain. Non-opioid analgesics may help, but patients often require narcotic preparations. Exogenous pancreatic enzymes are the cornerstone of therapy.

Endoscopic interventional therapies have been used to clear the ducts of calculi, relieve duct obstruction due to strictures or to divide the pancreatic duct sphincter. Surgery may be indicated to decompress the pancreatic duct and is more effective than endoscopic trans-ampullary drainage.

History:	• Alcohol abuse • Abdominal pain: upper abdomen, radiates to back • Weight loss • Steatorrhoea • Diabetes mellitus • Social sequelae in terms of employment, narcotic addition, problems with family

Investigations:	• Serum pancreatic enzymes
	• Pancreatic imaging:
	  – Abdominal X-ray
	  – Computed tomography (CT) scan
	  – Magnetic resonance imaging (MRI)
	  – Endoscopic retrograde cholangiopancreatography (ERCP), magnetic resonance cholangiopancreatography (MRCP)
	• Endoscopic ultrasonography (EUS)
	• Tube tests of pancreatic function
	• Faecal fat analysis—quantitative and qualitative

Management:	• Alcohol abstinence • Diet, nutrition, antioxidants • Pain therapy: analgesics, coeliac plexus neurolysis, EUS-guided coeliac axis block • Pancreatic enzymes • Octreotide • Diabetes mellitus treatment • Endoscopic interventional therapies • Surgery: pancreatic duct drainage, pancreatic resection
Complications:	• Pancreatic pseudocyst • Gastrointestinal haemorrhage • Pancreatic fistula • Pancreatic cancer

FIGURE 12.1: Chronic pancreatitis.

Major complications of chronic pancreatitis are pancreatic pseudocyst, gastrointestinal haemorrhage, pancreatic fistula (internal or external) and an increased risk of pancreatic cancer.

FURTHER READING

Ahlgren JD. Epidemiology and risk factors in pancreatic cancer. Semin Oncol 1996; 23:241–50.

Apte MV, Keogh GW, Wilson JS. Chronic pancreatitis: complications and management. J Clin Gastroenterol 1999; 29:225–40.

Cahen DL, Gouma DJ, Nio Y, et al. Endoscopic versus surgical drainage of the pancreatic duct in chronic pancreatitis. N Engl J Med 2007; 356:727–9.

DiMagno MJ, Di Magno EP. Chronic pancreatitis. Curr Opin Gastroenterol 2005; 21(5):544–54.

Friess H, Beger HG, Sulkowski U, et al. Randomized controlled multicentre study of the prevention of complications by octreotide in patients undergoing surgery for chronic pancreatitis. Br J Surg 1995; 82:1270–3.

Kim KP, Kim MH, Song MH, et al. Autoimmune chronic pancreatitis. Am J Gastroenterol 2004; 99(8):1605–16.

Lowenfels AB, Maisonneuve P, Cavallini G, et al. Pancreatitis and the risk of pancreatic cancer. International Pancreatitis Study Group. N Engl J Med 1993; 328:1433–7.

Malfertheimer P, Mayer D, Buchler M, et al. Treatment of pain in chronic pancreatitis by inhibition of pancreatic secretion with octreotide. Gut 1995; 36:450–4.

Scolapio JS, Malhi-Chowla N, Ukleja A. Nutrition supplementation in patients with acute and chronic pancreatitis. Gastroenterol Clin North Am 1999; 28(3):695–707.

Whitcomb DC. The spectrum of complications of hereditary pancreatitis. Is this a model for future gene therapy? Gastroenterol Clin N Am 1999; 28:525–42.

Chapter 13

CANCER OF THE PANCREAS AND PANCREATIC CYSTIC LESIONS

KEY POINTS

- Pancreatic cancer is an aggressive cancer with a low survival time: 10%–15% survival at 5 years.
- The major risk factors include smoking, chronic pancreatitis, hereditary pancreatitis and dietary factors.
- Most patients present with symptoms late in the course of the disease.
- The classical presentation is painless obstructive jaundice, weight loss and back pain.
- Imaging plays a vital role in diagnosis. Procedures include endoscopic ultrasound (EUS), contrast enhanced computed tomography (CE CT) scan, magnetic resonance imaging (MRI), magnetic resonance cholangiopancreatography (MRCP), endoscopic retrograde cholangiopancreatography (ERCP). It is often necessary to use a combination of modalities to obtain a diagnosis and select treatment.
- Early surgical resection is the only potentially curative treatment for pancreatic cancer.
- Gemcitabine is the choice of chemotherapeutic drugs.
- As a result of advances in imaging there is an increased prevalence of asymptomatic pancreatic cysts.
- Cysts are either inflammatory (pseudocysts), benign (serous cystadenomas), premalignant (mucinous cysts) or malignant (cystadenocarcinoma).
- Mucinous cystic neoplasms (MCNs) are considered premalignant and encompass intraductal papillary mucinous neoplasms (IPMN) and mucinous cystadenoma.
- Microcystic morphology is the hallmark of serous lesions.
- MCNs are characterised by proliferation of the epithelium of the pancreatic duct with various degrees of mucin hypersecretion and a dilated main pancreatic duct.

- The treatment of MCNs depends on the presence or absence of symptoms and the surgical risk to the patient.
- Patients are best managed in specialised centres.

PANCREATIC CANCER

Pancreatic cancer is an aggressive cancer with a low survival rate. It is the fifth most common cause of cancer related deaths in the USA. This is due to the advanced nature of the disease at diagnosis.

Risk factors

The major risk factors are: increasing age, smoking, chronic pancreatitis, hereditary pancreatitis (40% risk of developing cancer by the age of 70 years), recent onset of diabetes mellitus (particularly in patients over the age of 50 years) and dietary factors (a high intake of fat and/or meat),

Screening tests

For persons at high risk, screening should be initiated 10 years before the age at which pancreatic cancer was first diagnosed in families with syndromes and after the age of 35 in hereditary pancreatitis. At present, the strategy involves measurements of the tumour-associated antigen CA 19-9 and spiral CT followed by endoscopic ultrasound if CT results are not diagnostic.

Clinical features

Most patients present with symptoms late in the course of the disease. Tumours in the head of the pancreas present with symptoms earlier than those in the distal gland which are characterised by a 'silent' presentation, often with metastases. The classical presentation is painless obstructive jaundice, weight loss and back pain. Other presentations include nausea and vomiting, late-onset diabetes mellitus without obesity, acute/chronic pancreatitis, acute cholangitis, duodenal obstruction and deep vein thrombosis.

Clinical signs include evidence of weight loss, jaundice, hepatomegaly, a palpable gall bladder, Troisier's sign (enlarged left supraclavicular lymph nodes), an abdominal mass and ascites. In patients suspected of having a pancreatic malignancy, weight loss, hyperbilirubinaemia and an increased CA 19-9 may be highly predictive of pancreatic malignancy. Surgical exploration should be considered in these patients even in the absence of a preoperative diagnosis.

Diagnostic methods

Laboratory investigations

Laboratory investigations include a complete blood count, liver function tests, clotting profile and CA 19-9.

Imaging

Endoscopic ultrasound (EUS): has a high sensitivity and specificity. It can be combined with fine needle aspiration (FNA) to obtain biopsies. However, it is less effective in assessing nodal involvement.

Contrast-enhanced computed tomography (CE-CT) scan: the method of choice for diagnosis and staging. A correct diagnosis can be made in 97% of patients. Spiral CE-CT has almost 100% accuracy in predicting unresectable disease. Tumors involving critical structures (e.g. portal vein, hepatic or coeliac artery) are not resectable.

Magnetic resonance imaging (MRI): results in the same efficacy as CE-CT and is used if patients cannot tolerate intravenous contrast.

Magnetic resonance cholangiopancreatography (MRCP): provides images of the pancreatic and biliary duct systems. The procedure does not involve radiation and uses an iodine-free contrast agent.

Endoscopic retrograde cholangiopancreatography (ERCP): both diagnostic and therapeutic. Biopsies or brush cytology for diagnosis can be obtained and stents placed to relieve obstruction. At the initial ERCP, an attempt should be made to decompress the biliary tree, especially if the patient is symptomatic.

Positron emission tomography (PET): can differentiate inflammatory conditions from metastatic tumours.

Laparoscopy

Laparoscopy allows for direct observation of the pancreas and for biopsies and cytological washings to be taken. This is particularly important in cases where the other modalities are equivocal. It may also preclude unnecessary laparotomies. Laparoscopic ultrasound (LUS) is useful for liver and pancreas scanning.

In summary, it is often necessary to use a combination of modalities to obtain a diagnosis and select treatment.

Differential diagnosis

A pancreatic mass may be due to *autoimmune pancreatitis*. This is a rare disease. Elevated serum levels of IgG4, histology and response to steroids is diagnostic.

Treatment

Surgery

Early surgical resection is the only potentially curative treatment for pancreatic cancer and, even in the best circumstances, there is only a 10%–15% chance of surviving 5 years.

Contraindications to surgery include metastases in the liver, peritoneum, omentum, and extra-abdominal sites (see Table 13.1 for the TNM classification of tumours).

The most common operation is the Whipple pancreaticoduodenectomy. This is because the majority of tumours that are resectable occur in the head of the pancreas. Preoperative endoscopic stenting may facilitate planning of surgery. A modification of the Whipple procedure is the pylorus preserving partial pancreaticoduodenectomy. Overall mortality is less than 5% in specialised centres. Causes of death include haemorrhage, infection, myocardial infarction and multisystem organ failure. There is good evidence that this operation is effective for tumour clearance. Left pancreatectomy, accompanied by en bloc resection of the spleen and hilar lymph nodes, is reserved for tumours of the body or tail of the pancreas.

Octreotide (a somatostatin analogue) has been shown to reduce postoperative morbidity.

Complications of surgery include fistulae, delayed gastric emptying, bleeding and intra-abdominal abscess. Despite advances in surgical procedures, 5-year survival rates range from 10% to 25%. Unfortunately, approximately 88% of cancers are unresectable at diagnosis because of metastases. Good predictors of survival are small tumours (diameter less than 2 cm), negative lymph nodes, well differentiated histology and surgery in a high volume specialised centre. The difficulty in diagnosis is compounded by the fact that it may be difficult to differentiate benign chronic pancreatitis from pancreatic cancer. In a recent series 5%–15% of patients who underwent pancreaticoduodenectomy for suspected

TABLE 13.1: TNM classification of pancreatic cancer	
Tumour	
Tis	Carcinoma in situ
T1	Tumour limited to the pancreas, 2 cm or less in greatest dimension
T3	Tumour extends directly into any of the following: duodenum, bile duct peripancreatic tissues
T4	Tumour extends directly into any of the following: stomach, spleen, colon, adjacent large vessels
Lymph node metastases	
N0	No regional lymph node metastases
N1	Regional lymph node metastases
Distant metastases	
M0	No distant metastases
M1	Distant metastases

cancer of the head of pancreas or periampullary region were found to have benign disease.

Palliative procedures are used for relief of jaundice, duodenal obstruction and pain. Biliary bypass operations are effective but have a significant mortality and morbidity. Stents placed percutaneously or endoscopically can also be used for the relief of jaundice. Treatment of pain frequently requires the use of narcotics. Other methods used are percutaneous coeliac block and chemical intraoperative splanchnicectomy. Exocrine pancreatic insufficiency should be treated with pancreatic enzyme extracts.

Chemotherapy and radiotherapy

Chemotherapy is the primary therapeutic modality for patients with metastatic disease, the objectives of which are palliation of symptoms, improvement in the quality of life and to extend survival. Gemcitabine is used for its clinical-benefit response. Compared with fluorouracil, there is improvement in disease-related signs and symptoms. It demonstrated a statistically significant improvement in clinical benefit response as measured by weight gain, decreased pain medication need or increased performance status and a 5 week gain in median survival over that achieved with fluorouracil. An advance in therapy has been the use of a new agent, the epidermal growth factor receptor (EGFR) tyrosine kinase inhibitor erlotinib, combined with gemcitabine. Radiotherapy has not shown to be of any benefit compared to chemotherapy alone. As yet, there is no clear evidence that combined chemotherapy and radiotherapy is of significant benefit.

PANCREATIC CYSTIC LESIONS

Advances in radiologic technology and the more frequent use of abdominal imaging are resulting in an increasing prevalence of asymptomatic pancreatic cysts. The cysts are either inflammatory (pseudocysts), benign (serous cystadenomas), premalignant (mucinous cysts) or malignant (cystadenocarcinoma).

Mucinous cystic neoplasms (MCNs) encompass intraductal papillary mucinous neoplasia (IPMN) and mucinous cystadenoma.

Serous cystadenomas and MCNs account for more than 90% of the primary cystic neoplasms of the pancreas. IPMNs occur at a median age of 65 years with equal frequency in men and women.

Clinical presentation

Most patients have no signs or symptoms and the lesion is discovered incidentally due to imaging procedures for the evaluation of another condition (e.g. liver pathology). When symptoms are present, they comprise the symptoms of mild pancreatitis—recurrent abdominal pain, nausea and vomiting due to a lesion causing ductal obstruction or a connection with the main ductal system. Clinically, patients with a cystic malignancy may present the same as those with pancreatic cancer. Pseudocysts are associated with chronic abdominal pain. Large pseudocysts can mimic signs of a mass arising in other organs of the abdomen and, by their size, compress the stomach, duodenum or bile duct causing early satiety, vomiting or jaundice.

Differential diagnosis

Once a cystic lesion is observed, a pseudocyst should be excluded. This usually presents in a setting of acute or chronic pancreatitis. In addition, pseudocysts do not have an epithelial lining and are collections of pancreatic secretions that have arisen from a duct that has been disrupted from inflammation or obstruction. Imaging should confirm the diagnosis.

Once a pseudocyst has been excluded, differentiation between the different types of cystic neoplasms should be carried out. The hallmark of *serous* lesions is their characteristic microcystic morphology. They consist of numerous tiny cysts with a honeycomb appearance on cross section. Radiologically, large lesions often have a fibrotic or calcified scar but large lesions only occur in a minority of cases. The majority occur in the body or tail of the pancreas.

MCNs are considered premalignant and are characterised by proliferation of the epithelium of the pancreatic duct with various degrees of mucin hypersecretion and a dilated main pancreatic duct. IPMNs originate in the distal main pancreatic duct in most cases. Thus, they tend to produce obstruction with symptoms of pancreatitis or jaundice. As they are considered premalignant, on histologic examination their epithelium may demonstrate features of hyperplasia through to carcinoma within a single tumour. Pancreatic duct dilatation can be observed on imaging.

Imaging procedures to assess MCNs include CT scan, ERCP, MRCP and EUS with fine needle aspiration. Promising complementary studies in progress to aid diagnosis are Trucut biopsy examination, DNA analysis of cyst fluid and direct visualisation of peroral pancreatoscopy and biopsies.

Treatment

The treatment of MCNs depends on the presence or absence of symptoms and the surgical risk to the patient. With regard to the risk of malignancy, the true risk is not yet known and it is undecided whether observation or surgical resection is the best option. It is probably best for patients to be managed in specialised centres.

SUMMARY

Pancreatic cancer is an aggressive cancer with a low survival time. The major risk factors are increasing age, smoking, hereditary pancreatitis, chronic pancreatitis and dietary factors. The classical presentation is painless obstructive jaundice, weight loss and back pain (Figure 13.1). Laboratory investigations include a full blood count, liver function tests and CA 19-9. Imaging procedures appropriate for diagnosis and staging include CE-CT Scan, EUS (with fine needle aspiration), MRI, MRCP, ERCP and PET scan.

Laparoscopy allows for direct observation of the pancreas and laparoscopic ultrasound (LAS) can be performed.

Early surgical resection is the only potentially curative treatment for pancreatic cancer, but there is only a 10%–15% chance of survival at 5 years. The most common operation is a Whipple pancreaticoduodenectomy. Chemotherapy is the primary therapeutic modality for patients with metastatic disease. Gemcitabine is the drug of choice. An advance in therapy is the agent erlotinib combined with gemcitabine.

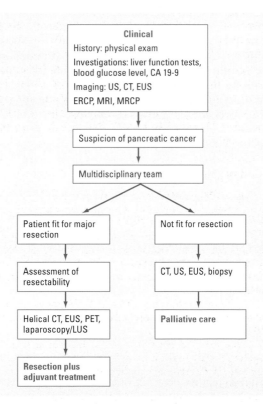

FIGURE 13.1: Diagnosis and management of pancreatic cancer.

CT = computed tomography; ERCP = endoscopic retrograde cholangiopancreatography; EUS = endoscopic ultrasound; LUS = laparoscopic ultrasound; MRCP = magnetic resonance cholangiopancreatography; PET = positron emission tomography; US = ultrasound.

Pancreatic cysts are either inflammatory (pseudocysts), benign (serous cystadenomas), premalignant (mucinous cysts) or malignant (cystadenocarcinoma). MCNs encompass intraductal papillary mucinous neoplasia (IPMN) and mucinous cystadenoma.

Most patients are asymptomatic and the cysts are discovered incidentally. When symptoms are present, they comprise the symptoms of mild pancreatitis. Clinically, patients with a cystic malignancy present the same as those with pancreatic cancer.

In the differential diagnosis, once a cystic lesion is discovered a pseudocyst should be excluded. Thereafter, differentiation between the different cystic lesions should be carried out. The hallmark of serous lesions is the characteristic microcystic morphology. MCNs are considered premalignant and encompass IPMNs and mucinous cystadenomas. They are characterised by proliferation of the epithelium of the pancreatic duct with various degrees of mucin hypersecretion and a dilated main pancreatic duct. Histologic examination of the epithelium may demonstrate hyperplasia to carcinoma within a single tumour. Imaging procedures to assess MCNs include CT scan, ERCP, MRCP and EUS with FNA. The true risk of malignancy is not as yet known.

FURTHER READING

Canto MI, Goggins M, Hruban RH, et al. Screening for early pancreatic neoplasia in high risk individuals: a prospective controlled study. Clin Gastroenterol Hepatol 2006; 4:766–81.

Canto MI, Kennedy T, Preczewski L, et al. Screening for pancreatic neoplasia in high risk individuals: who, what, when, how. Clin Gastroenterol Hepatol 2005; 3:S46–8.

Chak A. Pancreatic cysts: much ado or not enough? Clin Gastroenterol Hepatol 2005; 3:964–6.

Eloubeidi MA, Desmond RA, Wilcox CM, et al. Prognostic factors for survival in pancreatic cancer: a population based study. Am J Surg 2006; 192:322–9.

Kennedy T, Preczewski L, Stocker SJ, et al. Incidence of benign inflammatory disease in patients undergoing Whipple procedure for clinically suspected carcinoma: a single-institution experience. Am J Surg 2006; 191:437–41.

Khalid A, McGrath KM, Zahid M, et al. The role of pancreatic cyst fluid molecular analysis in predicting cyst pathology. Clin Gastroentrol Hepatol 2005; 3:967–73.

Levy MJ. Screening for pancreatic cancer: searching for the right needle in the haystack. Clin Gastroenterol Hepatol 2006; 4:684–7.

Chapter 14

CHALLENGING CONSTIPATION

KEY POINTS

- Constipation is a symptom not a diagnosis.
- There are three subtypes of functional constipation (no structural or biochemical cause): slow transit constipation, pelvic floor dysfunction and normal tests (normal transit and normal pelvic floor function).
- Irritable bowel syndrome may present as normal transit constipation but abdominal pain is characteristic.
- A detailed history should include ruling out constipating drugs.
- New-onset constipation in older age is a red flag and colon cancer should be excluded.
- A careful digital rectal examination should be performed to identify the presence of obstruction or abnormal pelvic floor function, as well as looking for evidence of rectal cancer.
- A colonic transit study by radio-opaque markers or scintigraphy provides a good assessment of colonic transit time.
- The balloon expulsion test is usually abnormal in pelvic outlet obstruction.
- Biofeedback therapy is efficacious in treating pelvic outlet obstruction.

INTRODUCTION

Constipation is a symptom not a diagnosis. Patients mean different things when they complain of constipation, but it is often defined as two or more of the following for at least 3 months:
- Excessive straining to pass stool
- Hard or lumpy stools
- Stool frequency less than three times per week
- A sensation of incomplete evacuation
- Sensation of anorectal blockage
- Use of manual manoeuvres such as digital evacuation.

It is important to take a detailed history from a patient presenting with constipation and, in particular, to decide whether it is a new symptom or the first presentation of a long-term complaint. Investigations and treatment will be determined by these factors.

CONSTIPATION IN ADULTS

The prevalence of constipation in the general population has been reported to be as high as 20%. The symptom is more common in women and some report they become more constipated in the premenstrual week. Constipation is also common in pregnancy, during periods of immobilisation, following surgery and in the elderly. Women in particular report becoming constipated when they travel. Many women are reluctant to use public toilets or empty their bowels at work and this can further complicate treatment.

Constipation is rarely a presenting symptom of colon cancer. However, the possibility should be considered in each and every patient. Colon cancer is a common malignancy, affecting one in 18 men and one in 24 women. A consultation concerning bowel habit can be a good time to discuss screening for bowel cancer (e.g. by colonoscopy) even if the symptoms don't warrant colonoscopy. Faecal occult blood testing is not an appropriate test for people with symptoms and should not be used to screen for bowel cancer in people who present with constipation.

There are a number of endocrine diseases that can present with constipation, including hypothyroidism and hypercalcaemia. Diabetes mellitus can also cause a change in bowel habit over time. Rarer conditions that can cause constipation include glucagon producing tumours, phaeochromocytoma and pseudohypoparathyroidism.

Constipation can also be associated with neurological disease, depression or anorexia nervosa. Very occasionally, a psychotic patient will complain that they haven't emptied their bowel for an improbable length of time, such as a year or two. It is important to be vigilant for these rare psychological associations.

It is important to differentiate between two important disorders of colonic motility:
- Slow transit constipation—slower than normal movement of contents from the proximal to the distal colon and rectum
- Pelvic floor dysfunction (dyssynergic defecation or anismus)— the primary failure is an inability to evacuate adequately contents from the rectum.

Combination syndromes are possible whereby elements of slow transit and disorders of evacuation coexist. Other patients with no structural or biochemical explanation for their constipation may have normal transit and normal pelvic floor function. Some of these cases also have abdominal pain related to their constipation, and are classified as having irritable bowel syndrome (IBS); others do not have IBS or any other explanation.

ASSESSMENT

A thorough medical history and physical examination, including rectal examination, is required. Enquiries should be made about general health, diet, psychological status and any medications being taken.

History

A detailed history should include exactly what the patient means by constipation. How often, what shape and consistency is the motion and with what difficulty or ease does defecation occur? Is there any abdominal pain or bloating? Is there any rectal bleeding? It is also important to take a detailed laxative history: what laxatives are used, how often and the dosage. The dietary history should include:

- Is cereal eaten for breakfast and what type of cereal is it? (Some commercial cereals contain almost no fibre.)
- What sort of bread is consumed and how many pieces are eaten per day?
- How many pieces of fruit are eaten per day?
- How many servings of vegetables are eaten per day?
- How much water, juice or tea is consumed per day? Patients are often surprised to hear that a couple of short black coffees are not sufficient fluid intake.
- Ask about exercise.

Simple suggestions on dietary modification can make quite a deal of difference.

Ask the patient to keep a diet diary for a few days. Most people overestimate the amount of fibre and underestimate the amount of fat they consume.

Medications

Constipation is a common side effect of many medications, particularly in the elderly. These include:

- aluminium-based antacids
- anticholinergic agents
- calcium supplements
- calcium channel blockers
- iron supplements
- tricyclic antidepressants
- narcotics.

It is often possible to substitute another medication for a possible culprit and assess the effect.

Physical examination

Every patient requires a thorough physical examination, including rectal examination, and neurological examination to exclude systemic illnesses that may cause constipation. The abdomen should be examined for masses. The thyroid status of the patient should be assessed.

Physical examination includes a check for perianal disease that might be complicating the constipation, such as haemorrhoids or anal fissures. People who consistently strain at stool are more likely to have haemorrhoids. If the haemorrhoids require banding, it is particularly important to alter the underlying bowel habit so that haemorrhoids don't recur. An anal fissure is not always preceded by constipation. However, once the fissure is present, anal spasm can make defecation very painful and difficult. The constipation in this situation may be difficult to treat until the fissure has been dealt with. Anorectal examination may also reveal skin tags and skin excoriation.

A careful digital rectal examination should be performed to exclude a rectal stricture or blood in the stool. During the rectal examination, the patient should be asked to bear down as if to defecate and the examiner should perceive relaxation of the external anal sphincter together with perineal descent. One should suspect dyssynergic defecation if this response is absent.

Some patients, particularly women, are troubled by rectal prolapse associated with long-term straining at stool. This is a symptom that is often not volunteered and direct enquiry and physical examination are required. Many women who have a degree of rectal prolapse will continue to strain at defecation because the sensation caused by the prolapse leads to the belief that there are still faeces in the rectum. A discussion of the mechanics of defecation with the aid of a diagram can be very helpful. Mucosal resection is indicated in some cases. Behaviour therapy, incorporating biofeedback, has a role in some long-term cases.

Neurological examination should screen for Parkinson's disease, multiple sclerosis, stroke, spinal cord injury or myotonic dystrophy. Look at the skin. Some people with scleroderma can have severe constipation whereas others are troubled by diarrhoea due to bacterial overgrowth in the small intestine. Appropriate management of these conditions is required as well as assessment and management of the constipation.

Investigations

Baseline investigations to exclude systemic diseases should be done initially. These include serum calcium, glucose and thyroid function tests.

A plain abdominal X-ray can be very helpful if there is doubt about the degree of constipation. Some patients will have marked faecal loading. Structural evaluation of the colon is appropriate and is done by carrying out a colonoscopy, or flexible sigmoidoscopy and barium enema. Colonoscopy is indicated if there has been a recent change in bowel habit or rectal bleeding. It may also be advisable if there is a family history of bowel cancer.

Further investigations

Colonic transit study (transit time): indicates the time for stool movement through the colon. The radio-opaque marker study may show one of three patterns: normal; slow transit; hold-up in the sigmoid and rectum suggesting, but not establishing, an obstructive defecation pattern.

In some patients with constipation, the colon transit time may be normal. In this scenario, it is important to exclude pelvic floor dysfunction. Similarly, if transit is slow this may be due to pelvic floor dysfunction, not colonic disease.

Balloon expulsion test: provides an assessment of the patient's ability to expel a water filled balloon. Most patients can expel the device within one minute. If the patient is unable to expel the balloon within 3 minutes, the clinician should suspect dyssynergic defecation.

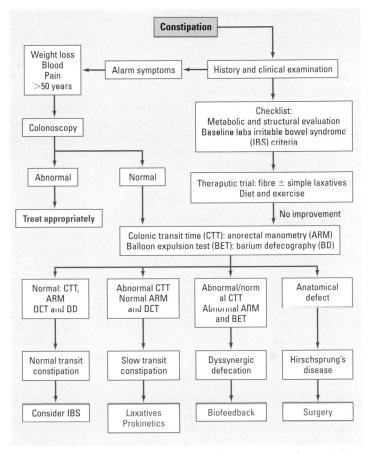

FIGURE 14.1: Algorithm for diagnosis and management of constipation.

Anorectal manometry: can confirm pelvic floor dysfunction, typically with absence or insufficient relaxation of the external sphincter pressure on straining, or poor propulsion, or both. Obstructed defecation may be associated with excessive straining, trouble letting go and a feeling of incomplete emptying. Patients may sit in a very peculiar position to try and empty the rectum. Some patients report splinting the perineum or even performing manual evacuations on themselves.

Hirschsprung's disease (congenital megacolon) is rare but presents with chronic constipation. During anorectal manometry, the anorectal inhibitory reflex is tested; failure of normal internal anal sphincter relaxation with distention suggests Hirschsprung's disease. Rectal biopsy looking for absence of ganglion cells is diagnostic.

Defecography: provides useful information about anatomical and functional changes in the anorectum. An alternative is MRI defecography. Such testing should be considered if anorectal manometry is equivocal or an anatomical obstruction (e.g. large rectocele) is suspected.

TREATMENT

It is rare for there to be a 'quick fix' in the treatment of chronic constipation. Many people benefit from a bowel program consisting of an improved diet, increased fluid intake and daily exercise. Others may require fibre supplementation or medications (Table 14.1). It is important to emphasise to some patients that they must take responsibility for their improvement by making time to go to the toilet in the morning or answering the call to stool when it comes without straining excessively.

TABLE 14.1: Drugs used to treat chronic constipation

Type of drug	Example
Bulking or hydrophilic laxatives	Psyllium (ispaghula), methylcellulose, bran, plantain derivatives, *Aloe vera*
Surfactant or softening or wetting agents	Docusate, poloxalkol
Osmotic laxatives	Sorbital, lactulose, milk of magnesia (magnesium hydroxide), polyethylene glycol (PEG) solutions
Peristaltic stimulants	Senna, bisacodyl, cascara
Prokinetics	Tegaserod
Chloride channel activator	Lubiprostone

Diet

Many people have insufficient fibre in their diet. Ideally, adults should consume about 30 g of fibre per day. Fibre should be increased gradually to avoid initial bloating and discomfort. It is important to give patients information as to what constitutes a high-fibre diet rather than just a figure of the amount of grams that need to be consumed. Pocket-sized books with information on the fat and fibre content of almost any food are widely available. It is useful to suggest a patient keep a diet diary in order to calculate their fibre intake over a couple of weeks.

Some people who do not respond to an increased dietary fibre intake still have benefit from adding psyllium to the diet. Adequate fluid intake is important to avoid dehydration, but increased fluids otherwise probably help very little. Exclude an eating disorder; anorexia nervosa will induce constipation because of inadequate dietary intake.

Laxatives

If fibre supplements have been unsuccessful it may be appropriate to try a regular laxative. Generally it is advisable to discover the lowest effective regular dose to control the patient's constipation. This is a matter of trial and error. Many constipated people will need laxatives for the rest of their lives and there is no clear evidence that this makes constipation worse over time. However, many clinicians avoid prescribing regular bowel stimulants such as senna or bisacodyl. Epsom salts are a cheap effective osmotic laxative for many people. The bitter taste can be masked by lemon juice. Sorbitol and lactulose are osmotic laxatives with a very sweet taste. However, they are relatively expensive. Polyethylene glycol is useful for more severe cases and can be taken regularly.

It is useful to give the patient an information sheet about constipation to take home, stressing that it is normal to empty the bowel between three times a day and three times a week, and making clear suggestions about what forms of therapy can be tried for that specific individual and how long they should persevere before asking for further clarification or help. A 'step-up' approach works well for many patients. For instance, a simple fibre supplement such as psyllium should be tried for a couple of weeks. If unsuccessful, the dose can be slowly increased or another fibre supplement such as sterculia should be tried for a couple of weeks. If unsuccessful, an osmotic laxative can be suggested. People who have difficulty with evacuation may benefit from glycerine suppositories or a faecal softener. If the constipation has been a very long-term problem, it is worthwhile asking the patient to come back for further evaluation and advice.

Other therapies

Lubiprostone is a bicyclic fatty acid that stimulates chloride channels in the intestines, increasing fluid secretion. It has been shown to be superior to placebo in the treatment of chronic constipation. Nausea is a common side effect.

Tegaserod is a 5-HT$_4$ agonist that has efficacy in treating constipation-predominant irritable bowel syndrome in women and chronic constipation in men and women under age 65. Side effects include diarrhoea and headache.

Patients with obstructed defecation may benefit from biofeedback techniques. The purpose of biofeedback therapy is to restore a normal pattern of defecation by using an instrument-based education program. The primary goals are twofold: to correct the underlying dyssynergia that affects the puborectalis and anal sphincter muscles, and to improve rectal sensory perception. Symptomatic improvement using this technique has been reported in approximately 70% of patients.

In patients with confirmed severe slow transit constipation, a colectomy and ileorectal anastomosis may be considered; localised colonic resections are not helpful. In this case, it is essential to exclude pelvic floor dysfunction and a more widespread motility disorder (e.g. small intestinal pseudo-obstruction) with appropriate testing at a specialised centre. Those patients with true colonic inertia typically have loss of the interstitial cells of Cajal, the pacemaker cells of the colon. A megacolon may develop, but is rare.

SUMMARY

Constipation is a very common problem with a wide spectrum of symptoms including excessive straining, hard stools, feeling of incomplete evacuation, use of digital manoeuvres, or infrequent defecation. An appropriate history and physical examination is required to be sure that the symptom of constipation is not the manifestation of some more serious underlying condition. Functional constipation consists of two major subtypes: slow transit constipation and pelvic floor dysfunction. Patients with irritable bowel syndrome have pain, and may exhibit features of both types of constipation. The condition can be managed in the vast majority of cases with simple advice on diet and lifestyle. Biofeedback therapy is an important advance for patients with dyssynergia.

FURTHER READING

American Gastroenterological Association medical position statement: guidelines on constipation. Gastroenterology 2000; 119:1761–78.

Bharucha A, Wald A, Enck P, et al. Functional anorectal disorders. Gastroenterology 2006; 130(5):1510–18.

Brandt L, Prather CM, Quigley EM, et al. Systematic review on the management of chronic constipation in North America. Am J Gastroenterol 2005; 100 Suppl 1:S5–21.

Wald A. Chronic constipation: advances in management. Neurogastroenterol Motil 2007; 9:4–10.

Chapter 15

ACUTE DIARRHOEA

KEY POINTS

- Acute infectious diarrhoea is common worldwide and is responsible for significant patient hospitalisation and mortality.
- Acute diarrhoea is defined as an increase of stool frequency (greater than three stools per day or at least 200 g of stool per day) lasting less than 14 days.
- The principal recognised causes of diarrhoea include viruses, bacteria and protozoa.
- Assessment should focus on the severity of illness, need for rehydration and the identification of the aetiology of the illness on the basis of history and clinical findings.
- Management of acute diarrhoea should include fluid resuscitation, empirical antibiotics or specific antibiotic therapy if the causative organism is isolated.

DEFINITION

Diarrhoea is a leading cause of death worldwide. It is defined as an alteration in normal bowel habit characterised by an increase in volume, water content and frequency of bowel movements, and must have a weight of at least 200 g stool per day.

A more practical approach for the definition of diarrhoea is the presence of three or more loose watery stools per day or a distinct change in a person's normal bowel routine. A working definition of diarrhoea is based upon the duration of symptoms:

- Acute—less than 14 days in duration
- Persistent—more than 14 days but less than 30 days in duration
- Chronic—more than 30 days in duration.

PATHOPHYSIOLOGY

The symptoms of acute diarrhoea vary according to the portion of the intestine that is involved in the disease process. Infectious diarrhoea is often associated with symptoms of nausea, vomiting and abdominal cramps.

The small intestine functions as a fluid and enzyme secretory organ and nutrient absorbing region. Therefore, a pathogen affecting this region will produce symptoms of watery diarrhoea, which is usually of large volume and is associated with abdominal cramping, bloating and weight loss.

The colon is involved in absorption of fluid and salt, as well as excretion of potassium. When this area is involved, the symptoms include frequent, regular small volume, often painful defecation. Fever and bloody mucoid stools are common.

AETIOLOGY

Infectious and non-infectious causes may be responsible for acute diarrhoea (Table 15.1).

Infectious causes include bacteria, viruses and protozoa.

TABLE 15.1: Agents that commonly cause acute diarrhoea	
Bacteria	*Viruses*
• *Campylobacter*	• Caliciviruses (norovirus and Norwalk-like and related viruses)
• *Salmonella*	
• *Shigella*	• Rotavirus
• *Escherichia coli* O157:H7	• Adenovirus types 40 and 41
• *Clostridium difficile*	• Astrovirus
Protozoa	
• *Cryptosporidium*	
• *Giardia*	
• *Entamoeba histolytica*	

Bacteria

- *Campylobacter*: most common bacterial cause usually from poultry, meat, dairy products and contaminated water.
- *Salmonella*: usually from poultry and livestock.
- *Shigella*: highly contagious spreads from person to person.
- *Escherichia coli*: O157:H7: usually from contaminated meat, can be associated with haemolytic uraemic syndrome.
- *Clostridium difficile*: major cause of nosocomial colitis occurring after antibiotic-induced alteration of bowel flora and subsequent proliferation of an endogenous strain. Can also be contagious.

Viruses

Viruses cause the vast majority of all cases of acute diarrhoea.

- Caliciviruses (norovirus/Norwalk): can be detected in vomitus and faeces as compared with bacterial causes of diarrhoea (which is usually shed in faeces alone). Contaminated food or water are the usual primary causes but person-to-person contact is a secondary cause.
- Rotavirus: usually occurs in young children (<2 years). Highly contagious.
- Adenovirus types 40/41: usually spread by person-to-person contact.
- Astrovirus: usually spread by person-to-person contact.

Protozoa

Protozoa are usually waterborne, but may spread from the faecal to oral route. Only need small inoculum for infection.

- *Cryptosporidium.*
- *Giardia.*
- *Entamoeba histolytica.*

Non-infectious causes

Non-infectious causes include drugs, food allergies, primary gastrointestinal diseases (e.g. inflammatory bowel disease) and other disease states, including thyrotoxicosis and carcinoid syndrome.

ASSESSMENT

A good clinical history is important and may allow empiric therapy to be started without the need for any further diagnostic investigation. Initial evaluation should focus on the need for rehydration, severity of illness and identification of a likely causative agent.

Assessment of the severity of dehydration is critical in the management of acute diarrhoea. Features suggestive of severe dehydration and subsequent need for hospital admission and intravenous fluid replacement include tachycardia, >20 mmHg decrease in systolic blood pressure, postural hypotension, poor skin turgor, severe dry mucosa and sunken eye balls. Other indications for consideration of hospital admission include stool frequency (>8/day), fever, significant constitutional symptoms, large amount of bloody diarrhoea, immunocompromised host, infants or the elderly.

Fever suggests infection with invasive bacteria (*Salmonella, Shigella* or *Campylobacter*), enteric viruses or a cytotoxic organism such as *Clostridium difficile* or *Entamoeba histolytica*.

Clostridium difficile should be suspected after recent antibiotic use or hospitalisation.

Food history is important.

- Symptoms that begin within 6 hours of ingestion suggest a preformed toxin of *Staphylococcus aureus* or *Bacillus cereus*.
- Symptoms within 16 hours suggests *Clostridium perfringens*.
- Symptoms emerging after 16 hours suggest viral or bacterial infection (e.g. enterotoxigenic or enterohaemolytic *Escherichia coli*).

INVESTIGATIONS

Stool culture

The diagnostic yield from stool culture is poor: 1.5%–5.6% positive in a number of large epidemiological studies. Routine culture can identify *Salmonella, Campylobacter* and *Shigella*.

Specifically request cultres for *Yersinia*, enterohaemolytic *E. coli* (EHEC), viruses and *Vibrio*.

Ova, cysts and parasites need to be specifically requested and are particularly useful for persistent diarrhoea, as well as in patients exposed to infants in daycare centres. However, cultures are not particularly cost effective as organisms are shed only intermittently.

Clostridium difficile toxin assay is particularly useful in people who have had prior antibiotic exposure.

Endoscopy

Not routinely required. However, it may be useful in distinguishing ischaemic colitis from infectious colitides.

Useful in immunocompromised patients when cytomegalovirus is in the differential diagnosis.

Faecal leucocytes and occult blood

Presence supports the diagnosis of a bacterial aetiology.

Faecal lactoferrin latex agglutination

Faecal lactoferrin latex agglutination (LFLA) is a marker for faecal leucocytes. It is more precise and less vulnerable to variations than faecal leucocytes.

TREATMENT

Symptomatic measures are generally all that are required and include hydration with solutions that contain water, salt and sugar. The composition of the oral rehydration solution recommended by the World Health Organization (WHO) consists of:

- 3.5 g sodium chloride
- 40 g sucrose (or 20 g glucose)
- 2.9 g trisodium citrate dehydrate or 2.5 g sodium bicarbonate
- 1.5 g potassium chloride in one litre of clean drinking water.

The use of an antimotility agent, loperamide, may be considered in patients with acute diarrhoea but is contraindicated in diarrhoea caused by invasive organisms because the intestinal stasis mediated by the medication may enhance invasion by the pathogen or delay clearance of the organism from the bowel. These patients often present with fever or bloody motions.

Empiric antibiotic treatment may be considered in those patients where there can be a significant reduction in diarrhoea and other symptoms. The group of patients in whom this should be considered include those with:

- moderate to severe travellers' diarrhoea
- more than 8 stools per day, volume depletion and symptoms lasting more than a week
- signs and symptoms of bacterial diarrhoea, such as fever and bloody diarrhoea.

The antibiotic of choice is an oral fluoroquinolone (ciprofloxacin 500 mg twice daily or norfloxacin 400 mg twice daily) for 3–5 days. Or, if fluoroquinolone resistance is suspected, erythromycin 500 mg twice daily is an acceptable alternative.

If nosocomial diarrhoea is suspected, discontinue the offending antibiotic, if possible, and start treatment with metronidazole 250 mg four times daily until *C. difficile* toxin assay is available.

Persistent diarrhoea from suspected *Giardia* infection should be treated with metronidazole 250–750 mg three times daily for 7–10 days.

Remember that if enterohaemorrhagic *E. coli* is suspected or proven, there is no benefit from the use of antibiotics and indeed antibiotic treatment may possibly increase the risk of the haemolytic uraemic syndrome by the increase in production or release of Shiga toxin.

When an intestinal bacterium or protozoon is isolated, specific antibiotic therapy can be prescribed (Table 15.2).

TABLE 15.2: Recommendations for therapy against specific pathogens

Organism	Recommendations for adults
Campylobacter species	Erythromycin 500 mg b.i.d. for 5 days
Salmonella (non-typhi species)	Not recommended in mild to moderate disease. For severe disease, sulfamethoxazole/trimethoprim if susceptible or fluoroquinolone antibiotic for 5–7 days
Shigella species	Trimethoprim sulfamethoxazole 160/800 mg respectively b.i.d. for 3 days (if susceptible) or fluoroquinolone antibiotic for 3 days
Escherichia coli Shiga toxin producing (O157:H7)	Supportive treatment only
Toxigenic *Clostridium difficile*	Offending antibiotic withdrawn if possible, treat with metronidazole 250 mg q.i.d. to 500 mg t.i.d. for 10 days
Cryptosporidium species	If severe, consider paromomycin, 500 mg t.i.d. for 7 days
Giardia	Metronidazole 250–750 mg t.i.d. for 7–10 days
Entamoeba histolytica	Metronidazole 750 mg t.i.d. for 5–10 days, plus either diiodohydroxyquin 650 mg t.i.d for 20 days or paromomycin 500 mg t.i.d. for 7 days

b.i.d. = twice daily; q.i.d. = four times daily; t.d.s. = three times daily.

SUMMARY

Infectious diarrhoea is common worldwide. The majority of infections are self-limiting. A patient's history is crucial as it may allow the early use of empiric antibiotic therapy (Figure 15.1). Clinical evaluation should identify if there is any evidence of volume depletion and oral rehydration solution can be started early to decrease the rate of hospitalisation. Stool cultures are often not required but should be considered in patients with severe illness, bloody diarrhoea or those with underlying inflammatory bowel disease in whom the distinction between a flare-up or coexisting infection needs to be excluded. Antimotility agents may be useful in symptomatic patients without evidence of fever or bloody stools.

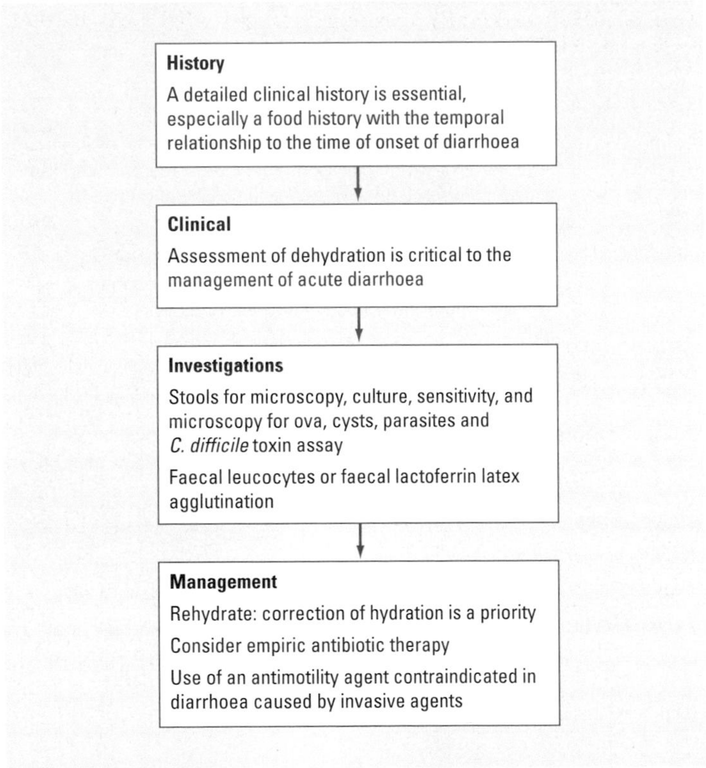

History

A detailed clinical history is essential, especially a food history with the temporal relationship to the time of onset of diarrhoea

Clinical

Assessment of dehydration is critical to the management of acute diarrhoea

Investigations

Stools for microscopy, culture, sensitivity, and microscopy for ova, cysts, parasites and *C. difficile* toxin assay

Faecal leucocytes or faecal lactoferrin latex agglutination

Management

Rehydrate: correction of hydration is a priority

Consider empiric antibiotic therapy

Use of an antimotility agent contraindicated in diarrhoea caused by invasive agents

FIGURE 15.1: Management of acute diarrhoea.

FURTHER READING

Bouza E, Burillo A, Munoz P. Antimicrobial therapy of *Clostridium difficile*-associated diarrhea. Med Clin North Am 2006; 90:1141–63.

Guerrant RL, Van Gilder T, Steiner TS. Practice guidelines for the management of infectious diarrhea. Clin Infect Dis 2001; 32:331–50.

Manatsathit S, Dupont HL, Farthing M, et al. Guideline for the management of acute diarrhea in adults. J Gastroenterol Hepatol 2002; 17:S54–71.

Musher DM, Musher BL. Contagious acute gastrointestinal infections. N Engl J Med 2004; 351:2417–27.

Thielman NM, Guerrant RL. Clinical practice. Acute infectious diarrhea. N Engl J Med 2004; 350:38–47.

Chapter **16**

INFLAMMATORY BOWEL DISEASE

KEY POINTS

Ulcerative colitis:

- In ulcerative colitis (UC), the rectum is always involved, which may lead to urgency and bleeding.

- The main parameters of disease activity are the number of bowel motions per day, the presence of blood and associated systemic symptoms.

- Patients may present in fulminant colitis—they require urgent assessment and treatment at specialist centres.

- Extraintestinal manifestations affect the skin, joints, eyes and/or the liver.

- Assess the patient's haemodynamic status for evidence of significant intravascular losses and their abdomen for distension, and/or signs of peritonism.

- C-reactive protein (CRP) is a more sensitive assay for inflammation than erythrocyte sedimentation rate (ESR).

- Sigmoidoscopy will show an abnormal rectal mucosa.

- The aims of therapy are to induce remission in active disease and to maintain remission/prevent relapse.

- Drugs that are effective in inducing remission are local or oral 5-aminosalicylates, local or oral corticosteroids, immunosuppressive agents including azathioprine and 6-mercaptopurine, and in special situations, cyclosporine and infliximab.

- Aminosalicylates should be continued indefinitely since they decrease the likelihood of recurrence.

- Azathioprine or 6-mercaptopurine are often useful in steroid-unresponsive patients or those who require high doses of steroids to remain in remission.

- In acute severe or fulminant colitis, if there is no clear improvement within 3–7 days surgery should be considered.

Crohn's disease:

- Crohn's disease has a multifactorial aetiology and there is a genetic predisposition (*NOD2/CARD15*) in 30%–50% of patients.
- Crohn's disease affects any part of the gastrointestinal tract.
- Diarrhoea and abdominal pain are common symptoms.
- Pain may be 'inflammatory' due to ulceration or inflammation or 'obstructive' from strictures.
- Left-sided colon involvement can present with symptoms similar to UC
- Perianal complications are common in Crohn's disease.
- Clinical assessment, laboratory investigations (haematocrit, CRP, ESR) endoscopy and radiology (small bowel series and barium enema) are the main modalities for assessing disease activity.
- Current therapeutic modalities include lifestyle modification (including cessation of smoking if a factor), drug therapy, nutritional support and surgery.
- Corticosteroids are the cornerstone of therapy to induce remission.
- Azathioprine/6-mercaptopurine are useful in both inducing remission and as maintenance agents.
- New 'biological' agents such as infliximab are increasingly being used to induce remission as well as for maintenance.
- Surgery is reserved for the treatment of complications or when medical therapy is ineffective.

INFLAMMATORY BOWEL DISEASE

Crohn's disease and ulcerative colitis are types of inflammatory bowel disease (IBD) characterised by inflammation leading to a disturbance of gut function and, to a greater or lesser degree, systemic symptoms. Therapy is empirical. Many patients require emotional support and contact with patient support groups is often very helpful. Although these conditions are sometimes hard to differentiate, there are sufficient differences between them to indicate distinct pathological processes. Some of these differences are listed in Table 16.1.

TABLE 16.1: Characteristics of Crohn's disease and ulcerative colitis

	Crohn's disease	**Ulcerative colitis**
Genetics	Identified susceptibility gene(s)	Weaker association
Distribution	Anywhere in the gut	Exclusively colonic
Perianal disease	Common	Uncommon
Pathology	• Full thickness of the intestinal wall • Macrophages (cell-mediated immunity) • Granulomata	• Superficial (epithelium) • Plasma cells (humoral immunity)

ULCERATIVE COLITIS

The diagnosis of ulcerative colitis (UC) is relatively easy since the inflammatory process almost always involves the rectum and generally causes urgency and bleeding. People generally present promptly when rectal bleeding is noted, but the onset may be insidious and the presentation delayed. The bleeding is persistent rather than intermittent as would be expected with local anal problems, such as haemorrhoids. Proctitis may also cause discomfort, increased frequency and a change in the consistency of the stools. Rarely, the presenting symptom may be constipation. As the disease extends more proximally and more of the mucosal surface area is involved, the symptoms become more severe: diarrhoea increases (with looser or more frequent stools) and pain may become more prominent. Systemic symptoms may also develop.

In a significant minority of patients, the presentation is as a fulminant colitis with features including fevers, anorexia and weight loss; such patients are at risk of developing life-threatening complications including toxic megacolon, perforation, peritonitis and haemorrhage, and require urgent assessment and treatment in specialist centres. Given the large surface area of the colon, it is not surprising that ulcerative pancolitis results in blood loss and consequent anaemia, protein loss, hypoalbuminaemia and fluid and electrolyte losses, and the associated metabolic disturbances.

The extraintestinal manifestations of UC may affect the skin, joints, eyes and/or the liver (Table 16.2). These may occur before, during or after the onset of gut symptoms and may be associated with disease activity. These are generally more common in UC than Crohn's disease.

TABLE 16.2: Extraintestinal manifestations of ulcerative colitis

Skin	Erythema nodosum
	Pyoderma gangrenosum
	Aphthous stomatitis
Joints	Type 1 peripheral osteopathy*
	Type 2 arthritis**
	Sacroileitis
Eyes	Iritis
	Uveitis
	Episcleritis
Liver	Primary sclerosing cholangitis

*Acute self-limiting inflammation affecting <5 joints, lasting <5 weeks and associated with symptom relapse and with other extraintestinal manifestations
**Chronic arthritis affecting five or more joints with a median duration of symptoms of 3 years, and associated with uveitis but not erythema nodosum.

When assessing patients with suspected UC, particular attention should be paid to the haemodynamic status for evidence of significant intravascular losses and the abdominal examination for distension, tenderness and/or signs of peritonism. There may also be signs of anaemia or significant weight loss. Sigmoidoscopy will show an abnormal rectal mucosa: there will be erythema, loss of the normal vascular pattern, contact bleeding and mucopus or blood in the lumen. In more severe disease there will be extensive ulceration and pseudopolyp formation.

The differential diagnosis is considered in Table 16.3.

The diagnosis depends upon the exclusion of infective and other causes of colitis and the demonstration of the typical endoscopic and histological features of UC. Stool cultures and microscopy and studies for *Clostridium difficile* toxin should be sent. If there is a history of overseas travel, a warm stool smear should be performed to exclude amoebic dysentery. Patients suffering from UC may also have relapses secondary to gastrointestinal infections or non-steroidal antiinflammatory drug (NSAID) usage.

Ulcerative colitis can generally be differentiated from Crohn's disease using endoscopic and pathological criteria (Table 16.1). UC

TABLE 16.3: Differential diagnosis of ulcerative colitis and Crohn's disease

- Infective causes:
  - *Campylobacter*
  - *Salmonella*
  - *Shigella*
  - *Clostridium difficile* (pseudomembranous colitis), especially in the hospital setting
  - *Entamoeba histolytica*
  - *Mycobacterium tuberculosis* (Crohn's disease)
  - *Yersinia* (Crohn's disease)
- Cytomegalovirus
- Others, e.g. Neisseriae, Herpes simplex, Chlamydiae, schistosomiasis, histoplasmosis

- Acute self-limited colitis
- Ischaemic colitis, especially in the elderly with evidence of widespread atherosclerosis or cardiac dysrhythmias, in particular atrial fibrillation
- Carcinoma and lymphoma (rarely)
- Appendiceal diseases including appendicitis and carcinoid tumours (Crohn's disease)
- Radiation enterocolitis
- Non-steroidal antiinflammatory drug (NSAID)-induced ulceration (Crohn's disease)
- Vasculitis (rarely)

affects the colon exclusively and almost always involves the rectum from which it extends proximally in continuity. Sigmoidoscopy will show evidence of proctitis although occasionally patients can have 'rectal sparing', particularly if there has been use of corticosteroid or 5-aminosalicylate enemas. Biopsies will show that the inflammation involves the more superficial layers of the mucosa, macrophages are less common and granulomata are not present. Sigmoidoscopic biopsies will help differentiate between UC and other causes of colitis, such as ischaemic colitis and radiation colitis.

Acute self-limited colitis

Some patients present with symptoms suggestive of UC, have no causative organisms grown on culture, resolve spontaneously and never have a subsequent attack. About one-half to two-thirds of patients with 'self-limited' colitis will develop recurrent symptoms characteristic of ulcerative colitis. The diagnosis of ulcerative colitis may be suspected after the initial presentaiion but is only confirmed after a subsequent attack.

Assessment and management of UC

Symptoms in patients suffering from UC characteristically remit and relapse. If gut or systemic symptoms do occur, investigations should be used to determine the activity of the disease, to determine how much of the bowel is involved and to decide whether or not complications have arisen.

The main parameters of disease activity in UC are the number of motions a day, the presence of blood and the associated systemic symptoms, including fevers, malaise and weight loss. Useful laboratory indices include haemoglobin, white cell count, ESR, C-reactive protein, electrolytes, creatinine and albumin. The C-reactive protein is generally a more sensitive assay for inflammation than the ESR. Sigmoidoscopy will demonstrate the changes of proctitis described above. Either endoscopy or radiology may be used to determine the extent of the disease; sigmoidoscopy and colonoscopy are regarded as more sensitive and are safe (as long as there is no evidence of toxic megacolon—see below). If the disease is restricted to the rectum or the sigmoid colon, the prognosis and clinical course is more favourable (although there is a subgroup of patients who are unresponsive to the standard treatment regimens). However 20% or more of these patients may develop disease extension over time but surgery is rarely necessary.

The aims of therapy are to induce remission in active disease and to maintain remission/prevent relapse. The severity of the disease and the site(s) of the affected colon are used to determine which agents may be used and their route of administration.

Proctitis and distal colitis

Patients with mild disease (less than four stools daily, no fever or weight loss) limited to the left side may respond to local therapy using 5-aminosalicylic acid and/or steroids as an enema, as a foam or as a suppository depending on the extent of the disease. There may be problems retaining the medication in the early stages of treatment because of urgency and diarrhoea. Side effects of topical steroids are minimal in the short term, but do occur if they are used long term. Local therapy is used once (or twice) a day until a response is achieved, and then decreased to every second or third day, generally at night before retiring. They are sometimes used in this fashion as maintenance therapy.

In moderate disease (4–8 bloody stools daily, low-grade fever, moderate abdominal pain) oral therapy is preferred. One agent is sulfasalazine, which consists of the active moiety, 5-aminosalicylic acid linked to a carrier molecule, sulfapyridine, which prevents it from being absorbed in the proximal gut. The azo bond joining the molecules is broken down by bacteria in the terminal ileum and colon. The majority of the 5-aminosalicylic acid remains in the colon and is excreted in the faeces. The sulfapyridine is absorbed and is responsible for the majority of the side effects. Since the side effects (especially nausea, anorexia and headache) are dose-related, sulfasalazine is generally introduced at a low dose and increased gradually over a week to 3–4 g/day. If these or other side-effects occur, there are alternative ways of administering the 5-aminosalicylic acid: olsalazine comprises two molecules of 5-aminosalicylic acid linked by an azo bond; various other formulations allow for the release of 5-aminosalicylic acid in the terminal ileum and colon by coating it in resins or encapsulating it in microspheres which result in pH-dependent release of the agent.

Disease proximal to the splenic flexure

If the disease extends proximally to the splenic flexure, oral therapy should be considered. If the disease is mild, the agent of choice is sulfasalazine or one of the other 5-aminosalicylates. A Cochrane meta-analysis showed that the newer 5-aminosalicylic acid preparations were superior to placebo and tended towards therapeutic benefit over sulfasalazine, which was not as well tolerated. However, considering their relative costs, a clinical advantage to using the newer 5-aminosalicylic acid preparations as first-line therapy in place of sulfasalazine appeared unlikely.

If there has been no response over 2–4 weeks, oral corticosteroids in doses of 30–60 mg/day may be commenced. Steroids are sometimes used as initial therapy because of a more rapid clinical response. After a response has been induced, the dosage can be reduced by 5 mg/week or 10 mg/fortnight. Once remission has been attained, steroids should be ceased.

Azathioprine or 6-mercaptopurine are often useful in steroid-unresponsive patients or those who require high doses of steroids to remain well. The dose of azathioprine is between 2 and 2.5 mg/kg body weight and 6-mercaptopurine 1–1.5 mg/kg. Adverse effects include bone marrow suppression, liver test abnormalities, pancreatitis and a clinical syndrome characterised by high fevers and/or myalgia. Blood counts should be performed weekly for the first month, then on a regular basis every 1–3 months.

Thiopurine methyltransferase (TPMT) testing can be considered to identify patients with low activity of this enzyme; they are at higher risk of bone marrow suppression and liver toxicity from azathioprine. The dose should be reduced if patients are on allopurinol therapy. If no response is seen within 3–6 months, azathioprine therapy should be withdrawn. Other approaches, including methotrexate, should be reserved for patients who are refractory to standard regimens.

The tumour necrosis factor (TNF) neutralising antibody, infliximab, has been also shown to be effective in inducing and maintaining remission in active ulcerative colitis, including fulminant colitis (see below). The major adverse events are infusion reactions and increased susceptibility to serious and/ or opportunistic infections (particular care is recommended to exclude latent infection with tuberculosis). There is concern about an increased risk of lymphoma and cancer (especially lung cancer in smokers). Patients may develop antibodies to double-stranded DNA but clinical features of systemic lupus erythematosis, especially end-organ damage, are very rare.

Maintaining remission

The aminosalicylates should be continued indefinitely since they decrease the likelihood of recurrence. In a Cochrane meta-analysis, the odds ratios were calculated for the trials in which sulfasalazine and 5-aminosalicylic acid were compared, revealing an odds ratio of 1.29 (95% CI: 1.05 to 1.57), with a negative number needed to treat (NNT) value (–19), suggesting a higher degree of therapeutic effectiveness for sulfasalazine. The newer 5-aminosalicylic acid preparations were superior to placebo in maintenance therapy, but sulfasalazine was significantly more effective than the newer 5-aminosalicylic acid preparations. Sulfasalazine and 5-aminosalicylic acid preparations had similar adverse event profiles, with odds ratios of 1.16 (0.62 to 2.16), and 1.31 (0.86 to 1.99), respectively. The number needed to harm (NNH) values were determined to be 171 and 78, respectively.

Acute severe or fulminant colitis and toxic megacolon

About 10%–15% of patients will develop acute severe or fulminant colitis, which is characterised by the presence of:
- >10 bloody bowel actions a day
- fevers greater than 37.8°C

- tachycardia >90 beats/min
- anaemia (haemoglobin <100 g/dL)
- leucocytosis
- elevated ESR
- hypoalbuminaemia.

Initial therapy is with bed rest, parenteral fluids, high-dose intravenous steroids (hydrocortisone 300–400 mg day or equivalent) and close monitoring (note: there is a significant risk of hypokalaemia if hydrocortisone is used). There is an increased risk of thromboembolic disease and appropriate prophylaxis should be considered for hospitalised patients. If there is no clear improvement within 3–7 days consideration should be given to surgery.

If fulminant colitis is present, there is a 10%–20% chance that there will be progression to toxic megacolon. This, in turn, carries a significant mortality. The main risk is from perforation, so patients should be monitored closely for evidence of deterioration as manifest by worsening signs of toxicity or increasing colonic dilatation on progress abdominal X-rays (diameter >6 cm in the transverse colon and/or >9 cm in caecum). Patients who have evidence of acute fulminant colitis should be managed in centres where there is expertise in the combined medical and surgical management of this problem. Cyclosporine or infliximab may avert the need for surgery in the short term and possibly the long term in such patients.

Dysplasia and the risk of colon cancer

There is an increased risk of developing epithelial dysplasia and colorectal cancer, particularly in patients who have long-standing pancolitis; oral aminosalicylates may decrease this risk. A colonoscopic surveillance programme is recommended (Chapter 18).

CROHN'S DISEASE

Crohn's disease is a chronic, often debilitating disease that affects any part of the gastrointestinal tract. Patients present in many ways, but diarrhoea, abdominal pain and weight loss are common symptoms. The condition is rarely fatal, but causes significant morbidity, particularly in young adults; the peak age of onset is in the second and third decades.

The diagnosis of Crohn's disease is often very hard to make: the symptoms may be non-specific and the disorder is rare, although it may be increasing in incidence. This difficulty in diagnosis is reflected in frequent delays—the mean time from onset of symptoms to diagnosis is in the order of three years in some studies.

When the left side of the colon is involved, the symptoms are similar to those described above for ulcerative colitis. When the right colon or terminal ileum is involved, there may be less disturbance of bowel function while pain may be more prominent. Pain may be 'inflammatory' due to ulceration or inflammation extending through the intestinal wall, or 'obstructive' from strictures (generally small intestinal colic). The strictures themselves may be either inflammatory when the disease history is of short duration or fibrotic if there has been long-standing Crohn's disease. Occasionally the presentation mimics acute appendicitis and the diagnosis of Crohn's disease is made at surgery.

The diarrhoea is often multifactorial, but generally reflects gut inflammation. It may be secondary to the many complications of Crohn's disease including fistula formation, bacterial overgrowth, bile salt malabsorption or fat malabsorption. A number of medications used for the treatment of Crohn's disease can also cause diarrhoea. Weight loss is also multifactorial: any of the factors listed above may cause significant loss of weight.

Systemic symptoms are often more prominent in Crohn's disease; patients often learn to recognise the fevers, anorexia, lethargy and malaise which herald a period of active Crohn's disease. A patient's 'well-being' may be used as a subjective measure of disease activity.

Another common association of Crohn's disease is the presence of perianal complications including anal fissures, abscesses and fistulae. The inflammation and ulceration in Crohn's disease is transmural and fistulae can occur between any of the viscera and cause symptoms including pneumaturia, faecal staining of urine or vaginal secretions, recurrent urinary tract infections, bleeding and dyspareunia.

Examination may demonstrate evidence of weight loss, localised tenderness or a mass in the right iliac fossa and perianal abnormalities, including anal induration.

The differential diagnosis of Crohn's disease is similar to that of UC, but includes mycobacterial and *Yersinia* infections and disorders of the appendix.

Assessment

Symptoms in patients suffering from IBD characteristically remit and relapse. If gut or systemic symptoms do occur, investigations should be used to determine the activity of the disease (which is not always easy), to determine how much of the bowel is involved (the extent of the disease will determine what treatment will be offered) and to decide whether or not complications have arisen.

Activity indices are available, but are complicated and are generally only used in clinical trials. Parameters include the number of bowel actions per day, the presence of abdominal pain, the sense of well-being, the presence of complications (e.g. fistulae, rashes, ocular manifestations, arthritis), the requirement of opiates to control diarrhoea, the haematocrit, the presence of an abdominal mass, and the degree of weight loss. An elevated ESR or C-reactive protein may also be an indicator of active disease.

Antibody testing remains of uncertain value, but patients who are antineutrophil cytoplasmic antibody (pANCA) negative but anti-*Saccharomyces cerevisiae* antibody (ASCA) positive or anti-OmpC antibody positive may be more likely to have Crohn's disease.

Endoscopic investigations (colonoscopy and terminal ileoscopy) and radiology (small bowel series and barium enema) are the main modalities used to determine the activity and extent of disease. Unlike patients with UC, sigmoidoscopy is not always helpful in determining the presence of recurrent disease. Abdominal ultrasound and CT scan may help determine whether or not there is active disease (thickening of the bowel wall, absent peristalsis, increased vascularity) and identify complications such as abscess or fistula formation. MRI may have a role in defining the extent of perianal disease and its response to therapy. The role of videocapsule endoscopy in the diagnosis of Crohn's disease and in the monitoring of its activity is still being defined. White cell scans use radiolabelled autologous leucocytes to demonstrate sites of active inflammation and may help to define the nature of strictures seen in a small bowel series (either inflammatory or fibrotic).

Management

Current therapeutic modalities include lifestyle modification, drug therapy, nutritional support and surgery.

There is evidence that relapse rates are lower in patients with Crohn's disease who are successful in giving up smoking compared to patients who continue to smoke. Patients should be counselled accordingly.

Drugs may be used to induce or maintain remission or both.

Corticosteroids (e.g. prednisone 40–60 mg/day) are the cornerstone of remission induction therapy; they may be successful in improving symptoms in 60%–70% of patients but have no effect on the endoscopic features or pathology of the disease. In contrast to UC where the dosage reduction is relatively rapid, steroids are withdrawn stepwise over a longer period of time—3 or 4 months or more. If symptoms recur on steroid reduction, the dosage may be increased to a level at which symptoms are controlled and then reduced at a slower rate. However, steroids should not be used as maintenance therapy because of the significant side effects, which include diabetes, hypertension, osteoporosis, increased susceptibility to infection, changes in mentation including insomnia, hypomania and psychosis, and many others.

There is an increased risk of thromboembolic disease and appropriate prophylaxis should be considered for hospitalised patients.

Azathioprine (2–2.5 mg/kg body weight) or 6-mercaptopurine (1–1.5 mg/kg) are useful for both inducing remission and as maintenance agents. They are also of benefit for the treatment of fistulae and perianal disease. As experience with these agents grows, they are becoming more widely used; there is good evidence that they are safe for use in pregnancy and in children. Particular care should be taken if there is evidence of sepsis (abdominal mass, ischiorectal abscesses, etc). Side effects include bone marrow suppression, liver test abnormalities, pancreatitis, myalgias, fevers and nausea. They are well tolerated in about 80%–90% of patients treated.

A Cochrane review (1998) provided the following data for the use of azathioprine and 6-MP in inducing remission in CD: the odds ratio of a response to azathioprine or 6-MP therapy compared with placebo in active Crohn's disease was 2.36 (95%

CI: 1.57 to 3.53). This corresponded to a NNT (number needed to treat) of about 5 to observe an effect of therapy in one patient. Treatment ≥17 weeks increased the odds ratio of a response to 2.51 (95% CI: 1.63 to 3.88), suggesting that there is a minimum length of time for a trial of therapy. A steroid sparing effect was seen with an odds ratio of 3.86 (95% CI: 2.14 to 6.96), corresponding to a NNT of about 3. Adverse events requiring withdrawal from a trial, principally allergy, leucopenia, pancreatitis and nausea, were increased on therapy with an odds ratio of 3.01 (95% CI: 1.30 to 6.96). The NNH to observe one adverse event in one patient treated with azathioprine or 6-mercaptopurine was 14.

Immunosuppressive agents are also effective as maintenance therapy, and, if tolerated, are generally used for years. After at least 4 years of continuous therapy, there is a 20% risk of relapse if treatment is ceased. Recommencement of therapy is generally effective in this context.

Sulfasalazine or the other oral aminosalicylates are sometimes used, particularly for mild colonic Crohn's disease, but are not much better than placebo. The dosage regimens are as described above for UC. It has a limited role in maintaining remission: meta-analyses indicate that the number needed to treat is in the order of 16.

Antibiotics such as metronidazole and ciprofloxacin may also have a role in the treatment of perianal disease or in the postoperative setting. They are not generally used for long-term maintenance therapy.

A number of new 'biologicals' have been developed. The first was infliximab, a monoclonal antibody directed against tumour necrosis factor alfa (TNF_α), an important cytokine involved in inflammation. About 60%–80% of patients will have an initial response to infliximab and more than half of these will benefit from regular infusions every 8 weeks over a period of a year or longer. Other anti-TNF agents that are effective for the treatment of Crohn's disease are adalimumab and certolizumab. Other biologicals using different strategies for the control of inflammation in Crohn's disease are in various stages of development.

Surgery is not curative, but is reserved for the treatment of complications or when medical therapy is ineffective. In historical studies, up to 70% of patients will require surgery at some stage; of these, 45%–50% will require more than one operation. It seems likely that the newer treatments and the use of effective maintenance therapy will reduce these figures in time.

Crohn's colitis is probably associated with an increased risk of colon cancer when longstanding, and colonoscopy surveillance is recommended (Chapter 18).

The agents that are generally regarded as being safe for use in pregnancy are the 5-aminosalicylates, corticosteroids, azathioprine and possibly infliximab. Metronidazole and methotrexate are teratogens.

Recent epidemiological studies suggest that mortality rates for IBD are similar to that of the general population for the majority of patients. However, older patients with IBD and newly diagnosed cases with severe disease are at increased risk of dying.

SUMMARY

UC almost always involves the rectum and causes urgency and bleeding. It has a remitting and relapsing course. Investigations focus on the activity of the disease, the distribution of the disease and to decide whether complications are present. The main parameters of disease activity are the number of motions per day, the presence of blood and associated constitutional symptoms (Figure 16.1). Extraintestinal manifestations affect the skin, joints, eyes and/or the liver. Endoscopy or radiology may be used to determine the extent of the disease. The aims of therapy are to induce remission in active disease and to maintain remission/ prevent relapse. The mainstay of therapy are the corticosteroids and 5-aminosalicylates. These agents may be administered either orally or as enemas, foams or suppositories. In acute, severe or fulminant colitis, parenteral fluids, high dose intravenous steroids and close monitoring is essential. Consider cyclosporine/infliximab or surgery if there is no clear improvement within 3–7 days.

Crohn's disease is a chronic, debilitating disease of multifactorial aetiology that affects any part of the gastrointestinal tract. There is a genetic predisposition (*NOD2/CARD15*) in 30%–50% of patients and other potential susceptibility genes are being assessed. Diarrhoea, abdominal pain and weight loss are common symptoms (Figure 16.2). Left-sided CD is similar in presentation to UC. Pain is a prominent symptom in right-sided CD. Systemic symptoms are often more prominent in CD than in UC. Perianal complications are prominent in CD. Activity indices are available but are generally only used in the research situation. A patient's well-being may be used as a subjective measure of disease activity.

Ulcerative colitis

Clinical
Persistent per rectum bleeding
Diarrhoea and change in consistency of stools
Abdominal pain—often tenesmus
Systemic symptoms
Anaemia
Extraintestinal symptoms

Investigations
Faeces: microscopy, culture. Exclude infective causes (e.g. *Clostridium difficile* toxin)
Haemoglobin, white cell count, ESR, C-reactive protein, electrolytes, creatinine, albumin
Sigmoidoscopy: erythema, loss of normal vascular pattern, contact bleeding, mucopus or blood in the lumen
Severe disease: extensive ulceration pseudopolyp formation
Colonoscopy—safe if no evidence of toxic megacolon

Management principles
i. Topical therapy: 5-ASA enemas or steroid enemas, foams or suppositories depending on extent of disease
ii. Oral therapy: sulfasalazine or 5-ASA
iii.Disease proximal to splenic flexure: oral therapy: mild disease, 5-ASA. No response, oral steroids 30–60 mg daily. Reduce following response. Continue 5-ASA as maintenance. Azathioprine/6-mercaptopurine or infliximab may be useful in steroid-unresponsive or dependent patients.
iv. Acute, severe or fulminant colitis and toxic megacolon: bed rest, parenteral fluids, high-dose IV fluids, close monitoring. Consider cyclosporine, infliximab or surgery if no clear improvement within 3–7 days.

FIGURE 16.1: Ulcerative colitis.

5-ASA = 5-aminosalicylates; ESR = erythrocyte sedimentation rate.

Crohn's disease

Clinical
Peak age onset: second to third decades
Diarrhoea
Abdominal pan
Weight loss
If left colon involved: symptoms similar to ulcerative disease
If right colon/terminal ileum involved: abdominal pain more prominent
Systemic manifestations
Perianal complications: anal fissures, abscesses, fistulae

Investigations
Exclude other causes of diarrhoea (as for ulcerative colitis)
Focus:

Activity of disease	How much bowel involved	Complications
Stool frequency	Endoscopy	Fistulae
Abdominal pain	Radiology (small bowel series)	Rashes
Sense of well-being		Arthritis
Haematocrit		Ocular manifestations
Abdominal mass	Abdominal ultrasound	
Degree of weight loss	CT scan, MRI	
↑ ESR, ↑ CRP		

CRP = C-reactive protein; CT = computed tomography;
ESR = erythrocyte sedimentation rate; MRI = magnetic resonance imaging.

Management
i. Lifestyle modification: stop smoking, if a factor
ii. Corticosteroids (40–60 mg daily) dose reduction stepwise (3–4 months). Do not use as maintenance
iii. Azathioprine or 6-mercaptopurine
iv. 5-aminosalicylic acid; mild colonic Crohn's disease
v. Antibiotics (metronidazole, ciprofloxacin): perianal disease, postoperative
vi. New 'biologicals': infliximab, adalimumab, certolizumab
vii. Surgery for complications or ineffective medical treatment

FIGURE 16.2: Crohn's disease.

FURTHER READING

Cohen RD, Woseth DM, Thisted RA, et al. A meta-analysis and overview of the literature on treatment options for left-sided ulcerative colitis and ulcerative proctitis. Am J Gastroenterol 2000; 95(5):1263–76.

Hanauer SB, Stromberg U. Oral Pentasa in the treatment of active Crohn's disease: a meta-analysis of double-blind, placebo-controlled trials. Clin Gastroenterol Hepatol 2004; 2:379–88.

Jess T, Loftus EV Jr, Harmsen WS. Survival and cause specific mortality in patients with inflammatory bowel disease: a long term outcome study in Olmsted County Minnesota, 1940–2004. Gut 2006; 55:1248–54.

Pearson DC, May GR, Fick G, et al. Azathioprine for maintenance of remission in Crohn's disease. Cochrane Database Syst Rev 2000; 2: CD000067.

Reese GE, Constantinides VA, Simillis C, et al. Diagnostic precision of anti-*Saccharomyces cerevisiae* antibodies and perinuclear antineutrophil cytoplasmic antibodies in inflammatory bowel disease. Am J Gastroenterol 2006; 101:2410–22.

Sandborn W, Sutherland L, Pearson D, et al. Azathioprine or 6-mercaptopurine for induction of remission in Crohn's disease. Cochrane Database Syst Rev 2000; 2: CD000545.

Siegel CA, Hur C, Korzenik JR, et al. Risks and benefits of infliximab for the treatment of Crohn's disease. Clin Gastroenterol Hepatol 2006; 4:1017–24.

Sutherland L, Roth D, Beck P, et al. Oral 5-aminosalicylic acid for induction of remission in ulcerative colitis. Cochrane Database Syst Rev 2006; 2: CD000544.

Chapter 17

COLORECTAL CANCER

KEY POINTS

- Colorectal cancer is a major health concern with more than one million new cases yearly, and an overall mortality rate of 50% worldwide.
- Surgery is the primary and definitive curative intervention.
- Adjuvant chemotherapy, following curative surgery, is essential in stage III.
- The new standard of adjuvant care is fluorouracil, folinic acid and oxaliplatin for 6 months.
- Combination chemotherapy with biological agents (bevacizumab) is the gold standard in advanced disease.
- Long-term survival for patients with resectable liver and lung metastasis is 30%–40%.
- Combination chemoradiotherapy is mandatory in patients with rectal cancer, preferably prior to surgery.

RISK FACTORS

Environmental and genetic factors can increase the likelihood of developing colorectal cancer (CRC) (Table 17.1). Although inherited susceptibility most strikingly increases the risk, the majority of CRCs are sporadic. Age is a very important risk factor. It rarely occurs before the age of 40, and the incidence begins to increase significantly in the sixth decade, with the highest rate between 65 and 75 years. The incidence rate is higher in industrialised regions, higher in African American than in whites, and it is nearly equal for males and females (M:F ratio1.3:1.0 for rectal tumours).

TABLE 17.1: Risk factors for colorectal cancer (CRC)

Risk factor	Examples	Risk
Genetic disorders	Familial adenomatous polyposis	I
	Hereditary non-polyposis colorectal cancer	I
	Peutz-Jeghers syndrome	I
	Hyperplastic polyposis	I
	Cowden's syndrome	I
	Juvenile polyposis syndrome	I
Personal history of CRC or adenoma		I
Family history of CRC or adenoma		I
Inflammatory bowel disease	Ulcerative colitis, Crohn's disease	I
Medications	NSAIDs, aspirin, calcium, vitamin D, statins, hormone replacement therapy (in postmenopausal women)	D
Endocrine disorders	Diabetes mellitus	I
	Insulin resistance	I
	Acromegaly	I
	Obesity	I
	Gastrin	I
Surgical interventions	Cholecystectomy	I
	Ureterocolic anastomoses	I
Environmental factors	Smoking	I
	Moderate physical activity	D
	Healthy diet (low calorie, rich in fruits and vegetables with low animal products)	D
	Alcohol (moderate and high amount)	I

D = decrease risk for CRC; I = increase risk for CRC; NSAIDs = non-steroidal antiinflammatory drugs.

SYMPTOMS

The majority of patients will present with change in the regular bowel habits, rectal bleeding (rarely melaena) and/or iron deficiency anaemia, abdominal pain, or a combination.

Symptoms may vary according to the site of the tumour. Approximately 25% of the patients have metastatic disease at the time of diagnosis. The most common metastatic sites are the regional lymph nodes, liver, lungs and peritoneum. Ovaries, adrenals, bone, skin and brain may be involved as well. Patients may present with signs or symptoms in any of these organs.

Patients who are symptomatic at the time of diagnosis have a somewhat worse prognosis.

Intestinal obstruction or colonic perforation carries a poor prognosis regardless of the stage of the tumour.

GENETICS

Cancers are all caused by abnormalities in genes, although most cancers are not caused by inherited genetic disorders. Cancer is the result of complex interactions between the fingerprints of the genome and interaction with the environment. For most cancers, the wide variations seen among different national groups appear to be explained almost entirely by environmental factors with familial factors playing a minor role. The exception to this is malignancy in the colon where genetics is much more important. CRC follows three major patterns:

- Sporadic—no family history. This type accounts for about 75% of the cases, and it is most common in subjects older than 50 years. Age, dietary and environmental factors are the most important known risk factors.
- Familial predisposition to CRC. This accounts for about 20% of the cases. Although there is a clear family history of CRC, the pattern is not consistent with any of the inherited syndromes described below. The relative risk for a single affected first-degree relative is 1.7. The risk is further increased if more relatives have CRC, or if affected relatives were diagnosed before 55 years of age.
- Inherited polyposis syndromes—5% of cases are due to these syndromes. This type includes familial adenomatous polyposis (FAP), hereditary non-polyposis colorectal cancer (HNPCC), hamartomatous polyposis syndromes (e.g. Peutz-Jeghers,

juvenile polyposis), hyperplastic polyposis and Cowden's syndrome. These conditions are associated with a very high risk of developing CRC (as well as other tumours outside the gastrointestinal tract), and the genetic mutations underlying many of them have been identified (Table 17.2).

TABLE 17.2: Inherited polyposis syndromes

Syndrome	Mutations	Risk of CRC (%)	Risk of other tumours (%)
FAP	*APC, MYH,* β-catenin	100	Small bowel (5–10), desmoid (10), stomach (0.5), thyroid (2), pancreas (2), CNS (1), osteomas, chondromas, epidermoid cysts, hepatoblastoma (1.6 of children)
HNPCC	*MLH1, MSH2, MSH3, MSH6, PMS1, PMS2*	85	Small intestine (1–4), stomach (13–19), urinary tract (4–10), ovaries (9–12), uterus (43–60), biliary tract (2–18), CNS (4)
Peutz-Jeghers	*STK11*	40	Small intestine (13), stomach (29), pancreas (36), oesophagus (<1), breast (54), ovarian (21), uterine (9), lung (15), testis (10–20)
Juvenile polyposis	*PTEN*	50	Stomach (rare), small intestine (rare)
Hyperplastic polyposis	Unknown	Increased	Stomach, small intestine
Cowden's syndrome	*PTEN*	10	Thyroid (3–10), breast (25–50), uterus (rare), ovaries (rare)

CNS = central nervous system; CRC = colorectal cancer; FAP = familial adenomatous polyposis; HNPCC = hereditary non-polyposis colon cancer.

MULTI-STEP MODEL OF CRC

Specific genetic mutations

The *APC* (adenomatous polyposis coli) gene on chromosome 5 is the most critical gene in the early development of CRC. Somatic mutations in both alleles are present in 80% of sporadic CRCs.

Most sporadic CRCs with wild-type *APC* have mutations in other genes of the Wnt signalling pathway, mostly in β-catenin.

The *K-ras* oncogene is found in up to 50% of sporadic adenomas and CRC. It encodes a family of G-proteins that regulate cellular signal transduction by acting as a one-way switch for the transmission of extra-cellular growth signals to the nucleus. Once mutations occur, they leave the ras in a constitutively active state that leads to a continuous growth stimulus.

The p53 gene located on chromosome 17p is the most commonly mutated gene in human cancer. It serves as the guardian of the genome. It is particularly critical when cells are under stress. Normally, cells arrest their growth in response to DNA damaging agents by induction or activation of p53. Once activated, p53 induces a variety of growth-limiting responses, including cell cycle arrest (to facilitate DNA repair), apoptosis, senescence and differentiation. In about 50%–70% of CRCs, p53 inactivation occurs by a mutation of one allele followed by loss of heterozygosity (LOH), as a late event in the transition from large adenoma into CRC. Patients who harbour p53 mutations have worse outcomes and shorter survival.

There are three candidate tumour suppressor genes on chromosome 18q. *DCC* (deleted in colon cancer), *SMAD4* and *SMAD2* genes were identified through studies of allelic loss. One copy of 18q was lost in 73% of sporadic CRC, and in 47% of advanced adenomas. For patients in stage II with *DCC* gene the prognosis is similar to that of patients with advanced stage III disease. The practical importance of this knowledge may be the identification of a subgroup of patients with stage II disease who may benefit from adjuvant chemotherapy.

Mismatch repair genes

Mismatch repair genes are the hallmark of HNPCC, but are also found in 15% of sporadic CRC. They are involved in correcting base mismatches and small insertions or deletions that occur during DNA replication. *MSH2* and *MLH1* are the most important ones followed by *MSH6*, *MSH3*, *PMS1* and *PMS2*. The prognosis in this setting is better and the response to chemotherapy is less favourable.

Cyclo-oxygenase 2 upregulation

Cyclo-oxygenase 2 (COX 2) is upregulated in 40%–50% of adenomas and in 85% of CRC cells. Overexpression of COX-2 plays a key role in the multi-step process of CRC. Inhibition of COX 2 may play an important role in preventing CRC. The protective effect of non-steroidal antiinflammatory drugs (NSAIDs), which are COX 2 inhibitors, has been demonstrated in epidemiological studies.

DIAGNOSIS

- CRC may be suspected based on one or more of the previously described symptoms, most commonly a change in bowel habit.
- The patient may be asymptomatic and CRC may be discovered by routine screening of average and high-risk subjects.
- Colonoscopy is the single best diagnostic test.
- If malignant obstruction precludes a full colonoscopy preoperatively, virtual colonoscopy or single-contrast barium enema should be performed. If none is possible, complete evaluation of the colon should be carried out 3–6 months after surgery.
- Distant metastases should be carefully investigated by chest X-ray, or computerised tomography (CT) and abdominal CT with contrast material. Positron-emission tomography (PET)-CT is the most sensitive method to detect metastasis, when there is a high level of suspicion for metastasis.
- Obtain carcinoembryonic antigen (CEA) levels before initiating any therapy. Elevated CEA is a poor prognostic factor after treatment. It is used for surveillance, and an elevated level is usually a sign of recurrence. It has low sensitivity and specificity, and should not be used for screening.

Laboratory findings

- The complete blood count (CBC) may reveal iron deficiency anaemia.
- Alkaline phosphatase can be elevated in case of liver or bone metastasis.
- Liver function tests may be normal if only a few liver metastases are present.

Pathology

- Adenocarcinoma occurs in 90%–95% of the cases of CRC.
- There are two separate and distinct major pathways leading to CRC: the chromosomal instability pathway (80%–85%), and the microsatellite instability pathway (15%–20%), which is implicated in HNPCC.
- Two important variants are mucinous adenocarcinoma with a variable amount of extracellular mucus, and signet-ring cell, which contains large portions of intracellular mucin with peripheral displacement of the nucleus.
- Rare types include squamous cell, carcinoid, adenosquamous, lymphoma, sarcoma and undifferentiated carcinomas.

Staging and prognosis

- The Dukes' staging system is still mostly used around the world, though the AJCC/TNM staging system is the preferred staging system in some countries (Table 17.3).
- Pathological stage is the single most important prognostic factor.
- Histological grade is not a major prognostic variable. Nevertheless, 5 years survival is better for grades I and II than for grades III or IV.
- Other adverse prognostic factors include: bowel obstruction, perforation, chromosome 18q allelic loss, high level of thymidylate synthase (TS) and mutations in p53.

THERAPY

The development of interdisciplinary diagnostic and therapeutic strategies has led to a moderate decline in mortality (2% per year). This is attributed to increased public and professional awareness, assimilation of recommended life style modification, screening and removal of polyps, better surgical techniques, better staging and use of adjuvant chemotherapy. Surgery will cure 50% of patients. More than 40% of the diagnosed patients will develop metastatic disease. Survival is directly related to the extent of disease at the time of diagnosis. If metastasis has occurred to distant sites, the 5-year survival rate is 5%–7%, but it increases to >90% when the cancer is diagnosed early. Long-term survival for patients with resectable liver and lung metastasis can be as high as 30%–40% with aggressive and novel therapy. Early detection of this surgically

TABLE 17.3: Different staging systems in colorectal cancer

T category describes the depth of penetration of the cancer through the different layers of the colonic wall. These layers include the mucosa, the muscularis mucosa (a thin layer of muscle tissue beneath the mucosa), the submucosa (connective tissue beneath this thin muscle layer), the muscularis propria (a thick layer of muscle that contracts to force the contents of the intestines along), the subserosa (a thin layer of connective tissue) and the serosa (a thin layer that covers the outer surface of some parts of the large intestine).

N category describes the number of involved lymph nodes. At least 13 nodes should be sampled.

M category describes the presence or absence of distant metastases.

Tis: The earliest stage. Tumour is confined only to the mucosa, the most inner layer. This stage is also known as carcinoma in situ or intramucosal carcinoma.

T1: The cancer has grown through the mucosa and extends into the submucosa.

T2: The cancer has penetrated the thick muscle layer.

T3: The cancer has spread into the subserosa, but not to any adjacent organs.

T4: The cancer has spread into nearby organs.

N0: No lymph node involvement.

N1: Cancer cells found in 1–3 regional lymph nodes.

N2: Cancer cells found in 4 or more regional lymph nodes.

M0: No distant metastasis.

M1: Evidence of distant spread.

TNM stage	TNM characteristics	Dukes' equivalent	Astler-Coller equivalent	5-year survival
0	Tis, N0, M0	–	–	
I	T1, N0, M0 T2, N0, M0	A	A and B1	93%
II	T3, N0, M0 T4, N0, M0	B	B2 and B3	IIA–85%
				IIB–72%
III	Any T, N1, M0 Any T, N2, M0	C	C1–C3	IIIA–83%
				IIIB–64%
				IIIC–44%
IV	Any T, Any N, M1	D	D	8%

curable disease and preventive interventions (e.g. polypectomy) is the single best modality. There is now compelling evidence that colon screening of asymptomatic, average risk individuals over 50 years of age can reduce CRC mortality by 15%–90%, depending on the screening programme (see Chapter 18).

Surgical management

Colectomy

Surgery is the primary and definite curative intervention. It consists of an en bloc resection of the intestinal segment containing the tumour along with adjacent mesentery, pericolic fat and the draining lymph nodes. A margin of 2–5 cm on either side of normal lower bowel is needed. The adequate number of lymph nodes that should be examined is at least 13. Sentinel lymph node biopsy aims to map lymph nodes that are most likely to contain metastatic disease. Even though it has gained popularity in breast cancer, it is rarely used in CRC. Type and extent of surgical resection depend on the location of the tumour. If the tumour is adherent to, or invades, another organ, an en bloc excision should be tried. Total abdominal colectomy with ileo-anal/rectal anastomosis is mandatory in FAP patients. Subtotal colectomy is usually recommended in HNPCC. Generally in the setting of obstructing or perforating tumour, a proximal protective colostomy is performed, followed by a second surgery after 4–8 weeks to establish colon continuity.

Laparoscopic colectomy

Laparoscopic colectomy is emerging as a novel and promising technology, although it is still considered investigational. In a large randomised study, quality of life, the rate of intraoperative complications, re-operation, 30-day mortality and hospital readmission were very similar between the two groups. The only advantages of laparoscopy were slightly shorter hospital stay and less use of postoperative pain medication that were needed with laparoscopy.

Adjuvant therapy

Fluorouracil: has been used since 1957 and remains the primary chemotherapeutic agent, with a response rate of 10%–12%. In 1990, an NIH consensus panel recommended adjuvant fluorouracil based chemotherapy in all stage III CRC. This was based on a large study in which fluorouracil and levamisole (an anthelmintic and immunostimulant agent), given for 12 months, achieved a 41% reduction in the relapse rate and a 33% decrease in mortality. Similarly, combining fluorouracil with folinic acid (calcium folinate) was shown to be effective as adjuvant therapy in stage III disease, and selected stage II cases. Fluorouracil and levamisole (given for 12 months) was as effective as fluorouracil and folinic acid (for 6 months), but more toxic. Consequently, the latter combination became the standard of care.

Capecitabine: an oral fluoropyrimidine that is converted by thymidine phosphorylase to active fluorouracil in the tumour tissue. It was shown to be as effective as fluorouracil, but less toxic, as an adjuvant therapy and in metastatic disease. Two major unique side effects are hand and foot syndrome and nonsignificant hyperbilirubinaemia.

Oxaliplatin: acts synergistically with fluorouracil, even in fluorouracil-refractory disease. The addition of oxaliplatin to fluorouracil and folinic acid appears to have a better outcome as adjuvant therapies in stage III. The new standard of adjuvant care is fluorouracil, folinic acid and oxaliplatin for 6 months. Fluorouracil is given in a continuous infusion or in a short drip. Oxaliplatin has a unique neurotoxicity—laryngopharyngeal dysaesthesia, cold hypersensitivity and cumulative, partially reversible peripheral neuropathy. Nausea, vomiting and myelotoxicity are also common.

Irinotecan: survival advantage had been shown as a second-line therapy for metastatic disease. Two forms of diarrhoea have been reported: early onset, which should be treated with atropine, and delayed onset (on days 3–5), requiring close monitoring and aggressive therapy (high dose loperamide, 4 mg initially and then 2 mg every 2 hours until diarrhoea stops for at least 12 hours). Neutropenia, alopecia, nausea and vomiting are also common. Adding irinotecan to folinic acid and fluorouracil failed to show an advantage in the adjuvant setting.

New biological agents

Cetuximab: a chimeric IgG monoclonal antibody that blocks epidermal growth factor receptor (EGFR) associating with its ligand, thus inhibiting the downstream signal transduction and preventing cell growth, differentiation and metastasis. It causes a typical acne-like rash, which is associated with a positive response.

Bevacizumab: a recombinant humanised vascular endothelial growth factor (VEGF) monoclonal antibody that blocks angiogenesis. Major toxicity includes proteinuria, hypertension, arterial thrombosis and intestinal perforation.

Addition of these new biological agents to oxaliplatin-based regimens is now being evaluated in the adjuvant setting.

Treatment of advanced disease

A combination of fluorouracil and folinic acid in continuous infusion, with irinotecan or oxaliplatin and bevacizumab is the most novel standard of care in first-line therapy. It confers a median survival of 20–24 months in metastatic disease. Oxaliplatin- or irinotecan-based chemotherapy can be given as second-line treatment. Cetuximab is active as third-line treatment in combination with irinotecan in irinotecan-resistant patients.

Treatment of rectal cancer

In contrast to colon cancer, 15%–20% of rectal tumours recur locally. Local recurrence can involve pelvic organs and bony structures, nerves and soft tissue. Radiotherapy has shown a protective, dose response curve, for preventing local recurrence in the rectum. Pelvic irradiation to the tumour bed and the pelvic lymph nodes is an integral component of the treatment in stages II and III.

Traditionally, postoperative radiotherapy was the gold standard in the USA, while the preoperative approach was preferred in Europe.

Currently, the most promising regimen worldwide is preoperative radiotherapy combined with fluorouracil in a continuous infusion (during radiation) 5 times a week for 6 weeks. This preoperative approach is advantageous since it improves compliance, pelvic recurrence, sphincter preservation and is associated with fewer radiation associated side effects to the small intestine.

Surgery is recommended following chemoradiotherapy.

Fluorouracil and folinic acid are given for an additional 4 months after successful surgery.

In cases when surgery was performed first, postoperative treatment includes fluorouracil (continuous infusion or bolus) during pelvic irradiation followed by four cycles of maintenance fluorouracil and folinic acid.

SUMMARY

Colorectal cancer (CRC) is a widespread and lethal disease in the Western world. It is the third most common malignancy after lung and breast cancer in women, and after lung and prostate in men. Approximately 75% of new cases occur among individuals at average risk. Adenocarcinomas account for 95% of cases, and synchronous adenocarcinoma can be found in 8%. Tumours of the proximal colon are now more common. CRC carcinogenesis is composed of a series of events that gradually (i.e. over 10–15 years) leads to transition from normal appearing mucosa, through adenoma (the pre-malignant lesion) into frank adenocarcinomas.

FURTHER READING

American Joint Committee on Cancer: Manual for staging of cancer, colon and rectum. 6th edn. New York: Springer-Verlag; 2002.

Kwak EL, Chung DC. Hereditary colorectal cancer syndromes: an overview. Clin Colorectal Cancer 2007; 6:340–4.

Levine JS, Ahnen DJ. Clinical practice. Adenomatous polyps of the colon. N Engl J Med 2006; 355:2551–7.

Pfister DG, Benson AB 3rd, Somerfield MR. Clinical practice: surveillance strategies after curative treatment of colorectal cancer. N Engl J Med 2004; 350:2375–82.

Smith RA, Cokkinides V, Eyre HJ. American Cancer Society guidelines for the early detection of cancer 2004. CA Cancer J Clin 2004; 54:41–52.

Chapter **18**

COLORECTAL CANCER SCREENING

KEY POINTS

- Colorectal (CRC) screening can reduce incidence and mortality from CRC by up to 90%.
- All average subjects aged 50 years and older should be screened.
- Colonoscopy is the best screening modality.
- The most prominent obstacle for CRC screening is the low compliance rate.
- Each of the current screening modalities is better than no screening and is effective in reducing mortality from CRC in the average risk population.
- Colonoscopy is the preferred screening tool for symptomatic patients and for moderate and high-risk groups.
- Recently developed screening modalities and technologies may replace current screening modalities.

BACKGROUND

The third millennium is witnessing the emergence of preventive medicine as a cornerstone in our concept of health. Colorectal cancer (CRC) is a major health concern (Chapter 17), and one that fits the criteria of a preventable disease. Approximately two-thirds of the cases involve average-risk men and women, with a sharp increase of its incidence starting from the fifth decade of life.

Detection and removal of colonic adenomas, the non-invasive neoplasm that are the precursors of CRC, could prevent up to 90% of CRC cases. The transition process between adenomas to carcinoma is estimated as 5–10 years and that of normal mucosa thorough adenoma to adenocarcinoma as 15–20 years. This interval provides a unique window of opportunity for screening and effective interventions to reduce CRC-associated mortality. The respective curative benefits that can be gained by detecting CRC at early stages, e.g. node-negative stages I and II, are as high as 90% and 75%, respectively, with surgery alone, while the 5-year survival rate is close to zero for metastatic CRC.

Most medical societies strongly recommend mass screening of the average-risk adult population starting at age 50 and earlier for individuals at higher risk due to family history or other predisposing factors. Several screening tests are available and are in common use.

FAECAL OCCULT BLOOD TESTING

Faecal occult blood test (FOBT) is a low-cost, non-invasive periodic procedure that detects faecal haemoglobin and does not require cathartic bowel preparation. Currently available approaches include a guaiac test, based on the peroxidase-like activity of haemoglobin, or immunochemical analysis. In the guaiac-based assay, accuracy of FOBT may be affected by stool re-hydration (which increases sensitivity but decreases specificity), haem degradation (reduced sensitivity), medications (false positives with non-steroidal antiinflammatory drugs [NSAIDS] and false negatives with vitamin C) and interfering dietary ingredients (such as peroxidases and meat haem). Recent professional guidelines have suggested that re-hydration is not recommended since the readability of the test is unpredictable, and the false positive rate is substantially increased. Newer guaiac-based and immunochemical tests are now available with improved sensitivity.

Support for the ability of annual FOBT to reduce the mortality from CRC emerged from several large prospective randomised trials. Mortality was reduced by 15%–33% if the test was done yearly, and when positive results were followed by colonoscopy. A meta-analysis that pooled the results of these studies estimated a 16%–23% reduction in CRC mortality. The estimated FOBT sensitivity for cancer ranges between 30% and 90% depending upon the test used. The major limitation of FOBT is its low sensitivity as a screening test, since some carcinomas and most adenomas do not bleed. Only 24% of advanced neoplasia cases had a positive FOBT result on the three consecutive days' samples obtained prior to bowel preparation. Proper FOBT testing requires examining three different bowel movements. Prerequisite compliance is difficult to achieve from both patients and physicians. In addition, the test gives an indirect result; hence, individuals who test positive have to undergo colonoscopy to confirm the presence of polyps, cancer or other pathology. Survival benefit may therefore reflect the benefit of colonoscopy, for detecting incidental lesions including those of subjects with false positive FOBT results. Lastly, upper gastrointestinal (GI) tract sources of occult bleeding, NSAID use or false positive results due to dietary ingredients may lead to unnecessary colonoscopies. There is often a low referral rate of patients with positive FOBT screening findings.

FOBT testing has no merit as a single test. It should definitely not be done when a patient has overt rectal bleeding (see Chapter 20) or any alarm symptoms. In such cases colonoscopy must be performed.

SIGMOIDOSCOPY

This method provides direct endoscopic visualisation of the distal part of the colon, preferably up to the splenic flexure, and enables biopsies to be taken and polyps resected. Sigmoidoscopy is considered less invasive than colonoscopy and requires a simple bowel preparation of only two fleet enemas, one hour prior to the procedure. It usually does not require sedation and can be performed by trained nurses. A finding of a neoplastic/dysplastic lesion mandates full evaluation of the entire large intestine by colonoscopy although, according to some guidelines, this decision should be individualised and be performed in high-risk subjects (e.g. age ≥65 years, villous histology in the large adenoma ≥1 cm or multiple adenomas). The currently published data on reducing CRC mortality by screening sigmoidoscopy are derived from non-prospective case-controlled trials which report that screening sigmoidoscopy can reduce the incidence and death rates of distal CRC by 59%–80% and lower overall CRC mortality by up to 40%–50%.

The main drawback of sigmoidoscopy is the limit of its extension, which is up to the splenic flexure at best. Unfortunately, the distance is often significantly shorter. Sensitivity actually depends on the varied experience of the examiners, and on patient discomfort, two factors that have a major impact on the depth of insertion and adequacy of mucosal inspection. Even in the hands of expert endoscopists, the sigmoidoscope was found to traverse the sigmoid colon in only 66% of cases. For more than 50% of proximal advanced lesions (i.e. advanced adenoma or carcinoma) there were no lesions in the distal colon, so those would have been missed by sigmoidoscopy. Sigmoidoscopy is even less rewarding in subjects aged 65–75 years, as a proximal shift of neoplasia in this age group is suggested.

COMBINED FOBT AND SIGMOIDOSCOPY

There is a lack of prospective data regarding the value of a combined approach of 5-year sigmoidoscopy and annual FOBT. Some evidence suggests that it may possess some advantage, as sigmoidoscopy is intended to screen the distal colon, and FOBT is more effective in detecting proximal lesions. Supporting data from case-control studies report that screening FOBT and sigmoidoscopy are individually associated with reduced CRC mortality after controlling for the other test. When both tests are to be done, the FOBT should be performed first because a positive result is an indication for colonoscopy, obviating the need for sigmoidoscopy. This combination may improve the relative efficacy of each test alone, and has been suggested as an alternative strategy for screening colonoscopy. The limitation of this combined approach is exposing individuals to inconvenience, cost and complications of both FOBT and sigmoidoscopy with an uncertain gain in efficacy.

COLONOSCOPY

Colonoscopy is the gold standard procedure to identify colorectal neoplasia. Skilled gastroenterologists perform the examination after a cathartic bowel preparation. Using back-to-back colonoscopies, it was shown that the sensitivity of a single colonoscopy is about 90%–95% for cancers and large adenomas and 75% for polyps <1 cm. The detection rates for adenomas ≥10 mm, 5–10 mm and 1–5 mm were found to be 98%, 87% and 74%, respectively. Colonoscopy miss rates are related to the skills of the endoscopist, withdrawal technique and, in particular, withdrawal time that reflects the time spent to inspect the colon. Although there are no published prospective studies on direct reduction of CRC mortality by primary screening colonoscopy, there is a large body of evidence to support it. The National Polyp Study has demonstrated a 76%–90% decrease in the incidence of CRC at 6 years after the index colonoscopy and polypectomy, compared with several appropriately selected control groups. A prospective 13-year follow-up demonstrated a relative risk of 0.2 for CRC in subjects who underwent colonoscopy with polyp removal compared with the control group. The prevalence of CRC in asymptomatic patients being screened aged 50–75 years in the USA is approximately 1%. Overall, the findings support the use of colonoscopy rather than sigmoidoscopy for screening in this age group.

The bowel preparation is inconvenient and poses a major obstacle. The myths of the discomfort of colonoscopy may be unjustified, since the examination is performed under conscious sedation and discomfort is rare. Indeed, patients who have undergone both endoscopic examinations report that non-sedated sigmoidoscopy is associated with a significantly higher recalled level of discomfort compared with conscious sedated colonoscopy. Studies on colonoscopy in the setting of ambulatory screening examinations have shown a considerably low risk of morbidity (0.1%–0.3%) with no procedure-related deaths. Colonoscopy costs more than FOBT and sigmoidoscopy. The true calculations, however, should be based on the long-term costs for a life-year saved. In a realistic model of a <50% compliance rate, the estimated cost per death prevented was similar for FOBT and endoscopy. Furthermore, if colonoscopy costs are below $750, once-in-a-life-time colonoscopy was found to be more cost effective than any other screening modality at every level of compliance.

Double-contrast barium enema
Double-contrast barium enema (DCBE) is not a viable contemporary screening modality for colorectal neoplasia because of its low sensitivity and specificity compared with other screening modalities.

RISK STRATIFICATION AND CURRENT SCREENING RECOMMENDATIONS

Screening for colonic neoplasia is important for individuals who are free of any signs or symptoms suggestive of CRC. A full colonoscopy is absolutely indicated in the presence of alarm symptoms. A key element for tailoring the most appropriate screening programme relies on the individual's level of risk, which is based primarily on age, as well as on personal, family and medical history. This risk status determines when screening should be initiated, at what frequency and by which modality.

Risk stratification can be determined by asking pertinent questions aimed at uncovering the risk factors for CRC (Table 18.1):

- Is there any personal or familial history of colon cancer, any familial polyposis syndrome or colonic polyps?
- Is there any personal history of inflammatory bowel disease?
- Is there any history of acromegaly or other cancers?

Asymptomatic individuals with any risk factors for CRC are then re-classified into 'moderate-risk' (personal and/or family history of CRC or adenoma), or 'high risk' for CRC (e.g. familial neoplastic syndromes or inflammatory bowel disease). Current CRC screening recommendations (based on recent professional guidelines) are shown in Figure 18.1.

TABLE 18.1: Risk factors for colorectal cancer that mandate colonoscopy as the screening tool

Genetic disorders	• Familial adenomatous polyposis • Hereditary non-polyposis colorectal cancer • Peutz-Jegher syndrome • Hyperplastic polyposis • Juvenile polyposis • Cowden's syndrome
Personal history of colorectal cancer or adenoma	
Family history of colorectal cancer or adenoma	First-degree relative diagnosed <60 years, or two first-degree relatives diagnosed at any age
Inflammatory bowel disease	After 8 years with pancolitis and 12 years with left-sided colitis
Endocrine disorders	Acromegaly
Other neoplasm	Breast cancer?

CRC screening in average-risk populations

Men and women at average risk should be offered screening with one of the following options beginning at the age of 50 years:

- Annual FOBT, with two samples from each of three consecutive stools examined without re-hydration
- Sigmoidoscopy every 5 years
- Colonoscopy every 10 years.

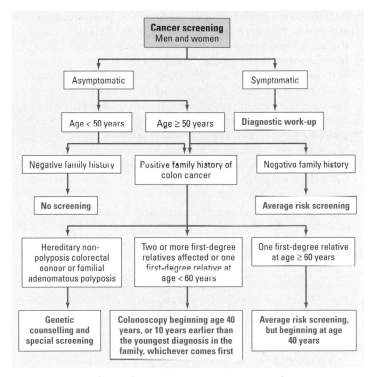

FIGURE 18.1: Colorectal cancer screening recommendations.
Based on Winawer S, Fletcher R, Rex D, et al. Colorectal cancer screening and surveillance: clinical guidelines and rationale—Update based on new evidence. Gastroenterology 2003; 124:544–60.

The rationale for presenting multiple options is that no single test is of unequivocal superiority and giving patients a choice may increase compliance. The strategies are different in terms of the evidence they provide and their specific degree of effectiveness, risk and costs. Clinicians should present the different features of each modality to their patients to enable them to make an informed choice about screening options.

CRC screening in moderate-risk populations

This subpopulation is defined by a personal or family history of adenoma/CRC. Professional guidelines recommend the following guidelines (Table 18.2):

- Colonoscopy (should be done every 5 years) starting at age 40 years or 10 years younger than the earliest diagnosis when the first-degree relative (parent, sibling or child) had CRC or adenomatous polyps diagnosed at age <60 years *or* if two first-degree relatives have been diagnosed with CRC at any age.
- Screening as for average-risk persons, but beginning at age 40 years when the first-degree relative with CRC or adenomatous polyp was diagnosed at age >60 years *or* if two second-degree relatives were diagnosed with CRC at any age.
- Screening as for average-risk persons when one second-degree relative (grandparent, aunt or uncle) with CRC or a third-degree relative (great-grandparent or cousin) has been diagnosed with CRC.

The rationale for beginning screening at age 40 years in persons with an affected first-degree relative is that the incidence of CRC for them parallels the risk in persons with no family history but precedes it by about 10 years.

TABLE 18.2: Guidelines for colorectal cancer (CRC) screening in a moderate-risk group
Colonoscopy* starting at age 40 years or 10 years younger than the earliest diagnosis if: • A first-degree relative (parent, sibling or child) with colorectal cancer (CRC) or adenomatous polyps diagnosed at age <60 years   • Two first-degree relatives diagnosed with CRC at any age
Screening as for average risk persons, but beginning at age 40 years, if: • A first-degree relative with CRC or adenomatous polyp diagnosed at age >60 years   • Two second-degree relatives with CRC of any age
Screening as for average risk persons if: • One second-degree relative (grandparent, aunt or uncle) with CRC   • One third-degree relative (great-grandparent or cousin) with CRC
* Colonoscopy should be done every 5 years.

High-risk groups for CRC screening

This group should undergo more intensive surveillance with colonoscopy only (see Table 18.1). These guidelines do not include screening for cancers outside the colon and, for the genetic syndromes, recommendations are based on phenotype only (Table 18.3).

- Familial adenomatous polyposis (FAP): annual sigmoidoscopy, beginning at age 10–12 years.
- Hereditary non-polyposis colon cancer (HNPCC): colonoscopy every 1–2 years beginning at age 20–25 years, or 10 years earlier than the youngest age of cancer associated with HNPCC (gastric, ovarian, uterine, small intestine) in relatives.
- Inflammatory bowel disease (IBD): colonoscopy every 1–2 years after 8 years of disease in patients with pancolitis or after 12–15 years in left-sided colitis. Biopsies should be taken every 10 cm in all four quadrants with additional sampling of strictures or any mucosal irregularities. This applies to both ulcerative colitis and Crohn's disease, since the cancer risk is similar in both diseases.
- Genetic testing for FAP or HNPCC should be offered to first-degree relatives of persons with a known inherited gene mutation. It should also be offered when the family mutation is not already known, but the clinical suspicion is high.

TABLE 18.3: Guidelines for colorectal cancer (CRC) screening in high-risk groups

Familial adenomatous polyposis	Annual sigmoidoscopy, beginning at age 10–12 years*
Hereditary non-polyposis colon cancer	Colonoscopy every 1–2 years beginning at age 20–25 years, or 10 years earlier than the youngest age of cancer associated with HNPCC (gastric, ovarian, uterine, small intestine)
Inflammatory bowel disease	Colonoscopy every 1–2 years after 8 years of disease in patients with pancolitis or after 12–15 years in left-sided colitis. Biopsies should be taken every 10 cm in all four quadrants with additional sampling of strictures or any mucosal irregularities

* This recommendation holds true based on phenotype only (without a definite genetic mutation).

SURVEILLANCE OF INDIVIDUALS AT INCREASED RISK

Patients who have had numerous adenomas, adenoma with invasive cancer, a large sessile adenoma or an incomplete colonoscopy should have a short-interval follow-up colonoscopy based on clinical judgment. Patients who have advanced or multiple adenomas (>3) should have their first follow-up colonoscopy in 3 years. Patients who have one or two small (<1 cm) tubular adenomas should have their first follow-up colonoscopy at 5 years. Patients with a CRC that has been resected with curative intent should have had a colonoscopy around the time of initial diagnosis to rule out synchronous neoplasm. If the colon is obstructed preoperatively, colonoscopy can be performed approximately 3 months after surgery. If this or a complete preoperative examination is normal, subsequent colonoscopy should be considered after 3 years, and then, if normal, every 5 years.

Emerging screening modalities

There are several newly developed screening tests for CRC, which have shown substantial promise, but none has been sufficiently developed or investigated to be offered as a routine.

Virtual colonoscopy (VC): the approach involves performing an abdominal computerised tomographic (CT) examination that is analysed by a computer to render an image resembling the one seen at optical colonoscopy. As in colonoscopy, the examination requires cathartic bowel preparation and air insufflations for intestinal distension, and the patients are not sedated. It is considered a minimally invasive procedure, although colonic perforation has been recognised as an associated complication. VC has the additional advantages of an abdominal CT scan, supplying information on tumour invasion, lymph node involvement and metastasis. In cases of suspected lesions, the examination should be followed by conventional colonoscopy. The sensitivity of VC for lesions ≥10 mm reportedly ranges from 81%–94%. The detection rate of polyps ≥6 mm ranges widely (39%–94%). Prepless VC using faecal tags to distinguish stool from true lesions is under evaluation.

Faecal DNA test: a stool-based molecular analysis of DNA markers in exfoliated colonocytes that are regularly shed in the stool. The rationale of the examination is that normal colonocytes are sparse and apoptotic (e.g. contain 'short' DNA fragments), while neoplastic colonocytes are abundant and harbour high molecular weight DNA ('long DNA'). Since CRC is a disease of mutations that occur as tissue evolves from normal to adenoma to carcinoma, these mutations can be detectable in the stool. Advantages of this test over the other screening modalities are their non-invasive nature and lack of bowel preparation or any dedicated procedural time. Testing can be performed on mailed-in specimens, whereby geographic access to stool screening is essentially unimpeded. Initial studies based on either single mutation or panels of genetic markers had a sensitivity of 91% and 82% for CRC and large adenomas, respectively, but controlled studies demonstrated less favourable results. Long DNA was the most frequent neoplastic marker in the stool. The most prevalent genetic alterations were mutations in K-*ras* and p53 genes, followed by microsatellite instability (MSI) and adenomatous polyposis coli (*APC*) gene mutations. The test seems promising with considerably higher sensitivity and specificity than FOBT, but has not yet been validated as a screening tool in large-scale prospective trials. At present, the high cost of faecal DNA testing is a major obstacle that reduces its cost-effectiveness. There is a promising future for this approach if sensitivity could be increased by additional markers (e.g. methylation) and if cost could be reduced.

Magnification high-resolution endoscopy: a development in endoscopy design. The new electronic videoendoscopes are equipped with charged couple device (CCD) chips of 100 K to 300 K pixels. The recent generation of videoendoscopes was introduced with 850 K-pixel density and referred to as high resolution endoscopes. In addition, some endoscopes, including the high-resolution types, are equipped with an optical zoom facility, which can provide a magnified image. The combination of both high resolution and magnification may become an important supplementary tool in CRC screening. High resolution can increase the detection rate of small and flat lesions while magnification can enhance details in the suspected lesions, thereby making endoscopic diagnosis more accurate.

Chromoendoscopy: a technique that consists of staining the mucosal surface of the GI tract in order to enhance the diagnostic yield of endoscopy. The main purpose is to screen for neoplastic or preneoplastic lesions (in particular flat or depressed lesions) and to direct endoscopic biopsies. Indigo carmine is a contrast stain that accumulates in pits and valleys between cells highlighting the mucosal architecture that becomes even more apparent with the use of magnification and/or high-resolution endoscopy. The technique only requires a special spraying catheter, making it simple and relatively inexpensive. Its only disadvantage is that it prolongs the overall procedural time. Currently, chromoendoscopy is reserved for high-risk subjects (i.e. patients with a personal history of neoplasia, inflammatory bowel disease or familial neoplastic syndromes).

New technologies on the horizon

The following new technologies are future screening approaches for CRC that have not yet been confirmed by large scale clinical trials.

Assisted colonoscopy: The FDA recently approved a device known as the ColonoSight® (Striker, USA). ColonoSight is ergonomically similar to currently existing colonoscopes. The device is covered by a disposable sleeve and the physician's hands remain clean. All channels within the device (insufflations, irrigation, suction/working) are completely disposable and no fibre-optics are necessary due to an incorporated LED light source. The air used for sleeve deployment adds a small amount of additional forward force just below the scope tip, which enhances device navigation and forward motion. Pilot studies are available with a mean examination time of 12.4 ± 10.8 minutes with a mean insertion length of 117 ± 26 cm.

Self-propelling self-navigating skill-independent colonoscopy: (The Aer-O-Scope™ GI View, Israel) This new disposable colonoscope is a skill-independent, anaesthesia-free, self-propelling, self-navigating miniaturised endoscopic device that moves along the entire length of the colon, transmitting video pictures of the colonic mucosa. This disposable product is based on a miniaturised self-propelling, self-navigating locomotion mechanism that contains a digital camera. The device is supplied with electricity, air, water and suction via a thin supply cable, which it drags behind it. The device has a novel optical system enabling a 360° view, and hence may decrease the polyp miss rate, particularly behind folds. So far the device has proven safe, without any complications in more than 60 subjects.

The PillCam™ COLON: (Given Imaging, Israel). This capsule is very similar to the oesophageal and small intestine camera capsules. It is slightly bigger (11 mm by 32 mm), has dual cameras, a wide field of view, automatic light control, four frames per second and a battery life of 10 hours. A meticulous preparation is absolutely necessary. The overall sensitivity for significant lesions was around 75%, specificity 70%, and positive and negative predictive values of 65% and 85%, respectively. False positive results were recorded in one-third of study cases.

SUMMARY

CRC is a major health concern and a largely preventable disease. A majority of CRC cases are preventable with screening. Early detection enables either detection of adenomas or diagnosis of CRC at an early stage, which carries a significantly better prognosis than advanced CRC. Screening modalities have developed substantially in recent years. Available modalities include FOBT, sigmoidoscopy, combination of FOBT and sigmoidoscopy and colonoscopy.

Each modality has its own pros and cons, though colonoscopy is the gold standard and is the mandatory screening modality for high-risk populations. There is now a consensus that any screening modality is better than nothing, and that each modality of screening is effective in reducing the mortality from CRC.

Emerging screening modalities include virtual colonoscopy, faecal DNA testing and advanced endoscopic techniques. The choice of screening modality depends upon the risk stratification of the patient. The age at which screening should start in the average risk population is 50 years of age. Higher-risk groups require earlier screening. The most prominent obstacle is low patient compliance rates.

FURTHER READING

Bernstein CN. Ulcerative colitis and low-grade dysplasia. Gastroenterology 2004; 127:950–6.

Levine JS, Ahmen DJ. Clinical Practice. Adenomatous polyps of the colon. N Engl J Med 2006; 355:2551–7.

Lindor NM, Petersen GM, Hadley DW, et al. Recommendations for the care of individuals with an inherited predisposition to Lynch syndrome: a systematic review. JAMA 2006; 296:1507–17.

Rex DK. Maximizing detection of adenomas and cancers during colonoscopy. Am J Gastroenterol 2006; 101:2866–77.

Schoen RE, Weissfeld JL, Pinsky PF, et al. Yield of advanced adenoma and cancer based on polyp size detected at screening flexible sigmoidoscopy. Gastroenterology 2006; 131:1683–9.

Walsh JM, Terdiman TP. Colorectal cancer screening; scientific review. JAMA 2003; 289:1288–96.

Winawer S, Fletcher R, Rex D, et al. Colorectal cancer screening and surveillance: clinical guidelines and rationale—Update based on new evidence. Gastroenterology 2003; 124:544–60.

Winawer S, Zauber AG, Fletcher RH, et al. Guidelines for colonoscopy surveillance after polypectomy: a consensus update by the US Multi-Society Task Force on Colorectal Cancer and the American Cancer Society. Gastroenterology 2006; 130:1872–85.

Chapter 19

FAECAL INCONTINENCE

KEY POINTS

- Faecal incontinence is the involuntary passage of stool through the anus.
- A detailed history and clinical examination is important. A special note on vaginal delivery and any complications should be noted.
- On rectal examination, it is important to ask the patient to strain to assess resting tone and squeeze tone.
- A flexible sigmoidoscopy or colonoscopy is mandatory.
- Medical treatment includes dietary changes, perineal exercises and, if needed, high doses of antidiarrhoeal drugs.
- There have been good results with biofeedback training.

DEFINITION

Faecal incontinence is the involuntary passage of stool through the anus.

PREVALENCE

The reported prevalence rates of faecal incontinence in the world vary from 0.7%–11%, depending on the definition and population group studied. This is demonstrated in Table 19.1.

Incontinence is such an embarrassing condition that few people speak of it. As a result, its true prevalence is believed to be higher than that reported.

AETIOLOGY

Table 19.2 lists the possible causes of faecal incontinence. Looser stool consistency is an important precipitating factor in those predisposed to faecal incontinence by anorectal abnormalities.

TABLE 19.1: International prevalence rates of faecal incontinence

Country	Population	Prevalence
Holland	Women >60 y	4.2% to 16.9% with rising age
France	All >45 y	11%, 6% to faeces, 60% women
UK	Community service	1.9%
USA	Market mailing	7% soiling, 0.7% to faeces
USA	Wisconsin households	2.2%, 63% women
USA	Wisconsin nursing homes	47%
New Zealand	>65 y	3.1%
Australia	Household survey	6.8% men 10.9% women >15 y
Australia	Postal survey Random selection from electoral roll (subjects ≥18 y)	Liquid incontinence 9% Solid incontinence 2%

Based on Continence Foundation of Australia. Incontinence: some key statistics and quotes clarified. Online.
Available: www.contfound.org.au/pdf/Keystatsquotsmay03.pdf.

TABLE 19.2: Classification of the aetiology of faecal incontinence

Altered stool consistency—diarrhoeal states

- Irritable bowel syndrome
- Inflammatory bowel disease
- Infectious diarrhoea
- Laxative abuse
- Malabsorption syndrome
- Short-gut syndrome
- Radiation enteritis

Inadequate reservoir capacity or compliance

- Inflammatory bowel disease
- Absent rectal reservoir
  - Sphincter-saving operations
    - Low anterior resection
    - Coloanal anastomosis
    - Ileorectal anastomosis
    - Ileoanal reservoir
- Rectal ischaemia
- Collagen vascular disease
  - Scleroderma
  - Dermatomyositis
  - Amyloidosis
- Rectal neoplasms
- Extrinsic rectal compression

TABLE 19.2: Classification of the aetiology of faecal incontinence
(continued)

Inadequate rectal sensation

- Neurologic conditions
  - Dementia
  - Cerebrovascular accidents
  - Tabes dorsalis
  - Multiple sclerosis
  - Injuries
    - Brain
    - Spinal cord
    - Cauda equina
  - Neoplasms
    - Brain
    - Spinal cord
    - Cauda equina
  - Sensory neuropathy

- Overflow incontinence
  - Faecal impaction
  - Encopresis
  - Psychotropic drugs
  - Antimotility drugs

Abnormal sphincter mechanism or pelvic floor

- Anatomic sphincter defect
  - Traumatic
  - Obstetric injury
    - Third-degree or fourth-degree lacerations
    - Episiotomy wound complications
    - Forceps injury
  - Anorectal surgery
    - Anal fistula surgery
    - Haemorrhoidectomy
    - Sphincterotomy
    - Dilatation or stretching injury
  - Neoplastic
  - Inflammatory

- Pelvic floor denervation
  - Primary ('idiopathic' neurogenic incontinence)
    - Pudendal neuropathy
    - Chronic straining at stool
    - Descending perineal syndrome
    - Vaginal deliveries
  - Secondary
    - Injuries to spinal cord/cauda equina/pelvic floor nerves
    - Diabetic neuropathy
- Congenital abnormalities
  - Spina bifida
  - Myelomeningocele
  - Imperforate anus
- Miscellaneous
  - Ageing
  - Rectal prolapse

Obstetric injuries

During vaginal delivery, perineal tears are common and complications of vaginal delivery are among the most common causes of incontinence seen by the surgeon. In fact one-third of vaginal deliveries lead to some form of sphincter injury. However, the majority of patients present with incontinence at a later stage when the muscles are unable to compensate.

The risk factors of vaginal delivery include primigravidas, babies with high birth weight and instrumental delivery, e.g. forceps delivery. The tear is not prevented by episiotomy. It is reported that 70% of women who experience a third or fourth-degree tear will report incontinence to flatus.

Another indirect mechanism of incontinence attributed to childbirth is stretch injury to the pudendal nerve during labour. This injury may then lead to denervation of the external sphincter, the internal sphincter and puborectalis muscle. The denervation injury may develop decades after the injury.

Ageing

A common form of anal incontinence is that associated with old age and general debilitation. It is usually a neurogenic incontinence.

Previous operations

Internal sphincterotomy

It is said that this operation may lead to incontinence to a variable extent. There are studies suggesting that incontinence to flatus could be up to 30%. The risk of incontinence is dependent on the amount of internal sphincter being divided. With tailored sphincterotomy, the risk of incontinence has been shown to be lower.

Anal fistula surgery

Anal fistula surgery may involve the division of part of the internal anal sphincter and/or external anal sphincter. As a result, incontinence may occur depending on the amount of sphincter divided. With the use of endoanal ultrasound to detect the anatomy of the fistula tract, especially in complex fistulas, the risk of incontinence has been shown to be lower.

Haemorrhoidectomy

With current surgical techniques for haemorrhoids, incontinence is a rare complication. However, if the anal sphincter is inadvertently divided, incontinence may result. With the use of a stapled haemorrhoidectomy, there is also a small risk of anal incontinence secondary to dilatation by the instrument. However, this form of incontinence usually resolves with time.

Manual dilatation of anus

Finger dilatation of the anal canal (Lord's procedure) for the treatment of anal spasm can result in incontinence to a variable degree. This procedure has mostly been abandoned in contemporary practice.

Sphincter-saving procedure

In a low anterior resection for rectal cancer, most of the rectum is usually excised. A 'new' rectum is usually created by using the descending colon. As the reservoir function of the rectum is lost and it takes time for the 'new' rectum to adapt to the function of the rectum, incontinence can occur during the interim period due to frequent bowel actions. However, this problem usually resolves after a few months.

Rectal prolapse

Rectal prolapse is a full thickness protrusion of the rectum through the anal sphincter.

Nearly 10% of women over 50 years old may have symptoms of pelvic organ prolapse, including urethral prolapse, vaginal prolapse, rectal prolapse or perineal descent.

Rectal prolapse is a distressing condition that is associated with faecal incontinence in 50%–70% of patients. The prolapse itself is socially embarrassing especially if it descends during normal activities. Per rectum bleeding and mucus discharge are common symptoms. It mainly affects females and the most common cause is vaginal delivery. When it occurs in males, there is usually some underlying predisposing factors such as straining at stool, constipation, neurological disorder or senile dementia.

In rectal prolapse, the incontinence may be related to chronic stretching of the anal muscles or partly due to nerve injury. Repair of the prolapse is said to result in improvement of incontinence in approximately 50% of patients.

Trauma

Traumatic injury to sphincters may occur during an accident. Serious forms of injury may require a temporary stoma. The anal sphincter is then re-assessed and appropriately treated prior to closure of the stoma at a later stage.

Primary disease

Diarrhoea from any cause, chronic inflammation in the rectum or carcinoma of the anal canal may present with incontinence. This obviously has to be treated according to the cause of the problem.

Radiotherapy

It has been shown that radiotherapy can increase the risk of anal incontinence. This is important as chemoradiation is commonly used as a pre-operative and post-operative treatment for rectal cancer. However, the incidence of incontinence is still quite low. Radiation proctitis can also lead to bleeding as well as incontinence.

Neurogenic causes

This includes myelomeningocele, demyelinating disease and diabetic patients with autonomic neuropathy.

Idiopathic incontinence

A large number of patients do not have any evidence of anorectal abnormality. However, they usually have problems with their pudendal nerve. It is probably related to stretching of the nerve during vaginal delivery or straining for any reason.

Congenital abnormalities

Various operations have been designed for treating an imperforate anus and they usually result in various extent of incontinence.

Miscellaneous causes

Overflow incontinence secondary to faecal impaction or pelvic floor disorders such as the solitary rectal ulcer syndrome (ulceration secondary to rectal prolapse or a non-relaxing puborectalis muscle) may be associated with varying degrees of incontinence.

HISTORY

A detailed history is absolutely necessary in the assessment of any pathological condition, paying particular attention to the characteristic cause and extent of the incontinence. It is important to determine the nature of incontinence—whether it is incontinence to solid, liquid or flatus—and to determine the frequency of the incontinence and the necessity to wear a protective pad. Other associated symptoms such as urgency need to be determined as well as social limitation as a result of the incontinence.

Direct questioning is necessary on the history of vaginal delivery and complications. The patient should also be asked about associated conditions such as urinary incontinence, rectal prolapse, diabetes mellitus, medications, radiation treatment or any congenital abnormalities. It is also important to determine whether the patient has had a previous anorectal operation, low colon anastomosis or trauma to the anorectal area.

There are many continence scoring systems available in the literature. Most of them are useful for research purposes but are not practical for day-to-day use. The St Mark's scoring system is listed in Table 19.3. A clue to the severity of incontinence is determining the frequency of the incontinence, the necessity to wear a protective pad and the effect on social function.

TABLE 19.3: St Mark's continence scoring system

Symptom severity	Score
Incontinence to solid stool	
Never	0
Less than once per month	1
Less than once per week	2
Most days	3
Incontinence to liquid stool	
Never	0
Less than once per month	1
Less than once per week	2
Most days	3
Incontinence to flatus	
Never	0
Less than once per month	1
Less than once per week	2
Most days	3
Ability to withhold defecation more than 15 min	
Yes	0
No	1

Symptom severity	Score
Difficulty cleaning after evacuation	
No	0
Yes	1
Soiling	
None	0
Minor	1
Major	2
0 = fully continent; 13 = regularly completely incontinent to all rectal contents.	

TABLE 19.3: St Mark's continence scoring system *(continued)*

PHYSICAL EXAMINATION

- The underpants and the perineum should be inspected for staining by stool, mucus or pus.
- On inspection of the perineum, a large patulous anus is suggestive of possible rectal prolapse. Scar from previous operations or episiotomies should also be carefully noted.
- The patient should be asked to strain. Perineal descent or mucosal/full thickness rectal prolapse may become obvious on straining.
- Per rectum examination:
  - Palpate for any sphincter defect
  - Palpation with the index finger can also detect any keyhole deformity of the anal canal, which may lead to soiling
  - Any tumour or the presence of blood can also be determined from the finger examination
  - Assess the resting and squeeze tones of the anal muscle. The tone is assessed both at rest (resting tone) and when the patient is asked to squeeze (squeeze tone). The resting tone assesses the function of the internal anal sphincter and the squeeze tone assesses the integrity of the external anal sphincter.
- Rigid sigmoidoscopy may reveal any internal rectal prolapse, inflammatory process or neoplasm contributing to the patient's complaint.

INVESTIGATIONS

Flexible sigmoidoscopy

It is important to exclude rectal tumour or inflammation in the rectum causing incontinence. This can be detected and biopsy taken with a flexible sigmoidoscopy.

Endoanal ultrasound

This is a procedure whereby an ultrasound probe is inserted into the anal canal for assessment of the integrity of the anal sphincters. It can detect a sphincter defect secondary to childbirth, trauma or previous operations. A sphincter defect usually implies that the problem is amenable to surgery.

Anorectal physiology

Anal manometry

A catheter is inserted into the rectum and the resting and squeeze pressure can be measured. The catheter is connected up to four to eight channels of fluids under a pressurised system. When the patient is at rest, the resting pressure is measured. The patient is then asked to squeeze on the catheter and the squeeze pressure is measured. The resting pressure is a measure of the function of the internal anal sphincter whereas the squeeze pressure is a measure of the function of the external anal sphincter. The rectoanal inhibitory reflex is measured in order to exclude the possibility of Hirschsprung's disease.

Pudendal nerve terminal motor latency

This procedure measures the conduction time for the pudendal nerve on each side. The pudendal nerve is the nerve supply to anal muscles. If the conduction time is prolonged, which is normally less than 2 ms, it indicates pudendal nerve neuropathy. This is usually performed with a finger electrode whereby electrical pulses are sent along the electrode to stimulate the pudendal nerve on each side. The conduction time is then recorded and measured once sizeable contraction of anal muscles occurs.

TREATMENT

Treatment of incontinence involves non-operative and operative procedures (see Figure 19.1).

Non-operative procedures

Medical treatment

Dietary changes and perineal exercises are often recommended for patients with faecal incontinence. There are also various antidiarrhoeal drugs that are available in the management of patients with incontinence. Drugs such as loperamide or diphenoxylate are used, which inhibit intestinal motility by a direct effect on the circular and longitudinal muscles of the intestinal wall. The majority of causes of faecal incontinence can be managed with medical treatment.

Biofeedback training

Biofeedback training involves at least three components: exercise of the external sphincter muscle, training in the discrimination of rectal sensation and training in synchrony of the internal and external sphincter responses during rectal distension. Selection of patients is very important for biofeedback training to be successful. The patients have to be well motivated and alert for the three-phase instructions on voluntary control mechanisms.

The method involves placing a balloon in the rectum and connecting pressure transducers to a graph to give the patient visual feedback corresponding to their sphincter responses to command. Initially, a large rectal balloon is used and the volume of distension of the balloon is gradually reduced until the patient can relax the external anal sphincter in response to a small distension. Finally, the visual feedback is eliminated and the patient is checked by a trained observer to see if they can respond to rectal sensation alone. This method improves contraction of the pelvic floor muscles, thereby increasing tone and reducing the chance of incontinence.

Operative procedures

It is important to bear in mind that the majority of patients with faecal incontinence can be treated with conservative management, i.e. diet change, medication, biofeedback training and continence advice. Only a minority of patients require operative intervention.

Overlapping sphincteroplasty

This operation is indicated for patients with a definite sphincter defect. The operation involves dividing the scar tissue and overlapping the sphincter complex (internal and external anal sphincters). The short-term results are good in about 80%–90% of patients. However, the results are not as good on long-term follow-up.

Postanal repair
This operation is now seldom performed and its success rate is said to be about 50%.

Graciloplasty
This operation involves using the gracilis muscle in the thigh to wrap around the anal canal and act as a new sphincter. It also involves stimulation of the gracilis muscle with a pacemaker via leads to the neurovascular bundle of the muscle. The gracilis muscle is constantly stimulated by the pacemaker to close the anus in the resting state. During defecation, the pacemaker can then be switched off with a remote control to relax the gracilis muscle so that the defecation process can occur. This operation carries a significant morbidity rate and almost 50% of patients require a stoma in the long term.

Artificial sphincter
This operation involves the insertion of an artificial sphincter around the anus. It is not often performed because of the high risk of infection of the prosthesis.

PTQ™ implant
PTQ™ implants are injectable tissue-bulking agents used for the treatment of faecal incontinence. They are made of small-refined solid particles of implantable silicone in a water-based carrier gel. It is injected into the sphincter defect or the intersphincteric space. The implant allows for the ingrowth of collagen tissues making it stay at the injected location permanently. It can be used for a small sphincter defect to fill the gap or for a weak thin internal anal sphincter to increase bulk in the anal canal.

The increase in bulk can then reduce the luminal size of the anal canal, thus improving incontinence. It is best injected under ultrasound control so that the placement of the implant is accurate.

Sacral nerve stimulation
This operation is indicated for patients who fail conservative management of faecal incontinence. It is divided into two stages.

The first stage involves testing the effect of stimulating the pelvic nerve—mainly S3. This is performed via insertion of lead wires into the S3 foramen to stimulate the S3 nerve. The wire is then connected to an external temporary pacemaker. The patient carries the pacemaker around for 7–10 days during this trial period to see whether the stimulation improves their continence. If continence does not improve over the trial period, the wires are then removed. If the continence improves, a permanent pacemaker is then inserted under the skin in either the buttock or the anterior abdominal wall. This stimulation of nerve leads to increase of anal tone and therefore improves continence. The result from the operation showed that 85% of patients have significant improvement—85% of patients have more than 50% reduction in incontinent episodes.

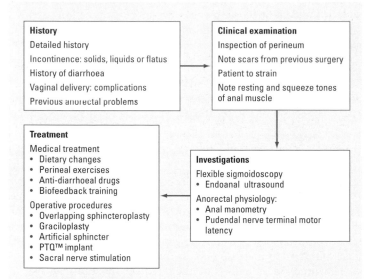

FIGURE 19.1: Diagnosis and treatment of faecal incontinence.

SUMMARY

Faecal incontinence is the involuntary passage of stools through the anus. The prevalence rates of faecal incontinence in the world vary from 0.7%–11%. Obstetric and operative injuries account for most cases of incontinence. Incontinence is common with ageing and debilitation.

A detailed history and clinical examination is important with special emphasis on vaginal delivery and any complications (Figure 19.1). On per rectum examination, assess resting tone and squeeze tone. Investigations include flexible sigmoidoscopy, which is mandatory, endoanal ultrasound, anal manometry and pudendal nerve terminal motor latency.

The mainstays of medical treatment are diet, perineal exercises and anti-diarrhoeal drugs. There have been good results with biofeedback training. Operative procedures include overlapping sphincteroplasty and sacral nerve stimulation.

FURTHER READING

Kalantar JS, Howell S, Talley NJ. Prevalence of faecal incontinence and associated risk factors; an underdiagnosed problem in the Australian community? Med J Aust 2002; 176(2):47–8.

Madoff RD, Parker SC, Varma MG, et al. Faecal incontinence in adults. Lancet 2004; 364:621–32.

Norton C. Behavioral management of fecal incontinence in adults. Gastroenterology 2004; 126(1 Suppl 1):S64–70.

Rao SS. Pathophysiology of adult fecal incontinence. Gastroenterology 2004; 126(1 Suppl 1):S14–22.

Wald A. Clinical practice. Fecal incontinence in adults. N Engl J Med 2007; 356:1648–55.

Chapter 20

RECTAL BLEEDING AND HAEMORRHOIDS

KEY POINTS

Rectal bleeding:

- Initial management of massive rectal bleeding always involves assessment and resuscitation.

- Colonoscopy, radiolabelled red cell scan, selective mesenteric angiography, and computed tomography angiography can be used to identify the site of bleeding. Angiographic embolisation can stop localised bleeding. In stable patients, capsule endoscopy is useful to detect vascular lesions.

- On-table gastroscopy, colonoscopy, and enteroscopy should be considered if the site of massive rectal bleeding is in doubt. Partial or total colectomy may be required if bleeding is not controlled.

Haemorrhoids:

- First-degree haemorrhoids do not prolapse, second degree prolapse on defecation but return spontaneously, third degree prolapse but require manual reduction, and fourth degree prolapse and are not reducible.

- Conservative treatment includes advice to avoid prolonged straining and fibre supplementation. Injection sclerotherapy and rubber band ligation are the two most common interventional treatment options for first- and second-degree haemorrhoids. Haemorrhoidectomy is usually reserved for third- and fourth-degree haemorrhoids.

RECTAL BLEEDING

Causes

Bleeding per rectum can originate from the stomach, duodenum, small intestine, colon or anorectum (Table 20.1). The diagnosis of colorectal neoplasia should be entertained in most cases: 1 in 20 patients over the age of 45 years of age who present with new onset rectal bleeding have colon cancer. The colour of the blood may indicate the source of the bleeding but the rate of bleeding

TABLE 20.1: Causes of rectal bleeding

Region	Causes
Anorectum	• Haemorrhoids • Anal fissure • Rectal prolapse/solitary rectal ulcer • Anal fistula • Anal varices • Anal cancer
Colonic	• Diverticular disease • Angiodysplasia • Colitis (inflammatory, ischaemic, infective, pseudomembranous, radiation) • Neoplasia/polyp • Post-polypectomy/anastomosis bleeding
Other (stomach, small intestine)	• Upper gastrointestinal sources (peptic ulcer, erosions, Mallory-Weiss tear, oesophagitis, varices, neoplasia) • Small intestine angiodysplasia • Meckel's diverticulum and ulcer

needs to be taken into account. Haematochezia is the passage of bright red blood per rectum and usually indicates bleeding from the distal colon, rectum or anal canal. Dark red blood mixed in with bowel motions usually originates from the small intestine or proximal colon. Melaena, the passage of black tarry stools with characteristic odour, occurs with bleeding proximal to the ligament of Treitz.

Other symptoms are useful to help localise the site of bleeding. Epigastric pain, heartburn and haematemesis or melaena are symptoms associated with bleeding from the upper gastrointestinal tract. Significant weight loss is associated with malignancy and inflammatory bowel disease. Change in bowel habit, tenesmus (feeling of incomplete evacuation) and blood mixed in with faeces are consistent with colonic pathology. Bloody diarrhoea indicates the possibility of colitis. Bright red rectal bleeding not mixed with faeces, blood on the toilet paper and anal pain or discharge are symptoms more indicative of an anorectal source. Personal and family history of colonic polyps, cancer and inflammatory bowel disease are important to elicit.

The site and cause of bleeding can be identified by appropriate investigations such as proctoscopy, sigmoidoscopy, colonoscopy and upper endoscopy. In stable patients, capsule endoscopy is useful to detect vascular lesions. Small intestine endoscopy is worth considering in difficult diagnostic cases with recurrent bleeding (e.g. double-balloon enteroscope).

Causes of massive rectal bleeding

Common causes of massive rectal bleeding include colonic diverticular disease and angiodysplasia. Diverticula in the colon are caused by increased intraluminal pressure together with segmentation of the colon resulting in herniation of mucosa through the muscle wall. Bleeding from diverticular disease is usually a large amount because it results from direct trauma to the adjacent penetrating vessels. It is uncommon for patients to present with diverticulitis and bleeding because the pathogenesis of the two is different. Diverticulitis results from micro-perforation of colonic diverticula. The inflammation is located on the outside of the colon with minimal intraluminal involvement. Ischaemic colitis is a more likely diagnosis if a patient presents with abdominal pain, fever, and rectal bleeding. Angiodysplasia are venous ectasia at the submucosal level and are more frequently found in the right side of the colon. They can be treated with electrocautery or argon plasma coagulation.

Other less common causes include colorectal cancer, colitis, Meckel's diverticulum, small intestine angiodysplasia and upper gastrointestinal sources. Bleeding from radiation proctitis can be treated with sucralfate enemas, topical formalin or argon plasma coagulation. Bleeding associated with Meckel's diverticulum is due to ulceration secondary to heterotopic gastric mucosa. Bleeding from an upper gastrointestinal source can be the cause of haematochezia in 10%–15% of cases.

Management

Management of rectal bleeding is shown in Figure 20.1. Initial management involves assessment and resuscitation. Any clotting abnormalities and other medical conditions should be corrected and optimised. Any evidence that the bleeding may be coming from the upper gastrointestinal tract should be looked for.

Bleeding stops spontaneously in most cases. Intervention is required for continual bleeding. Colonoscopy (after rapid cleansing in 12 hours), radiolabelled red cell scan, selective mesenteric angiography and computed tomographic angiography can be used to identify the site of bleeding. Red cell scan and angiography can localise the site of bleeding if it is faster than 0.5–1 mL/minute. Colonoscopic intervention or angiographic embolisation can be used to stop bleeding if an active site is identified. A Meckel's scan (^{99}Tc pertechnetate) can be useful in younger patients to exclude a bleeding Meckel's diverticulum from ectopic gastric mucosa.

In cases where preoperative localising information is available via a red cell scan or angiographic embolisation is unsuccessful, partial colectomy can be performed. However if the patient

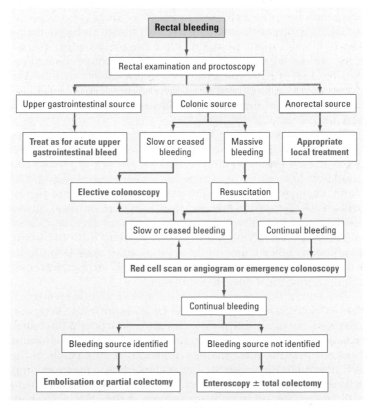

FIGURE 20.1: Management of rectal bleeding.

remains haemodynamically unstable despite resuscitation and if preoperative localising studies have not been performed, total colectomy may be required as a last resort. On-table gastroscopy and colonoscopy should be considered if the site of bleeding is in doubt. Intraoperative enteroscopy may be required if there are any concerns that the site of bleeding is from the small intestine.

HAEMORRHOIDS

Haemorrhoids are vascular cushions of submucosal tissue in the right anterior, right posterior and left lateral positions. They keep the anal canal closed to prevent flatus incontinence. They become symptomatic when these cushions prolapse out secondary to degeneration of the supportive suspensory (Treitz) muscles—the sliding anal lining theory. The haemorrhoidal cushions derive a rich blood supply from the superior, middle and inferior rectal arteries with venous drainage via the corresponding veins. Prolapse leads to impediment of the venous drainage from the haemorrhoid by anal closure on the rectal tributaries. This results in engorgement of the haemorrhoid making it difficult to reduce, which predisposes to thrombosis.

Bleeding and prolapse are the most common symptoms. Haemorrhoids are classified according to degree of prolapse. First-degree haemorrhoids do not prolapse, second-degree prolapse on defecation but return spontaneously, third-degree prolapse but require manual reduction and fourth-degree prolapse and are not reducible. Other symptoms include discomfort or pain, mucus discharge and itch. Bleeding is usually bright red in colour (from arteriovenous communications) and is separate from the stools. The blood is noted either on the toilet paper or splattered on the toilet bowl. These symptoms are not specific for haemorrhoids and other investigations may be required.

The dentate line separates internal haemorrhoids from external haemorrhoids. Thrombosis of external haemorrhoids (otherwise called perianal haematomas) most commonly occurs from repeated trauma to the anal verge associated with a diarrhoeal illness. If a patient presents early, the best treatment is evacuation of the clot after infiltration with local anaesthesia. If the presentation is delayed for more than five days, then conservative management with analgesia is sufficient because most of the pain would have abated by then. Patients may be left with a residual anal skin tag.

Treatment

Fibre for the treatment of haemorrhoids

Treatment of haemorrhoids depends on the frequency and severity of symptoms. Conservative treatment includes advice to avoid prolonged straining, increased fluid intake and fibre supplementation. Fibre increases bowel frequency as well as faecal bulk. A meta-analysis of randomised trials showed a beneficial effect of fibre in the treatment of symptomatic haemorrhoids. However, fibre supplementation does not improve the degree of prolapse and can cause bloating.

Drug treatment of haemorrhoids

The prime objective of drug treatment is to control acute symptoms such as bleeding so that definitive treatment can be scheduled at a more convenient time. There are a number of drugs that are used in the treatment of symptomatic haemorrhoids (Table 20.2).

TABLE 20.2: Drug treatment of haemorrhoids	
Type	**Action**
Flavonoids	Improve venous tone and lymphatic drainage, reduce capillary hyperpermeability
Ginkgo	Increase venous tone and vessel wall resistance, decrease permeability, encourage venous blood return
Heparin sulfate	Normalisation of hyperaemia and mucoid secretions
Calcium dobesilate	Opposes breakdown of collagen, reduces blood hyperviscosity improving flow
Local application (nitrates, local anaesthetic preparations)	Nitrates reduce anal spasm via nitric oxide action. Local anaesthetic/corticosteroid/antibacterial combinations reduce pain and bleeding
Herbal and other extracts	Standardised blood leech extract reduces inflammation. Horse chestnut seed extract (aescin) fosters normal venous tone, improves venous flow, and is antiinflammatory. Other traditional remedies have astringent antiseptic, antiinflammatory and laxative properties

Micronised purified flavonoid fraction (MPFF) is an oral drug made up of 90% micronised diosmin and 10% flavonoids expressed as hesperidin. It improves venous tone and lymphatic drainage, and reduces capillary hyperpermeability by protecting the microcirculation from inflammatory processes. Trials have shown MPFF drugs to be effective in relieving acute symptoms (pain, inflammation, congestion, prolapse and use of analgesics and topical medications) as well as reducing the duration of bleeding.

Interventional treatment

Injection sclerotherapy and rubber band ligation are the two most common interventional treatment options for first- and second-degree haemorrhoids (Table 20.3). Injection sclerotherapy with phenol in almond oil causes fibrosis of the haemorrhoid at the submucosal level. Rubber band ligation involves ligation of haemorrhoidal tissue above the dentate line resulting in ischaemia of the banded tissue, with subsequent sloughing of the tissue in 7–10 days. A major secondary bleed can occur at this time if a large vessel is at the base of this banded tissue. The best treatment is to tamponade the bleeding site by insertion of a 50 mL balloon on an indwelling catheter and application of mild traction.

TABLE 20.3: Interventional treatment of haemorrhoids	
Type	**Action**
Injection sclerotherapy	Fibrosis at submucosal level
Rubber band ligation	Strangulation of haemorrhoids above dentate line and subsequent sloughing
Infrared coagulation, cryotherapy, and electrocautery	Tissue destruction and fibrosis at submucosal level
Haemorrhoidectomy	Excision of haemorrhoids with preservation of sphincters and skin/mucosal bridges
Stapled haemorrhoidopexy	Excision and stapling of circumferential rectal mucosal cuff above haemorrhoids to elevate prolapse and interrupt blood supply
Other treatment: HAL (haemorrhoidal artery ligation)	Ligate haemorrhoidal vessels with ultrasound guidance

Other complications include vasovagal syncope, pain and, rarely, sepsis. Rubber band ligation has been found to be more effective than sclerotherapy in a meta-analysis. Infrared coagulation and electrocautery cause tissue destruction and submucosal fibrosis.

Haemorrhoidectomy is usually reserved for third- and fourth-degree haemorrhoids. It involves surgical excision of the haemorrhoids with protection of the internal anal sphincter and preservation of mucosal and skin bridges between the wounds. The preservation of bridges prevents anal stenosis. Residual small haemorrhoids in these areas can be removed submucosally or left for future treatment, usually by rubber band ligation. The wounds can be left opened, closed or semi-closed by leaving the external portion of the skin wound open. Pain is the most common problem after this operation. The use of metronidazole has been shown in prospective, double-blind randomised trials to reduce pain after open haemorrhoidectomy but not with the closed operation.

New ways to treat haemorrhoids have been devised. The LigaSure™ (Valleylab) instrument uses bipolar diathermy and the Harmonic Scalpel® (Johnson & Johnson) relies on high frequency ultrasonic waves to seal blood vessels. Less blood loss and postoperative pain may occur with these new techniques. Stapled haemorrhoidopexy involves resuspending the internal haemorrhoids by excising a circumferential cuff of rectal mucosa proximal to the dentate line with a circular stapler. Complications of this technique include bleeding, faecal urgency, residual skin tags, incontinence and sepsis. Haemorrhoidal artery ligation involves direct ligation of haemorrhoidal vessels localised by an endoanal Doppler ultrasound.

SUMMARY

Rectal bleeding can originate from the stomach, duodenum, small intestine, colon or anorectum. Colorectal neoplasia should be considered and excluded particularly in any patient over the age of 40 years.

The site and cause of bleeding can be identified by appropriate investigations. Common causes of massive rectal bleeding include colonic diverticular disease and angiodysplasia. Ischaemic colitis should be considered if the patient presents with abdominal pain, fever and rectal bleeding.

Initial management involves assessment and resuscitation. Bleeding stops spontaneously in most cases. Intervention is required for continual bleeding.

Haemorrhoids are vascular cushions of submucosal tissue in the right anterior, right posterior and left lateral positions. Bleeding and prolapse are the most common symptoms. Haemorrhoids are classified according to degree of prolapse. The prime object of drug treatment is to control acute symptoms such as bleeding. Drugs used include micronised purified flavonoid fraction (MPFF) and calcium dobesilate and local applications. Injection sclerotherapy and rubber band ligation are the two most common interventional treatment options. Haemorrhoidectomy is usually reserved for third- and fourth-degree haemorrhoids.

FURTHER READING

Alonso-Coello P, Guyatt G, Heels-Ansdell D, et al. Laxatives for the treatment of hemorrhoids. Cochrane Database Syst Rev 2005; 4: CD004649.

Brandt LJ. Bloody diarrhea in an elderly patient. Gastroenterology 2005; 128:157–63.

du Toit J, Hamilton W, Barraclough K. Risk in primary care of colorectal cancer from new onset bleeding: 10 year prospective study. Brit Med J 2006; 333:69–70.

Farrell JJ, Friedman LS. Review article: the management of lower gastrointestinal bleeding. Aliment Pharmacol Ther 2005; 21:1281–98.

Hewett PJ, Maddern GJ. Haemorrhoids: evidence? ANZ J Surg 2004; 74:679–80.

Misra MC, Imlitemsu. Drug treatment of haemorrhoids. Drugs 2005; 65(11):1481–91.

Chapter 21

ANAL PAIN

KEY POINTS

- The differential diagnosis of anal pain includes anal fissure, abscess and proctalgia fugax. Haemorrhoids rarely cause pain unless they are complicated by thrombosis.
- Patients with thrombosed external haemorrhoids (perianal haematoma) present with severe pain associated with a tense bluish lump adjacent to the anal verge.
- Patients with perianal haematoma present with severe pain and a tense bluish lump adjacent to the anal verge.
- Thrombosed internal haemorrhoids can occur when prolapse becomes irreducible. Conservative treatment involves bed rest, elevation, ice, analgesia and aperients.
- When an anal fissure is not situated in the posterior or anterior positions, a secondary aetiological factor such as Crohn's disease, infection or malignancy should be considered.
- Proctalgia fugax is a benign fleeting pain in the perineum that often wakes patients.
- Pruritus ani results in distressing itching and excoriation around the anus.

CAUSES OF ANAL PAIN

There are many causes of anal pain (Table 21.1). Patients usually attribute anal pain to haemorrhoids. However, haemorrhoids rarely cause pain unless they are complicated by prolapse and thrombosis. There is usually some delay in presentation because of patient embarrassment. A thorough history and careful examination can usually elicit the diagnosis without need for further investigations (Figure 21.1). Occasionally, other investigations are required and may include examination under anaesthesia, biopsy and pathological analysis, sigmoidoscopy, endoanal ultrasound and magnetic resonance imaging (MRI).

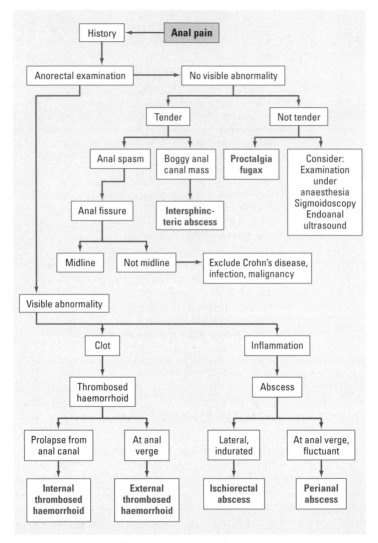

FIGURE 21.1: Diagnosis of anal pain.

TABLE 21.1: Causes of anal pain	
Frequency	**Causes**
Common	• Anal fissure • Anorectal abscess/fistula • Thrombosed external haemorrhoid • Thrombosed internal haemorrhoid • Proctalgia fugax • Pruritus ani • Postoperative (anal procedures)
Infrequent	• Rectal prolapse • Foreign body • Faecal impaction • Hidradenitis suppurativa • Crohn's disease • Low pilonidal abscess • Bartholin's abscess
Rare	• Anal tumours (squamous cell carcinoma, melanoma, Bowen's disease, Paget's disease, basal cell carcinoma) • Rectal cancer • Tumours of pelvic bones or organs (prostate, cervix, vulva, vagina or urethra) • HIV and other sexually transmitted infections • Tuberculosis and actinomycosis

Anal fissure

Anal fissure is caused by a tear in the mucosa of the anal canal, usually from a hard stool. It causes anal pain worse on defecation, lasting for several hours and associated with a small amount of bright red rectal bleeding. Physical examination may reveal the triad of internal anal papilloma, anal fissure and external sentinel skin tag. Sphincter muscle is present in the base of the fissure. Of all anal fissures, 90% are located in the posterior region, 5% in the anterior region and 5% in other areas. When an anal fissure is not situated in the posterior or anterior positions, a secondary aetiological factor (e.g. Crohn's disease, infection or malignancy) should be entertained. Delay in healing of anal fissures has been attributed to impaired blood supply, demonstrated on ultrasound Doppler studies and postmortem studies.

Conservative treatment with addition of aperients, increased fibre and fluid intake and warm baths after each bowel motion is effective. The addition of topical ointments can help relieve pain. Topical glyceryl trinitrate has been shown in some studies to promote healing by its effect on nitric oxide to enhance sphincter muscle relaxation. Botulinum toxin and other drugs (e.g. calcium antagonists) have been used with varying success.

Lateral internal anal sphincterotomy is the most effective surgical treatment for anal fissures. However there is a risk for future incontinence because some sphincter muscle is divided. It is unclear how much internal anal sphincter needs to be divided: some surgeons advocate division to the height of the fissure and others advocate minimal division. Posterior internal anal sphincterotomy and anal dilatation are rarely performed now because of the risk of keyhole deformity and uncontrolled sphincter tears, respectively. Other surgical options include fissurectomy (excising the edges of the fissure to stimulate healing) and advancement flaps to cover the defect.

Anorectal abscess/fistula

Anorectal abscess results from infection in the anal glands, which are situated in the intersphincteric plane. The infection can spread downwards to present a perianal abscess, laterally to present as an ischiorectal abscess, upwards rarely to present as a supralevator or pelvic abscess, or remain to present as an intersphincteric abscess. Symptoms include throbbing pain, sometimes associated with fever or swelling. Perianal abscesses are situated adjacent to the anal verge and are usually fluctuant. Fever and other constitutional symptoms may be absent. Ischiorectal abscesses usually present as a more indurated infection lateral to the anal verge and are frequently associated with systemic toxicity. Intersphincteric abscesses are frequently missed unless a rectal examination is performed and a tender boggy mass is palpated.

The treatment for anorectal abscesses is incision and drainage. Antibiotics are not always required. Pus drained should be sent for microbiological analysis. If skin organisms are cultured, there is minimal chance of recurrence. If enteric organisms are cultured, there is a 50% chance of developing a fistula and recurrent symptoms.

Anal fistula is a tract from the anal canal to the perianal skin. They are classified as intersphincteric, transsphincteric (most common), suprasphincteric and extrasphincteric. Patients with anal fistulas present with persistent discharge of pus and/or blood from the external opening. If the external opening closes over, recurrent abscess formation will occur. Assessment of anal fistulas includes identifying the internal and external openings, the primary track, secondary extensions, and other associated diseases.

Treatment of anal fistula involves defining the anatomy, draining associated sepsis, eradicating the fistula, preventing recurrence and preserving continence. The best treatment of low anal fistulas is fistulotomy. Fistulotomy involves laying open the fistula tract to allow healing by secondary intention. If the fistula is high, more sphincter muscle is involved and division would result in incontinence. Females are at higher risk of faecal incontinence because they have shorter anal sphincter lengths than males and may have sustained occult obstetric sphincter injuries. There are many operations available for high fistula-in-ano, each with varying cure and incontinence rates (Table 21.2). The best treatment is probably mucosal advancement flap, which has high cure and low incontinence rates.

TABLE 21.2: Treatment options for high anal fistulas

Treatment	Cure rate	Incontinence rate
Mucosal advancement flap	60%	5%
Draining seton	20%	<1%
Fibrin glue/plug	20%	<1%
Cutting seton	95%	Up to 30%
Fistulotomy	95%	Up to 30%
Anocutaneous flap	60%	5%
Fistulectomy	55%	Up to 30%

Thrombosed external haemorrhoids

Thrombosed external haemorrhoids or perianal haematomas result from a sudden increase in venous pressure or direct trauma usually from diarrhoea. Patients present with severe pain associated with a tense bluish lump (haematoma) adjacent to the anal verge. If the patient presents in the first few days, the best treatment is evacuation of the clot under local anaesthesia. If the presentation is delayed, it is often better to leave it untreated because pain would have largely subsided by then. Patients are usually left with a residual anal tag if it is untreated.

Thrombosed internal haemorrhoids

Thrombosed internal haemorrhoids can occur when prolapse becomes irreducible and the sphincter muscles restrict venous return. This can involve one haemorrhoid or be circumferential. This condition is not uncommon during pregnancy. Treatment is either conservative or surgical excision. Conservative treatment involves bed rest, elevation, topical ice to reduce swelling, analgesia and aperients. The aim of conservative treatment is to reduce the swelling and allow return of the prolapse and natural dissolution of the clot. Subsequent treatment may only require rubber band ligation of the offending haemorrhoid. Surgical excision is sometimes required during the acute event. This requires a general anaesthesia and a formal haemorrhoidectomy. Drainage under local anaesthesia is ineffective.

Proctalgia fugax

Proctalgia fugax is a sharp, deep stabbing, fleeting pain in the perineum that often wakes patients from sleep. Duration ranges from several minutes to one hour. It is more common in young men. The aetiology is unknown but may be related to spasm of the pelvic floor or internal sphincter muscle. The history is typical and simple reassurance is often sufficient. Treatment aims to relax the pelvic floor or internal sphincter. Warm baths, topical nitrates, calcium antagonists and botulinum toxin have been used for treatment.

Pruritus ani

Pruritus ani results in distressing itching around the anus and results in excoriation of the skin secondary to scratching. The causes include systemic conditions, local anal pathology and psychological disturbances (Table 21.3). Certain drugs and foods can precipitate symptoms. Drugs such as colchicine and quinidine have been implicated. Foods that induce histamine release have also been implicated, including caffeine, milk, beer, tomato and lemon.

Local causes should be identified and treated. If no cause is readily identifiable, the patient should be reassured and simple

TABLE 20.3: Causes of pruritus ani	
Systemic	• Diabetes mellitus • Jaundice • Leukaemia • Aplastic anaemia • Thyroid disease • Renal failure
Local	• Haemorrhoids • Anal fissure • Anal fistula • Loose stool (incontinence/diarrhoea) • Anal tumours (malignant or premalignant) • Drug reaction • Dermatological conditions (psoriasis, dermatitis) • Infections (sexually transmitted infections, bacterial, fungal, scabies)

measures taken to alleviate the symptoms. Exacerbating foods should be avoided and a high fibre diet instigated. Simple hygiene is important with removal of any particles after bowel movements with warm water or baths (not wiping with toilet paper). Use of soap should be avoided because its slightly alkaline pH can react with the slightly acidic environment of the perianal skin. Prolonged use of topical ointments should be avoided. Loose cotton underwear may ameliorate symptoms. In severe intractable cases, subcutaneous injection of methylene blue has been used to anaesthetise the skin.

SUMMARY

Patients usually attribute anal pain to haemorrhoids. However haemorrhoids rarely cause pain unless they are complicated by prolapse and thrombosis. A detailed history and careful examination can usually elicit the diagnosis.

Anal fissure is caused by a tear in the anal canal mucosa. Treatment is with aperients, increased fibre and fluid intake and warm baths. Lateral internal anal sphincterotomy is the current surgical treatment of choice.

Anorectal abscess results from infection in the anal glands. Symptoms include throbbing pain associated with fever or swelling.

Anal fistula is a tract from the anal canal to the perianal skin. Treatment involves defining the anatomy, draining associated sepsis, eradicating the fistula and preserving continence.

Perianal haematoma results from a sudden increase in venous pressure or trauma. Patients present with severe pain and a tense bluish lump adjacent to the anal verge.

Thrombosed internal haemorrhoids can occur when prolapse becomes irreducible. Treatment is either conservative or haemorrhoidectomy. Conservative treatment involves bed rest, elevation, ice, analgesia and aperients.

Proctalgia fugax is a benign fleeting pain in the perineum that often wakes patients from sleep.

Pruritus ani results in distressing itching and excoriation around the anus. Causes include systemic conditions and anal pathology. Simple hygienic approaches can often provide relief.

FURTHER READING

Bharucha AE, Wald A, Enck P, et al. Functional anorectal disorders. Gastroenterology 2006; 130:1510–18.

De Parades V, Etienney I, Bauer P, et al. Proctalgia fugax: demographic and clinical characteristics. What every doctor should know from a prospective study of 54 patients. Dis Colon Rectum 2007; 50:893–8.

Steele SR, Madoff RD. Systemic review: the treatment of anal fissure. Aliment Pharmacol Ther 2006; 24:247–57.

Rickard MJ. Anal abscesses and fistulas. ANZ J Surg 2005; 75:64–72.

Zuccati G, Lotti T, Mastrolorenzo A, et al. Pruritus ani. Dermatol Ther 2005; 18:355–62.

Chapter 22

HIV/AIDS: GASTROINTESTINAL AND LIVER MANIFESTATIONS

KEY POINTS

- In acquired immunodeficiency syndrome (AIDS), reduction in oral intake is a critical factor in malnutrition and cachexia. Nutritional supplementation is important in treatment and comprises appetite stimulants, enteral alimentation and total parenteral alimentation.

- The CD4 lymphocyte count facilitates the assessment of chronic diarrhoea. If the CD4 lymphocyte count is <200/mm³ (μ/L), check for *Cryptosporidium*, *Microsporidium* and *Clostridium difficile*. If <100/mm³, check for cytomegalovirus infection and *Mycobacterium avium* infection. Panendoscopy will increase the diagnostic yield if stool tests are negative.

- The spectrum of hepatobiliary disease includes viral hepatitis and opportunistic infections.

- In the presence of hepatobiliary disease, a CD4 count of >500/mm³ suggests a liver-specific process. If the CD4 cell count is <200/mm³ it suggests that the liver is involved as part of a systemic opportunistic infection.

- AIDS cholangiopathy presents with upper abdominal pain and diarrhoea; endoscopic retrograde cholangiopancreatography is diagnostic.

INTRODUCTION

Acquired immunodeficiency syndrome (AIDS) has become a pandemic, resulting in 25 million deaths and 40 million persons infected with the AIDS virus. The disease prevalence is particularly high in developing countries. The enormity of the problem is highlighted in the sub-Saharan African continent, which represents only 10% of the world's population, but constitutes 77% of AIDS deaths.

Clinical advances have evolved in consonance with a greater understanding of the virologic and immunologic markers of disease stage, mechanisms of viral transmission and the problem of viral resistance to antiretroviral drugs. Gastrointestinal and hepatobiliary complications are important components of the HIV/AIDS syndrome. They are common and affect most patients with AIDS during the course of their illness.

MALNUTRITION AND CACHEXIA

Survival in AIDS patients is strongly associated with nutritional status. Weight loss is a cardinal feature of AIDS. The factors contributing to weight loss include anorexia, inadequate oral intake, intestinal malabsorption and alterations in metabolism and endocrine dysfunction.

Reduction in oral intake allied to anorexia is a critical factor in weight loss. Malnutrition also has deleterious effects on the immune system. Careful assessment of the patient and the diagnosis, with treatment of systemic illness or upper gastrointestinal disease, usually results in weight gain.

Nutritional supplementation in the form of appetite stimulants and enteral alimentation often leads to a greater feeling of well-being. Total parental nutrition may be indicated in some cases.

CHRONIC DIARRHOEA

Because of the wide spectrum of potential infections that may cause diarrhoea (Table 22.1), it is appropriate to have a systematic approach in investigating the aetiologic agent/s (Figure 22.1; Table 22.2). Weight loss and diarrhoea suggest an opportunistic infection, malabsorption or small bowel bacterial overgrowth. Severe watery diarrhoea suggests cryptosporidiosis. Diarrhoea with nausea and abdominal pain may indicate *Giardia*, *Isospora belli* or *Mycobacterium avium*. Rectal bleeding may indicate viral or bacterial colitis or Kaposi's sarcoma.

A clinical caveat is to assess whether the patient is at risk for an opportunistic infection. The CD4 lymphocyte count is critical to answer the question (see Figure 22.1). If the CD count is less than $100/mm^3$ (μ/L), opportunistic infections are probable.

Appropriate tests on faeces can facilitate a diagnosis. The initial laboratory investigation is an assessment of microscopy, culture

TABLE 22.1: Common causes of diarrhoea in AIDS	
Protozoa	*Microsporidium; Cryptosporidium; Isospora belli, Giardia lamblia, Blastocystis hominis; Pneumocystis carinii; Entamoeba histolytica*
Bacteria	*Mycobacterium tuberculosis; Mycobacterium avium* complex (MAC); *Clostridium difficile; Salmonella, Shigella, Campylobacter*
Viruses	Cytomegalovirus; herpes simplex; adenovirus; rotavirus
Fungi	Candidiasis; *Cryptococcus*; Histoplasmosis; Coccidioidomycosis
Neoplasms	Lymphoma, Kaposi's sarcoma
Drug-induced	HIV protease inhibitors
Idiopathic	AIDS enteropathy
Pancreatic disease	Pancreatitis; infectious pancreatitis; drug-induced pancreatitis

and parasites. Three sampling tests are recommended. If the CD4 lymphocyte count is <200/mm^3, then check for cryptosporidia, microsporidia and *Clostridium difficile*. Blood cultures should be done in febrile patients with a CD4 <100/mm^3, including mycobacteria.

Patients are at risk for cytomegalovirus (CMV) when the CD4 count <100/mm^3. The diagnosis is established by doing a mucosal biopsy at endoscopy.

The risk for small intestine *Mycobacterium avium* infection is increased when the CD4 count is <100/mm^3. Duodenal biopsy is required to establish the diagnosis. However, if blood cultures are positive for mycobacteria, biopsy is unnecessary and antimicrobial therapy should be initiated. Table 22.3 lists treatment options for diarrhoea as a result of specific pathogens.

Drug-induced diarrhoea due to the highly active antiretroviral treatment (HAART) regimen is frequent but is usually mild. If no cause of diarrhoea is found, symptomatic therapy is indicated.

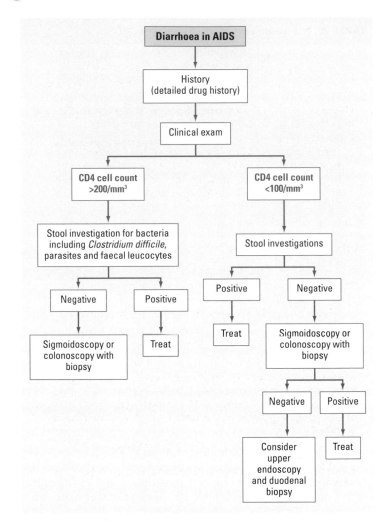

FIGURE 22.1: Assessment of diarrhoea in AIDS.

Based on Wilcox CM. AIDS and the gut. In: Weinstein WM, Hawkey CJ, Bosch J, eds. Clinical gastroenterology and hepatology. Philadelphia: Mosby; 2005:8331–6, with permission.

TABLE 22.2: Assessment of diarrhoea in AIDS

- History including detailed drug history
- Physical examination
- Stool specimen for bacterial culture: *Salmonella, Shigella, Campylobacter*
- Stool assay for *Clostridium difficile* toxin
- Examination for parasites and faecal leucocytes: 3–6 separate specimens including acid fast stain
- Endoscopy:
  - If rectal bleeding or faecal leucocytes are present, flexible sigmoidoscopy or colonoscopy with colon biopsies
  - If diarrhoea and weight loss persist and above evaluation is negative, then upper endoscopy including small bowel biopsy

TABLE 22.3: Treatment of diarrhoea

Protozoa: treatment duration 14–28 days
- Microsporidia: albendazole; metronidazole, atovaquone
- Cryptosporidia: paromomycin
- *Isospora belli:* ciprofloxacin or pyrimethamine or sulfamethoxazole/trimethoprim
- *Cyclospora:* sulfamethoxazole/trimethoprim or ciprofloxacin

Bacteria
- *Mycobacterium tuberculosis:* isoniazid, rifampicin, pyrazinamide, ethambutol. Treatment duration: 9–12 months
- *Mycobacterium avium* complex (MAC): multidrug regimen—combinations of clarithromycin, azithromycin, ethambutol, amikacin, ciprofloxacin. Treatment duration: 9–12 months
- *Salmonella, Shigella, Campylobacter:* fluoroquinolone. Treatment duration: 10–14 days
- *Clostridium difficile:* vancomycin, metronidazole. Treatment duration: 14 days

Viruses
- Cytomegalovirus: ganciclovir, foscarnet, cidifovir. Treatment duration: 14–28 days
- Herpes simplex: aciclovir. Treatment duration: 5–10 days

TABLE 22.3: Treatment of diarrhoea *(continued)*

Fungi
- Histoplasmosis: amphotericin B for 14 days; then chronic suppression with itraconazole
- Coccidioidomycosis: amphotericin B then fluconazole. Treatment duration: 28 days
- Cryptococcus: amphotericin B; then fluconazole. Treatment duration: 28 days

N.B. Prior to the advent of HAART, diarrhoea occurred in 90% of AIDS patients. However, with the inception of HAART, diarrhoea is still frequent but is most often drug-induced or caused by disorders unrelated to HIV infection.

HEPATOBILIARY DISEASE

The diagnosis of liver disease should encompass history, physical examination, liver tests and CD4 lymphocyte count (Figure 22.2).

Table 22.4 details the spectrum of hepatobiliary disease in AIDS. Opportunistic infections and neoplasms usually involve the liver secondarily through lymphohaematogenous dissemination. Therefore, initial evaluation of blood or bone marrow specimens may provide important information towards a diagnosis.

Hepatitis B, C and D viruses commonly coinfect with HIV and treatment with interferon results in a poor response. It is appropriate to screen HIV-positive patients for hepatitis B and C infection.

With regard to CMV infection, hepatitis and biliary tract disease may be manifestations of the infection. Another important cause of liver function test abnormalities is drug-induced liver injury. The drugs involved include antiretroviral (highly active antiretroviral treatment or HAART) medications, isoniazid, rifampin and trimethoprim-sulfamethoxazole.

Causes of hepatobiliary disease depend on the extent of immunocompromise. If the CD4 count is >500/mm^3, hepatic complications usually represent liver specific processes. When the CD4 cell count is <200/mm^3, then the liver is usually involved as part of a systemic opportunistic infection due to *M. avium* complex, fungi or CMV.

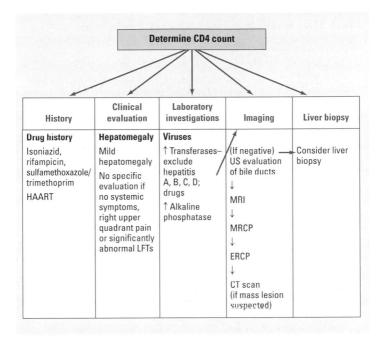

FIGURE 22.2: Evaluation of hepatobiliary disease in AIDS.

CT = computed tomography; ERCP = endoscopic retrograde cholangiopancreatograph; HAART = highly active antiretroviral treatment; LFTs = liver function tests; MRCP = magnetic resonance cholangiopancreatography; MRI = magnetic resonance imaging; US = ultrasound.

Imaging provides further opportunities for establishing a diagnosis. Ultrasonography is a non-invasive imaging procedure for evaluation of the biliary system. Other tests that can be used include magnetic resonance imaging (MRI), magnetic resonance cholangiopancreatography (MRCP) and endoscopic retrograde cholangiopancreatography (ERCP). CT scan is indicated if a mass lesion is suspected.

Liver biopsy should be considered in patients in whom a treatable cause of parenchymal liver disease is suspected, and when blood cultures and other non-invasive tests do not reveal a cause.

TABLE 22.4: Spectrum of hepatobiliary disease in AIDS	
Hepatobiliary disease	**Example**
Viral hepatitis	Hepatitis A, B, C and D, cytomegalovirus, Epstein-Barr virus, herpes simplex virus, human immunodeficiency virus
Opportunistic infections	*Mycobacterium avium* complex (MAC), *Cryptosporidium*, *Candida albicans*, *Mycobacterium tuberculosis*, *Coccidioides immitis*, *Pneumocystis carinii*, *Cryptococcus neoformans*, *Histoplasma capsulatum*
AIDS cholangiopathy	Acalculous cholecystitis, sclerosing cholangitis, papillary stenosis, lymphoma of the biliary tree, Kaposi's sarcoma
Neoplasms	Kaposi's sarcoma, non-Hodgkin's lymphoma
Drug-induced hepatitis	

AIDS cholangiopathy presents with epigastric or right upper quadrant pain as well as diarrhoea. It can result in four types of pathology:

1 Papillary stenosis with dilatation of the common bile duct
2 Sclerosing cholangitis
3 A combination of papillary stenosis and sclerosing cholangitis
4 A long extrahepatic stricture formation.

The CD4 count is usually below $100/mm^3$. Typically alkaline phosphatase and gamma-glutamyl transpeptidase are elevated, but these can be normal in 20% of cases. ERCP is diagnostic. If cholangitis or jaundice develops, sphincterotomy at ERCP is helpful.

TREATMENT OF HIV

Initiation therapy is recommended in all symptomatic persons and in asymptomatic persons after the CD4 cell count falls below $350/mm^3$ and before it declines to $200/mm^3$. A non-nucleoside reverse transcriptase inhibitor or a protease inhibitor boosted with low-dose ritonavir each combined with two nucleoside (or nucleotide) reverse transcriptase inhibitors is recommended with choice based on the individual patient profile. Therapy should be changed when toxicity or intolerance mandate it, or in the event of treatment failure. The virologic target for patients with treatment failure is a plasma HIV-1 RNA level below 50 copies/mL.

SUMMARY

Gastrointestinal and hepatobiliary complications are important components of the HIV/AIDS syndrome, and affect most patients with AIDS during the course of their illness. Anorexia is a frequent risk factor for weight loss, which is a cardinal feature of AIDS. Chronic diarrhoea is frequent. If the CD4 lymphocyte count is less than 100/mm^3, opportunistic infections are probable.

Hepatitis B, C and D viruses commonly coinfect with HIV, and treatment with interferon results in a poor response. It is appropriate to screen HIV-positive patients for hepatitis B and C infection. Drug induced injury is an important cause of liver function test abnormalities. If the CD4 cell count is >500/mm^3, hepatic complications usually represent liver-specific processes whereas a CD4 cell count <200/mm^3 usually indicates that the liver is involved as part of a systemic opportunistic infection.

FURTHER READING

Campbell MS, Reddy RK. HIV and the liver. In: Friedman LS, Keefe EB, eds. Handbook of liver disease. 2nd edn. Philadelphia: Churchill Livingstone; 2006:317–27.

Hammer SM, Saag MS, Schechter M. Treatment of adult HIV infection: 2006 recommendations of the International AIDS Society–USA Panel. JAMA 2006; 296:827–43.

UNAIDS/WHO. AIDS epidemic update: December 2005. Report. Online. Available: http://www.unaids.org/epi/2005/doc/report.asp

Wilcox CM, Rabeneck L, Friedman S. AGA technical review: malnutrition and cachexia, chronic diarrhea, and hepatobiliary disease in patients with human deficiency virus infection. Gastroenterology 1996; 111:1724–52.

Wilcox CM. AIDS and the gut. In: Weinstein WM, Hawkey CJ, Bosch J, eds. Clinical gastroenterology and hepatology. Philadelphia: Mosby; 2005:8331–6.

Chapter 23

OCCULT GASTROINTESTINAL BLEEDING AND IRON DEFICIENCY ANAEMIA

KEY POINTS

- The source of gastrointestinal bleeding is undetected in up to 30% of patients in whom adequate and timely gastroscopy and colonoscopy have been performed.

- Gastrointestinal bleeding may present obviously with melaena, haematemesis or haematochezia, but may also present more subtly, with iron deficiency anaemia, with or without blood in the stools.

- Occult gastrointestinal bleeding may be intermittent or continuous and range from oozing to massive bleeding.

- Most causes of occult gastrointestinal bleeding derive from the small intestine.

- In patients aged 40 years or younger, small intestine tumours, Meckel's diverticulum, polyposis syndromes and Crohn's disease are more common causes of occult gastrointestinal bleeding. In patients over 40 years of age, arteriovenous malformation, neoplasia and Dieulafoy's malformation are more common causes.

- The most common cause of occult small intestinal bleeding, accounting for 80% of cases, is arteriovenous malformation or angiodysplasia.

- Coeliac disease is the most common cause of malabsorption in the Western world and frequently presents with iron deficiency anaemia.

- Non-steroidal antiinflammatory drugs may cause small intestinal inflammation, which may, in turn, result in blood loss.

This chapter concentrates on unexplained or occult gastrointestinal bleeding from the upper gastrointestinal tract and small intestine.

CLINICAL PRESENTATION

If bleeding is overt, patients may present with melaena or haematochezia. Most patients do not have overt bleeding and are observed to have iron deficiency anaemia of varying severity. Some patients are profoundly anaemic, but others may have a more subtle persistent anaemia. Depending on the severity and the rapidity of onset of anaemia, some patients complain of significant lethargy. If the gastrointestinal bleeding is more acute, patients may present with signs and symptoms of hypovolaemia and shock.

AETIOLOGY

Most causes of occult gastrointestinal bleeding derive from the small intestine. In patients aged 40 years or younger, small intestine tumours, Meckel's diverticulum, polyposis syndromes and Crohn's disease are more common. In patients over 40 years of age, arteriovenous malformation (the most common cause overall), neoplasia and Dieulafoy's malformation are more prevalent. Some of the specific causes of gastrointestinal bleeding are listed below.

Arteriovenous malformations

Arteriovenous malformations (AVMs) or angiodysplasias are idiopathic, discrete vascular lesions. AVMs are classically described as occurring in the right colon, but they also occur in the stomach and small intestine. They are the most common cause of small intestinal bleeding, accounting for 80% of cases. The cause of angiodysplasias is not known but they occur with increased frequency in the elderly and in association with other chronic medical conditions such as chronic renal failure, valvular heart disease (particularly aortic stenosis, although this is controversial), scleroderma, von Willebrand's disease and chronic pulmonary disease.

Bleeding may be occult or severe. The most common presentation is with haematemesis or melaena. The diagnosis of gastric AVMs is made with upper endoscopy and in the small intestine using capsule endoscopy. The lesions are bright red and well circumscribed and they may be flat or raised. It is frequently difficult to determine whether a visualised AVM is the actual bleeding site. Generally, evidence for bleeding is required, as indicated by active bleeding from the lesion or an affixed clot.

Treatment of AVMs focuses on controlling bleeding. Therapeutic endoscopy with a thermal probe or laser therapy is the accepted first-line therapy. Angiographic therapy with Gelfoam embolisation is also appropriate when bleeding is severe and cannot be controlled endoscopically.

Cameron erosions

Linear gastric erosions located at or near the level of the neck of a large diaphragmatic hernia are referred to as Cameron erosions. The diagnosis is made endoscopically following a thorough examination of the hiatal hernia sac. Patients with Cameron ulcers present with acute upper gastrointestinal bleeding (haematemesis or melaena) or chronic blood loss (faecal-occult-blood-test-positive stools or iron deficiency anaemia). The pathogenesis of these lesions is postulated to involve mechanical trauma; with respiratory excursions, the gastric mucosa at the level of the

TABLE 23.1: Aetiology of occult gastrointestinal bleeding	
Hiatal hernia Cameron erosions	*Small intestine* • Portal hypertensive intestinal vasculopathy • Neoplasias (leiomyoma, leiomyosarcoma, carcinoma) • Crohn's disease • Arteriovenous malformation (angiodysplasia) • Aorto-enteric fistulas • Radiation ileitis • Meckel's diverticulum • Polyposis and Peutz-Jeghers syndrome • Medication-induced mucosal lesions (non-steroidal antiinflammatory drugs) • Jejunal diverticula • Adenocarcinoma • Carcinoid tumours
Stomach • Portal hypertensive gastropathy • Dieulafoy's disease • Gastric antral vascular ectasia (GAVE; watermelon stomach) • Arteriovenous malformation (AVM; angiodysplasia)	
Biliary tree Haemobilia (trauma or stone)	
Pancreas Aneurysm (haemosuccus pancreaticus)	*Colon* Arteriovenous malformation (angiodysplasia)

neck of the hernia rub against adjacent mucosa. The mainstay of medical treatment is acid suppressive therapy. If blood loss is severe or persistent, or if the ulceration of hernia is complicated, surgical repair of the hernia should be considered.

Gastric antral vascular ectasia

Gastric antral vascular ectasia (GAVE), or watermelon stomach, results from ectatic mucosal and submucosal capillaries. Typically, patients present in their 70s (age range 50–90 y) with occult or slow gastrointestinal bleeding. Endoscopically, GAVE appears most commonly as raised, convoluted, red antral folds radiating in a spoke-like pattern towards the pylorus. This appearance of GAVE has been likened to the stripes on a watermelon rind. A more diffuse involvement of the stomach is also recognised in which many ectasias coalesce to form a large red lesion resembling honeycomb.

Endoscopic thermal ablation therapy using heater probes or Argon plasma coagulator is accepted first-line therapy for control of gastrointestinal bleeding due to GAVE. Treatment coagulates the lesion, with success rates of 90% achievable.

Portal hypertensive gastropathy

Portal hypertensive gastropathy (PHG) is a vascular disorder, which is recognised to be a complication of advanced liver disease. Although its pathogenesis is directly related to portal hypertension, the exact mechanisms involved in the development of this condition remain unclear. On endoscopy, the characteristic lesion is a mosaic pattern of small, raised erythematous areas outlined by a white or yellowish reticular pattern resembling that of snakeskin. PHG is more commonly localised to the proximal stomach.

Mild PHG is generally of no clinical significance and can be considered an incidental endoscopic finding in patients with portal hypertension. In contrast, severe PHG is associated with a high risk of gastrointestinal bleeding. Bleeding characteristically presents as chronic mucosal oozing with the development of iron deficiency anaemia, but may occasionally be acute.

The treatment of PHG consists of addressing the underlying portal hypertension. Unlike variceal bleeding, this condition cannot be treated with band ligation. Effective treatment requires a reduction in portal pressure. This can be accomplished with β-blockers, such as propranolol, portal decompression using radiological placement of a transjugular, portosystemic intrahepatic shunt, or surgical shunting. Somatostatin infusion is routine first-line treatment for actively bleeding cirrhotic patients with PHG.

Dieulafoy's disease

Dieulafoy's disease is characterised by a bleeding or clot-bearing artery protruding into the intestinal lumen, usually without ulceration. It occurs mostly in the stomach, usually on the lesser curvature and within 6 cm of the cardio-oesophageal junction. The disease is thought to be caused by an area of necrosis in an unusually large artery with a relatively superficial location in the gastric submucosa. The appearance is that of a tiny necrotic spot with or without a slightly protruding vessel stump, with minimal or no surrounding erosion. While bleeding is usually significant, producing haematemesis and/or melaena, the condition is nevertheless notoriously difficult to diagnose. Quite often, multiple endoscopies are necessary before the lesion is recognised. Treatment consists of endoscopic local injections of adrenaline 1:10,000 and coagulation using heat probes.

Small intestine neoplasms

Small intestine neoplasms are rare. Although the small intestine provides about 80% of the luminal surface area of the entire alimentary canal, only 2% of alimentary cancers involve this anatomical site. Nevertheless, small intestine tumours account for 5%–10% of all cases of small intestinal bleeding. Patients with small intestine tumours are generally younger. Small intestine tumours may present with chronic blood loss and, overall, are the second most common cause of occult small intestinal bleeding. Early use of endoscopy, capsule endoscopy and radiological evaluation is essential to make a preoperative diagnosis.

Benign small intestine tumours are more common than malignant tumours. Of these, the leiomyomas are most frequently associated with bleeding. Frequently, abdominal pain and nausea are associated presenting symptoms. Leiomyomas are diagnosed endoscopically and, in recent times, increasingly using capsule endoscopy. Arteriography demonstrates a well circumscribed tumour blush in most lesions. Treatment for all symptomatic leiomyomas is surgical resection, because they are macroscopically indistinguishable from malignant leiomyosarcomas. Adenomas are the most common mucosal tumour of the small intestine, typically occurring in the periampullary region. Bleeding may occur in large polypoid lesions. All adenomas should be removed, usually endoscopically, because of the risk that they may progress to carcinoma. Other small intestine tumours such as carcinoids, adenocarcinomas, lymphomas and metastatic disease can also present with chronic blood loss.

Malignant small intestinal tumours account for less than 2% of all gastrointestinal cancers. Adenocarcinomas are the most common type of malignant small intestine neoplasm and may present with occult gastrointestinal bleeding as well as abdominal pain and weight loss. Most adenocarcinomas are diagnostically accessible by gastroscopy, push enteroscopy or capsule endoscopy. Metastatic lesions in the small intestine (e.g. from malignant melanoma, carcinoma of the lung and renal carcinomas) can present with chronic blood loss.

Peutz-Jeghers syndrome

Peutz-Jeghers syndrome is a dominantly inherited disorder characterised by mucocutaneous pigmentation and gastrointestinal hamartomas. It is important to consider this diagnosis in young patients with unexplained gastrointestinal bleeding. Polyps are generally small (<1 cm), but can grow larger and cause occult gastrointestinal bleeding. There is an increased risk of malignancy arising from the polyps. The polyps may be visualised endoscopically but, because they are usually multiple, endoscopic polypectomy is not possible and segmental surgical resection should be performed.

Aorto-enteric fistulas

Aorto-enteric fistulas are a rare source of chronic blood loss but frequently present with massive haemorrhage, usually in the form of haematemesis, melaena or haematochezia. Consequently, this condition is life-threatening. Think about this possibility in anyone who has had an aortic graft or a diagnosed aortic aneurysm. Most fistulas communicate with the third or fourth portion of the duodenum. Fistulas may be primary and associated with aneurysms, or secondary, following aortic reconstructive surgery. Characteristically, the bleeding is intermittent, often starting with a 'herald bleed' and subsequently (usually within 1–3 weeks) presenting with an exsanguinating haemorrhage. Ultimately the diagnosis is made at laparotomy, although endoscopic visualisation with upper endoscopy or push enteroscopy and aortography can make the diagnosis in up to 50% of cases.

Meckel's diverticulum

Meckel's diverticulum of the terminal ileum occurs in about 2% of the population and is located 100 cm from the ileocaecal valve. It is the cause of bleeding in two-thirds of men under the age of 30 years presenting with small intestine bleeding. The ectopic gastric epithelium within the diverticulum may lead to peptic ulceration of the diverticulum, with consequent haemorrhage. Bleeding is invariably brisk. The diverticulum is identified by means of a technetium-99m pertechnetate scan. Parietal cells in the ectopic gastric mucosa take up the radioisotope. A superior mesenteric arteriogram may help identify the anomaly.

Jejunal diverticula

Jejunal diverticula can cause small intestine bleeding. These are acquired pseudodiverticula that develop on the mesenteric border of the intestine at sites of perforating blood vessels. Although they may give rise to gastrointestinal bleeding, jejunal diverticula are mostly an incidental finding on a small bowel series. Nevertheless, when bleeding does occur it is usually massive and associated with a mortality rate as high as 20%.

Coeliac disease

Coeliac disease is the most common cause of malabsorption in the Western world and frequently presents with iron deficiency anaemia. This condition is discussed in more detail in the chapter on malabsorption syndromes.

Crohn's disease

Gross bleeding is unusual in Crohn's disease—occurring in 4%–10% of patients with ileitis. Transmural inflammation can erode submucosal vessels, causing massive bleeding at times. Usually the patients do not present with bleeding as the sole symptom.

Treatment-induced mucosal lesions

Non-steroidal antiinflammatory drugs may cause small intestinal inflammation, ulceration and web-like structures, which, if sufficiently severe, may result in blood loss presenting as haemoccult-positive stools and iron deficiency anaemia. Such medication-induced mucosal lesions are best diagnosed with capsule endoscopy.

Radiation injury to the small intestine can cause vasculitis and subsequent bleeding. Since the ileum is most frequently affected, this condition is often referred to as radiation ileitis.

Haemobilia

Haemobilia is a rare cause of obscure gastrointestinal tract bleeding. The term describes any bleeding originating in the liver, biliary tree or pancreas and passing through the ampulla of Vater. Haemobilia usually follows abdominal trauma, surgical treatment of biliary disease or liver biopsy. Gastroscopy may reveal obvious bleeding from the ampulla of Vater. Angiography can confirm haemobilia, since it permits visualisation of the hepatic artery and its branches. Vascular tumours and aneurysms may require surgical intervention or selective angiographic embolisation using Gelfoam coils.

Haemorrhage through the pancreatic duct, or haemosuccus pancreaticus, is an uncommon cause of gastrointestinal bleeding. Patients present with haematemesis or melaena in combination with epigastric pain and hyperamylasaemia. The source of bleeding is secondary to an aneurysmal bleed from a splenic artery aneurysm. The diagnosis is made angiographically.

INVESTIGATION OF UNIDENTIFIED GASTROINTESTINAL BLEEDING

The discussion is based on the premise that the patient has already had a gastroscopy and colonoscopy, which have not been able to identify the source of bleeding (see Table 23.2).

Laboratory studies

Initially, it is routine to request a full blood count to evaluate the degree of anaemia, coagulation parameters to exclude associated coagulopathy, and clinical chemistry to evaluate renal function. There is a higher prevalence of AVM in patients with renal failure.

Small bowel series and enteroclysis

Positive findings on routine small bowel series are rare in patients presenting with bleeding of obscure origin. While Crohn's disease is often diagnosed with the use of this standard examination, only around 5% of small bowel follow-through examinations detect an intestinal bleeding site. Overall, therefore, a small bowel series is regarded as a poor test for elucidating the source of occult gastrointestinal bleeding.

Enteroclysis can increase the yield from small bowel radiography to 10%. In this procedure, a tube is positioned radiographically in the duodenum and a mixture of barium, air, water or methylcellulose is instilled. The radiographs obtained are comparable to double-contrast studies of the colon. This technique has a greater chance of demonstrating intraluminal pathology than single-column barium radiography of the small bowel. Diagnosis of angiodysplasias cannot be made on barium radiographic studies. Increasingly, small intestine barium studies are being done with the assistance of computed tomography (CT) and magnetic resonance imaging (MRI) scanning technologies in an effort to obtain better results.

Nuclear scans

Radioisotope bleeding scans may be diagnostic when bleeding is distal to the ligament of Treitz. Their ready availability, low cost and absence of complications have led to universal acceptance. In technetium-99m-labelled bleeding scans, red blood cells are labelled either in vitro or in vivo with a radionuclide tag. During an acquisition period of 1–2 hours, detection of as little as 5 mL of intraluminal blood is considered a 'positive' scan. Another advantage of red blood cell scans is that erythrocytes have an intravascular half-life of 24 hours, thereby permitting sequential scans.

Although radionuclide scanning can confirm haemorrhage originating in the small intestine segments distal to the ligament of Treitz, it does not accurately detect the exact location of the bleeding.

A Meckel's scan using technetium-99m pertechnetate is used to identify a Meckel's diverticulum.

Angiography

Angiography can detect bleeding at a rate of 0.5 mL/min and can localise a site of bleeding in 50%–70% of patients with massive haemorrhage. However, the yield decreases to around 25% when active bleeding has slowed or stopped. In addition to demonstrating active bleeding, angiography can diagnose non-bleeding lesions such as angiodysplasias and small bowel tumours. When haemorrhage is active, the site of bleeding is usually identified rapidly by technetium-labelled red blood cell scan and/or mesenteric angiography. If no diagnosis can be made, and the patient continues to bleed profusely, exploratory surgery is sometimes essential. Intraoperative enteroscopy is frequently performed initially as an aid to making a diagnosis.

Enteroscopy

Small intestine enteroscopy is performed most often using push enteroscopy, a technique in which a flexible endoscope is passed orally under direct vision into the more distal small bowel in a manner similar to that used in conventional gastroduodenoscopy. The depth of insertion allows excellent visualisation of about 50% of the small intestine mucosa. In addition to its diagnostic capabilities, push enteroscopy offers the possibility of endoscopic treatment of bleeding lesions and access to tissue specimens. Lesions that may be detected by this technique include AVMs, ulcerative jejunitis and small intestine tumours.

Intraoperative enteroscopy is an alternative. Some perform an enterotomy, through which an endoscope is placed. With the advent of video-endoscopy, both the surgeon and the endoscopist can see the intraluminal view.

Capsule endoscopy

The development of capsule endoscopy (CE) has been a significant advance that has allowed for more complete evaluation of the small intestine. The capsule is a disposable, 27 mm × 11 mm video capsule containing its own optical dome, light source, batteries, transmitter and antenna and is swallowed with water after a 12 h fast. It captures 2 images per second, and has a battery life of approximately 8 hours. Images are transmitted to a data recorder via digital radio frequency communication, and downloaded to a workstation computer, where it can be read by a gastroenterologist.

The capsule is propelled via peristalsis through the gastrointestinal tract, capturing about 55,000 digital images and is excreted in the faeces. CE has become an important investigative tool in patients with occult gastrointestinal bleeding, suspected small intestine tumours and other abnormalities. Its interplay with the new technique of double balloon enteroscopy enables the small intestine to receive proper attention, similar to other parts of the gastrointestinal tract.

Double-balloon enteroscopy

Double-balloon enteroscopy (DBE) is a new endoscopic tool that allows both the diagnostic workup of small bowel diseases and also makes it possible to carry out therapeutic interventions. DBE enables visualisation of the entire small intestine and also allows for interventional therapy in the small intestine. This method can be used from either an oral or an anal insertion.

TABLE 23.2: Diagnostic tips

- Patients who present with massive haemorrhage require prompt hospital referral whereas those with anaemia and faecal occult blood test-positive stools can be investigated as outpatients
- Routine studies in patients with unidentified gastrointestinal bleeding include a full blood count, coagulation parameters and clinical chemistry to evaluate renal function
- A small bowel series is generally a poor test for elucidating the source of occult gastrointestinal bleeding
- Radioisotope bleeding scans are readily available, inexpensive, have a low complication rate and may be diagnostic when bleeding is distal to the ligament of Treitz; their disadvantage is that they do not accurately detect the exact location of the bleeding
- Angiography can localise a site of bleeding in 50%–70% of patients with massive haemorrhage but the yield decreases to around 25% when active bleeding has slowed or stopped
- Capsule endoscopy is now regarded as the most accurate and useful diagnostic test to investigate the small bowel, particularly where no cause for blood loss has been detected with a gastroscopy and colonoscopy
- Push enteroscopy is used to evaluate the small intestine in patients with unexplained gastrointestinal bleeding. Double balloon enteroscopy is increasingly being utilised as an investigative tool in unexplained iron deficiency. This form of endoscopy permits the complete visualisation of the small bowel and has the advantage of allowing targeted therapeutic interventions. It is usually used when capsule endoscopy has identified a specific lesion in the small intestine that warrants endoscopic therapeutic intervention
- Exploratory surgery, often with intraoperative enteroscopy, may be essential if a diagnosis can be made and profuse bleeding continues

---

SUMMARY

Patients presenting with obscure gastrointestinal haemorrhage represent a difficult diagnostic and management problem. This patient group frequently requires sophisticated investigations in an effort to make a specific diagnosis. Patients with anaemia and faecal occult blood test-positive stools can be investigated as outpatients (Figure 23.1). However, patients who present with massive haemorrhage certainly require prompt hospital referral for resuscitation and further investigation (Figure 23.2). When gastroscopy and colonoscopy fail to identify a source of bleeding, it may be necessary to investigate the small intestine. While radiological techniques are still frequently utilised, the advances in technology such as capsule endoscopy and double-balloon enteroscopy are now incorporated into clinical practice.

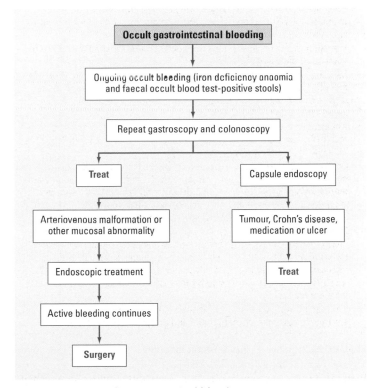

FIGURE 23.1: Occult gastrointestinal bleeding.

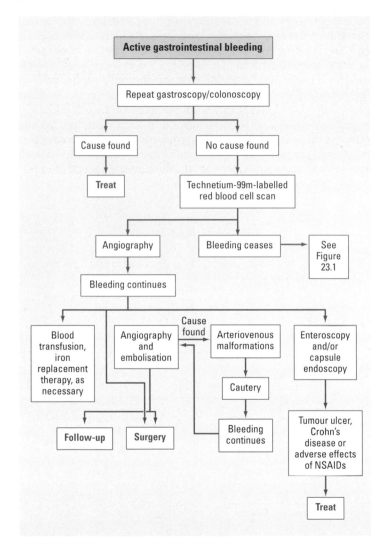

FIGURE 23.2: Active gastrointestinal bleeding.
NSAIDs = non-steroidal antiinflammatory drugs.

FURTHER READING

Carey EJ, Leighton JA, Heigh RI, et al. A single-center experience of 260 consecutive patients undergoing capsule endoscopy for obscure gastrointestinal bleeding. Am J Gastroenterol 2007; 102:89–95.

Eliakim AR. Video capsule endoscopy of the small bowel (PillCam SB). Curr Opin Gastroenterol 2006; 22:124–7.

Martins NB, Wassef W. Upper gastrointestinal bleeding. Curr Opin Gastroenterol 2006; 22:612–19.

May A, Nachbar L, Pohl J, et al. Endoscopic interventions in the small bowel using double balloon enteroscopy: feasibility and limitations. Am J Gastroenterol 2007; 102:527–35.

Rockey DC. Occult gastrointestinal bleeding. Gastroenterol Clin North Am 2005; 34:699–718.

Chapter 24

WEIGHT LOSS

KEY POINTS

- Weight loss is defined as >5% loss of usual body weight over a period of 6–12 months.
- Body mass index (BMI) is defined as body weight in kg divided by height in metres squared (kg/m^2).
- Weight loss in elderly people is largely caused by a reduction in food intake and contributes to morbidity and mortality.
- Potential causes of weight loss are strongly influenced by the age at presentation.
- A cause for weight loss can be established in at least 75% of patients.
- Management is determined by the cause. Depression is the most common treatable cause.

INTRODUCTION

The major influences on body weight are caloric intake, intestinal absorption and utilisation. The purpose of this chapter is to outline an approach to the diagnosis and management of weight loss, particularly in adults.

An important message is the need for greater attention to undernutrition as a cause of weight loss. In the elderly, weight loss is strongly associated with functional decline and mortality.

Definitions

In research studies, weight loss may be defined as a weight loss of >5% of usual body weight over a period of 6–12 months. Weight loss >10% is usually associated with protein–energy malnutrition while weight loss >20% implies severe protein–energy malnutrition and significant organ dysfunction. One quantitative measure of nutritional status is that of body mass index (BMI). This is defined as body weight in kg divided by height in metres squared (kg/m^2). A BMI lower than 17 is consistent with undernutrition. Other anthropometric measures include arm circumference and triceps skin fold thickness, but these are affected, at least to some extent, by skin changes associated with ageing.

Prevalence

Features of undernutrition or significant weight loss have been documented in at least 10% of elderly patients attending outpatient clinics, 25% of elderly inpatients needing acute care and 40% of patients in nursing homes and other institutions.

PATHOPHYSIOLOGY

The weight loss that occurs with ageing is largely caused by a reduction in food intake. This has been attributed to a variety of factors including age-related losses in taste and smell, age-related decreases in opioid receptors and enhanced sensitivity to the satiating effects of cholecystokinin. Other factors may include changes in the secretion of leptin and sex hormones and age-related changes in intestinal absorption, sometimes mediated by changes in gastrointestinal motility. In the setting of acute and chronic disease, anorexia and weight loss can be caused by a variety of factors including ill health, weakness and side effects from medication. Some of these effects may be mediated by elevated levels of cytokines such as interleukins and tumour necrosis factor and by elevated levels of corticotrophin-releasing factor. At a practical level, at least 20% of inpatients in acute hospitals have a nutrient intake of <50% of their calculated maintenance energy requirements.

CAUSES OF WEIGHT LOSS

Potential causes of weight loss are strongly influenced by the age at presentation. For example, in young adults, unintentional weight loss is often due to psychiatric disorders such as depression, anorexia nervosa, bulimia, psychoses and substance abuse. In contrast, weight loss in the elderly is often due to multiple factors including social isolation, bereavement, dementia, depression, poor dentition and side effects from drugs. In middle age, there may be a greater contribution from cancer, alcoholism, endocrine disorders and chronic inflammatory disorders. Cancer is diagnosed in up to 25% of patients with weight loss over the age of 50 years. Some of the factors that contribute to weight loss are outlined below and are summarised in Figure 24.1.

- *Anorexia*. Many acute and chronic disorders are associated with a decrease in appetite. These include infections, cancer, peptic ulceration, renal impairment, liver disease, alcoholism and cardiac failure. Anorexia can also be a side effect of medication.
- *Oral disorders*. Eating may be impaired by oral factors such as absent or ill fitting dentures, dental decay, periodontal disease and a dry mouth. The latter can be caused by an age-related reduction in salivary secretion, Sjögren's syndrome and side effects from drugs with anticholinergic activity.
- *Swallowing disorders*. Swallowing may be impaired by weakness in pharyngeal muscles, by motility disorders of the oesophagus or by benign or malignant strictures of the oesophagus. Of these, the most common is pharyngeal weakness following a cerebrovascular accident.
- *Non-malignant gastrointestinal disorders*. This group includes disorders such as peptic ulceration, biliary disorders, chronic inflammatory bowel disease, coeliac disease, chronic pancreatitis and bacterial overgrowth in the small intestine.
- *Cancer*. The most common primary sites are colon, stomach, lung and pancreas.
- *Endocrine disorders*. These include thyrotoxicosis and hyperparathyroidism.
- *Miscellaneous causes*. These include chronic infections such as tuberculosis, lung abscess and osteomyelitis and chronic inflammatory disorders such as rheumatoid arthritis, systemic lupus erythematosus and polyarteritis nodosa.
- *Psychosocial factors*. Psychiatric disorders include depression, anorexia nervosa, bulimia, psychoses and drug addiction. Dementia is also important and may be aggravated by social isolation, bereavement, poverty and insufficient assistance with feeding.

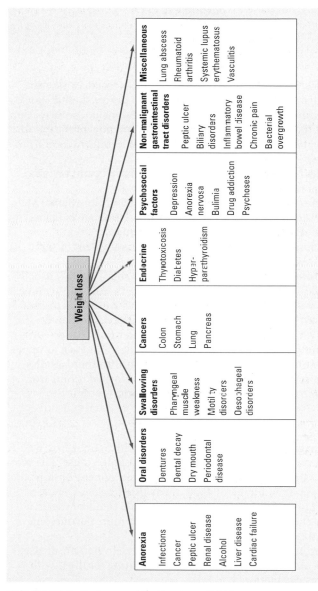

Anorexia	Oral disorders	Swallowing disorders	Cancers	Endocrine	Psychosocial factors	Non-malignant gastrointestinal tract disorders	Miscellaneous
Infections	Dentures	Pharyngeal muscle weakness	Colon	Thyrotoxicosis	Depression	Peptic ulcer	Lung abscess
Cancer	Dental decay	Motility disorders	Stomach	Diabetes	Anorexia nervosa	Biliary disorders	Rheumatoid arthritis
Peptic ulcer	Dry mouth	Oesophageal disorders	Lung	Hyperparathyroidism	Bulimia	Inflammatory bowel disease	Systemic lupus erythematosus
Renal disease	Periodontal disease		Pancreas		Drug addiction	Chronic pain	Vasculitis
Alcohol					Psychoses	Bacterial overgrowth	
Liver disease							
Cardiac failure							

Weight loss

FIGURE 24.1: Factors contributing to weight loss.

ASSESSMENT

A cause for weight loss can be established in at least 75% of patients. This is achieved by history, physical examination and a limited number of targeted diagnostic studies.

- *History:* should include documentation of weight loss and a detailed review of symptoms relevant to cancer, mental illness and gastrointestinal disease. It should also include information about diet, use of alcohol, prescription and non-prescription medication, social details and, if applicable, information from care-givers.
- *Physical examination*: focus on the oral cavity and on areas commonly affected by cancer.
- *Psychosocial tests*: may include the Folstein Mini-Mental State Exam, depression questionnaires and questionnaires related to nutrition, depending on the clinical setting.
- *Functional evaluation*: may include an assessment of sight, gait, hearing and ability to self-care.
- *Laboratory evaluation*: screening laboratory tests will usually include a blood count, chemistry profile, thyroid stimulating hormone (TSH), urine tests and a chest X-ray. A low plasma albumin can reflect severe protein deficiency. Additional tests will be influenced by symptoms and results from screening studies but may include investigations such as upper gastrointestinal endoscopy, colonoscopy, ultrasound studies and computed tomography (CT) scans. Normal results from screening tests should be highly reassuring.

MANAGEMENT

The management of individual patients with weight loss will be largely determined by the established or presumed cause. The most common treatable cause is depression. Management options that may increase the intake of food are as listed below.

- *Diet*. Food intake may increase with more frequent meals, a wider choice in foods or by making food more flavoursome and attractive.
- *Assistance with meals*. This can include delivered meals (e.g. Meals on Wheels) and assistance with eating for those with various disabilities.

- *Oral nutritional supplements*. A variety of supplements are available that appear to be helpful in at least undernourished older people.
- *Micronutrient supplements*. Multivitamin supplements are of potential but unproven benefit. Thiamine supplements should be provided for alcoholics and individual patients may need supplements of folic acid, and vitamins B_{12}, C and D.
- *Enteral feeding*. This should be considered when swallowing is difficult or unsafe. Feeds can be provided by fine-bore nasogastric tubes or by gastric or jejunal tubes after percutaneous endoscopic gastrostomy (PEG).
- *Drugs for anorexia and nausea*. A variety of drugs have been used for anorexia including corticosteroids, progestogens, serotonin antagonists, anabolic agents and anticatabolic agents.

PROGNOSIS

High mortality rates have been observed in patients in nursing homes who lose 10% or more of body weight over 0.5–3 years. In relation to morbidity, malnourished patients in acute care hospitals have more complications, longer hospital stays and require longer periods of convalescence.

SUMMARY

The major influences on body weight are caloric intake, intestinal absorption and utilisation. Weight loss may be defined as weight loss of greater than 5% of usual body weight over a period of 6–12 months. BMI provides a quantitative measure of nutritional status. It is defined as body weight in kg divided by height in metres squared (kg/m^2). A BMI lower than 17 is consistent with undernutrition.

The weight loss that occurs with ageing is largely caused by a reduction in food intake. Up to 40% of patients in nursing homes and other institutions have features of undernutrition or significant weight loss.

The causes of weight loss include anorexia, oral disorders, swallowing disorders, cancer, endocrine disorders and psychosocial factors (Figure 24.1). A cause for weight loss can be established in 75% of patients.

Assessment should include history, clinical examination, psychosocial tests, functional evaluation and laboratory evaluation.

The various options available for treatment include diet, assistance with meals, nutritional supplements, micronutrient supplements, enteral feeding and drugs for nausea and vomiting.

High mortality rates have been observed in patients in nursing homes who lose 10% or more of body weight over 0.5–3 years.

FURTHER READING

Bouras EP, Lange SM, Scolapio JS. Rational approach to patients with unintentional weight loss. Mayo Clin Proc 2001; 76:923–9.

Gazewood JD, Mehr DR. Diagnosis and management of weight loss in the elderly. J Fam Pract 1998; 47:19–25.

Lankisch P, Gerzmann M, Gerzmann JF, et al. Unintentional weight loss: diagnosis and prognosis. The first prospective follow-up study from a secondary referral centre. J Intern Med 2001; 249:41–6.

Morley JE. Anorexia of aging: physiologic and pathologic. Am J Clin Nutr 1997; 66:760–73.

Rolland Y, Kim MJ, Gammack JK, et al. Office management of weight loss in older persons. Am J Med 2006; 119:1019–26.

Chapter 25

EATING DISORDERS: ANOREXIA NERVOSA

KEY POINTS

- Anorexia nervosa (AN) is characterised by a refusal to maintain a healthy body weight; resistance to gain weight, an intense fear of gaining weight, disturbance in the way in which shape or weight is experienced and denial of the seriousness of an individual's current low body weight.
- Assess carefully for protein–calorie restriction.
- Medical complications can include non-alcoholic steatohepatitis.
- Refeeding syndrome may occur if calorie intake is increased too rapidly, leading to sudden death.
- The overall mortality of AN is 5%.

INTRODUCTION

Eating disorders have been the focus of increasing community and professional awareness in recent years. They form a heterogeneous group of illnesses that affect adults, adolescents and, more rarely, children. Anorexia nervosa (AN) is a specific eating disorder and the third most common chronic illness in adolescent females. It affects one in 200 girls between the ages of 15 and 19 years. Males develop AN less commonly, with the male to female ratio between 1:10 and 1:20. The increasing incidence of eating disorders and their impact on the health of a new generation of young people are of particular concern.

Clinicians need to think about eating disorders in patients presenting with weight loss, anorexia or malnutrition.

The key diagnostic features of AN are:

- Refusal to maintain a healthy body weight and resistance to weight gain. There can be a history of weight loss to less than 85% of expected weight for age, sex and height, or a failure to gain expected weight during a period of growth.

- An intense fear of gaining weight or becoming fat even though underweight.
- Disturbance in the way in which body shape or weight is experienced and reported, or denial of the seriousness of the current low body weight.
- Amenorrhoea in post-menarchal patients (i.e. the absence of at least three consecutive menstrual cycles).
  The subtypes of AN are:
- Restricting type—during the current episode the patient has not engaged in binge eating or purging behaviour (i.e. self-induced vomiting or the misuse of laxatives, diuretics or enemas)
- Binge-purge type—during the current episode the patient has regularly engaged in binge eating or purging behaviour, on at least three occasions a week, for at least 3 months.

ASSESSMENT

History

After noting the cause for presentation, it is important to take a full history of how the low weight has occurred. This includes the change in weight, particularly noting the maximum and lowest weights, or alternatively change in clothes size. It is important to inquire about dietary intake and eating or purging behaviour. Additionally, the amount and intensity of exercise regimens should also be recorded as a significant minority of patients with AN use strenuous exercising as a major strategy to manipulate their weight.

An inquiry should also be made as to how the patient perceives their body shape, weight and health. Body dissatisfaction—if the patients feels their body is fat or would want to change aspects of their body in which fat is deposited—should also be recorded.

Menstrual history, including the duration of amenorrhoea, and sexual history are important. Bone size and mineralisation are influenced by the duration of amenorrhoea as well the severity of malnutrition.

Family structure and history, as well as history of comorbid psychiatric or medical conditions, are also important information to record at the time of initial assessment.

Physical findings

The protein–calorie malnutrition (PCM) that accompanies AN affects every organ in the body. The clinical presentation may have a number of features in common with hypothyroidism (Table 25.1); mentation and locomotion are slowed, hypothermia, constipation, pretibial oedema may be present, however patients do not have a goitre and thyroid hormones (thyroid stimulating hormone [TSH] and thyroxine [T_4]) remain within normal parameters. Triiodothyronine (T_3; measured by radioimmunoassay) is depressed commensurate with the degree of PCM, and recovers with correction of the malnutrition.

TABLE 25.1: Medical differential diagnosis of anorexia nervosa

- Hypothyroidism
- Inflammatory bowel disease
- Type 1 and 2 diabetes
- Addison's disease
- Systemic lupus erythematosus
- Brain tumour

On initial inspection, the patient has a wasted appearance with lanugo (fine downy hair) present over the torso and limbs. There is often a generalised pallor with peripheral cyanosis. Capillary refill is delayed (more than 2 seconds). The hands are cool and peripheral pulses are slow and low in volume. Although the circulating volume and red cell mass is decreased, pallor is usually not observed in the palmar creases or conjunctiva. Blood pressure is maintained though there is often a postural drop in excess of 15 mmHg with moderate or severe protein–calorie malnutrition.

Heart sounds tend to be soft. Pericardial effusions are reported in severe PCM, and occur particularly in those patients with very low thyroid hormone (T_3).

The abdomen is scaphoid and skin over the anterior abdominal wall is lax. Muscles of the anterior abdominal wall are typically decreased permitting palpation of abdominal organs easily. An enlarged fatty liver (with a soft, smooth, non-tender lower border) is commonly detected. Stool in the sigmoid colon is also easily palpable in the left lower quadrant.

Oedema around the sacrum and pretibial areas may be present, though this usually occurs with refeeding rather than at initial presentation. Inspection of the feet is also important. The decreased peripheral circulation, particularly in patients who exercise excessively, may lead to signs of peripheral vascular insufficiency as well as poor hygiene (and a potential for sepsis).

Clinical findings may vary with patients who have more chronic AN and have adapted to the long standing PCM. These patients are haemodynamically compensated.

Investigations

Baseline investigations are useful in screening for micronutrient deficiencies as well as excluding differential diagnoses, particularly for atypical presentations. A low erythrocyte sedimentation rate (ESR) is typical of anorexia nervosa and distinguishes the eating disorder from malignancies, as well as inflammatory and autoimmune conditions.

Specific evaluation for micronutrient deficiency (e.g. iron, vitamins, trace elements) are unlikely to be clinically useful at initial evaluation.

- Blood tests
  - Full blood count
  - Erythrocyte sedimentation rate
  - Urea, electrolytes, creatinine
  - Liver function tests
  - Blood sugar level
  - Calcium, magnesium, phosphate
  - Follicle stimulating hormone, luteinising hormone, oestradiol
  - Thyroid stimulating hormone, thyroxine, triiodothyronine (measured by radioimmunoassay)
- Cardiac investigations
  - Electrocardiograph
- Imaging
  - Dual energy X-ray absorptiometry (DEXA)
  - Cerebral computed tomography

Criteria for medical admission

These criteria vary broadly.

- Weight and BMI (body mass index, kg/m²) are important indicators though evidence of medical instability is usually a prerequisite for inpatient admission.
- Alterations in vital signs are key indicators. Lowering of temperature (<35.5°C), heart rate (<40 beats/min) or blood pressure (<70 mmHg systolic, <40 mmHg diastolic) are commonly used cut points. Patients who have lost weight rapidly, but who are not at low weights (i.e. still above the 25th centile BMI) may present with alteration of vital signs, as with very low weight patients (i.e. <5th centile BMI).
- Disturbances in heart rhythm and electrical conduction, as well as heart rate, are criteria for admission. Prolongation of the QT corrected interval above 470 ms should be managed in an inpatient setting, with 450–470 ms being a 'grey zone'.
- Electrolyte disturbances from manipulation of weight by water loading, restriction or purging should also be managed through inpatient admission. Metabolic disturbance from comorbid illness, such as diabetes, should also be considered as criteria for medical admission.

RESUSCITATION

Medical stabilisation involves replacement of fluid, energy, electrolytes, protein and micronutrients; monitoring of vital signs; and containment of exercising or purging behaviours. Nasogastric feeding provides a practical and efficient means for fluid and nutrient replacement. Intravenous access may be required to manage acute fluid and electrolyte changes, or if there is any gastrointestinal disturbance.

Measures to support the circulation are of the highest priority as invariably neither the airway nor breathing is compromised. Care must be taken not to use fluid replacement routinely, as cardiac failure is relatively easily induced in patients with PCM by volume overload. In particular, for those patients who have been chronically malnourished (i.e. over 6 months) circulatory changes should be induced slowly; and the adaptive physiological changes producing a low volume, low pressure circulation corrected over several days to a week or so depending on the severity of the PCM at presentation.

A continuous infusion of energy is optimal, and periods of 'fasting' such as occur during overnight sleep avoided until vital signs can be maintained (see cut points indicated above). For patients with less than 1000 kcal intake prior to admission or those with severe PCM, caloric replacement should commence at ~1200 kcal per 24 hours. (This is estimated to be about 30% greater than resting energy expenditure.)

Strategies to maintain body temperature above 35.5°C such as space blankets or overhead heating are used.

Vitamin supplements are also commenced. There is great variability here with some units prescribing a multivitamin preparation and other units prescribing individual vitamins such as thiamine on admission. Supplementation of phosphate (e.g. sodium acid phosphate 500 mg) is recommended, particularly if serum levels are decreased on admission. The dose is empirically adjusted from serial measurements of serum phosphate.

Monitoring of vital signs should occur every 6 hours. Serial measurements of electrolytes, blood sugar and phosphate should continue daily until levels are within normal ranges. Mental state should also be assessed daily for mood symptoms as well as the development of delirium, associated with the refeeding syndrome, described below.

REFEEDING

Once medically stable, weaning of nasogastric feeds and increases in regular food can occur. Total daily energy content of regular food or nasogastric feeds should be gradually increased to around 2700 kcal. Increases of 500–1000 kcal per week can be safely made. Sudden death and delirium—the 'refeeding syndrome'—may occur if the increase in daily caloric intake is too rapid. A weight gain of one kilogram per week can be safely maintained. Patients who have a chronic or relapsing course with AN may be treated less aggressively. Maintaining the serum phosphate level above 1.0 mmol/L is recommended.

In addition to having sufficient energy, the daily intake needs to contain a balance of macronutrients. High-quality proteins are important for rebuilding lost lean tissue mass. It is also important that nutritional rehabilitation be supported by healthy (resistance) exercising. A supervised and graded programme offers potential benefit, though these have not been scientifically investigated to date.

MEDICAL COMPLICATIONS

The protein–caloric malnutrition that occurs with anorexia nervosa affects all body organs. Further medical complications arise from purging behaviours, such as vomiting, strenuous exercise and the use of laxatives, as well as other 'fat burning' strategies. The resultant effects on pubertal development, growth and bone mineralisation can have a profound effect on survivors.

Fluids and electrolytes

The cardinal feature associated with fluid and electrolyte disturbances in patients with eating disorders is intravascular volume contraction. Vital sign instability with abnormalities in heart rate and blood pressure and skin manifestations are more commonly seen. Serum sodium tends to be in the upper limit of normal range, and blood urea nitrogen (BUN) and creatinine are usually elevated, despite a low muscle mass.

Serum phosphate levels fall in a significant minority of patients during nutritional rehabilitation. Typically this occurs in the first week of refeeding, in over a quarter of patients. Hypophosphataemia is the hallmark of the refeeding syndrome, a well known complication of nutritional rehabilitation in anorexia nervosa.

Endocrine

Delayed puberty is one of the cardinal features of anorexia nervosa during adolescence. It is defined as deviating two standard deviations (SD) below the mean for age and gender.

The presence of amenorrhoea in an adolescent female should prompt the clinician to evaluate other possible causes for this situation. Pregnancy, even though a rare event in a young female with anorexia nervosa, needs to be excluded by obtaining a detailed clinical history including health risk behaviour and, more specifically, sexuality issues.

Amenorrhoea is considered one of the clinical criteria to establish the diagnosis, by DSM-IV criteria. Secondary amenorrhea is hypothalamic in origin, and it is due in part to suppression of the hypothalamic–pituitary–gonadal axis. Other factors include stress, the additive effects of malnutrition, weight loss, starvation and strenuous exercise. A weight of approximately 90% of standard body weight (50th centile for age, sex and height), on average, is required for resumption of menses to occur, and serum oestradiol levels at follow-up best track this process. However, the weight at which an individual patient with anorexia nervosa may resume menses is variable. The use of ancillary methods such as measures of body composition and serum oestradiol may be used to predict this significant landmark in the treatment of patients with eating disorders.

Bone

Up to 50% of bone mass is attained during adolescence in females and 67% for males. The timing of peak bone mineral content velocity and menarche were closely related and followed peak height velocity by approximately a year.

Osteopenia and bone health improves with nutritional rehabilitation, weight restoration and the return to a normal physiology of the endocrine-skeletal homeostasis. To date the gold standard method to evaluate bone mass as it relates to tissue composition is dual energy X-ray absorptiometry (DEXA).

Prevention of osteopenia and optimising bone growth and mineralisation in adolescents with anorexia nervosa may be achieved by a two-track approach. Firstly, with nutritional rehabilitation through weight restoration (promoting development of the muscle-bone unit) and, secondly, by facilitating resumption of normal menstrual physiology. Moderation in weight-bearing exercise should be encouraged, and resistance exercising promoted.

Cardiovascular

Mortality rates associated with eating disorders are noted to be the highest among psychiatric disorders, with sudden death resulting from ventricular dysrhythmias being responsible for up to 50% of deaths. The increase in body weight and basal metabolic rate place a considerable strain on the cardiovascular system. Additional stress is placed on the myocardium as a result of electrolyte abnormalities, hypothermia and autonomic nervous system instability. These changes in association with hypophosphataemia are recognised as the refeeding syndrome, and account for the mortality seen in early nutritional rehabilitation in anorexia nervosa.

Haematological

Bone marrow hypoplasia and its implications in this population have been described. In children and adolescents with anorexia nervosa, the most commonly seen haematological changes include normal or marginally low haemoglobin and haematocrit with abnormal erythrocyte indices, showing increased mean corpuscular volume (MCV), mean corpuscular haemoglobin (MCH), and mean corpuscular haemoglobin concentration (MCHC). These macrocytic changes are rarely associated with folate or vitamin B_{12} deficiency in this patient population; but need to be considered when present. Other abnormalities include leucopenia and thrombocytopenia. All of these changes are reversible with weight restoration and nutritional rehabilitation.

Microcytic, hypochromic anaemia due to iron deficiency is considered one of the most common nutritional deficiencies for growing adolescents, with a peak prevalence (3.5%–14.2%) between 11 and 19 years of age for both genders. Iron deficiency anaemia is rarely seen in the initial stages of anorexia nervosa in female patients. Low ESR is a common feature of malnourished patients with anorexia nervosa. This parameter may be used to aid in the differential diagnosis of anorexia nervosa from other ominous causes of malnutrition (infectious processes, chronic inflammatory and systemic illnesses).

Neurological
Abnormal enlargement of cortical sulci and subarachnoid spaces has been reported in anorexia nervosa. Cerebrospinal fluid volume is increased, and reductions in cerebral grey and white matter volumes have been described. In weight-recovered patients with anorexia nervosa, grey matter volume deficit, but not white matter changes, persist.

Renal
Impairment of renal function occurs in anorexia nervosa from pre-renal and renal factors. In the former, dehydration and low circulating blood pressure and volume contribute to the pre-renal effects. Persistent and severe protein calorie malnutrition results in a diffuse glomerular sclerosis. This is a non-reversible insult to the kidney leading to a progressive decline in glomerular filtration rate and eventually renal failure should nutritional rehabilitation not occur.

Should there be persistent hypokalaemia, as a result of chronic vomiting or diuretic abuse, as in bulimia nervosa and patients who purge in anorexia nervosa, vacuolation of the renal tubules has been observed resulting in impaired tubular function affecting fluid and electrolyte balance.

Liver

Non-alcoholic steatohepatitis (NASH syndrome) occurs in a significant minority of patients with anorexia nervosa. Typically the transaminase levels are in the several hundreds, but not thousands. The raised enzyme levels persist for several weeks at the beginning of nutritional rehabilitation. These changes are usually asymptomatic and uncomplicated. These changes resolve with nutritional rehabilitation.

GOALS FOR THERAPY

The goals for therapy are to achieve nutritional and psychological recovery. Weight goals are linked to reestablishing a healthy body composition such that spontaneous resumption of menses occurs along with increases in lean tissue mass to support increases in bone size and mineralisation. Goal weight can be calculated from weight for age, sex and height centile charts. Endocrine measures can also be used to identify a minimum healthy weight range. Leuteinising hormone, then follicle stimulating hormone and finally oestrogen levels return to adult levels in postmenarchal patients. For premenarchal patients, estimation of fat mass from anthropometry (skinfolds) or DEXA may be used to identify a healthy minimum weight. A body fat percentage of at least 18% is required among adolescent females to sustain pubertal development.

PROGNOSIS

AN has the highest mortality of any psychiatric condition. A crude mortality rate of 5.1% has been consistently reported with a mortality rate of 20%, 20 years after diagnosis.

Most adolescents make a recovery from AN over a three- to five-year period after diagnosis. A significant minority of those who develop AN in adolescence, about one quarter, continue to have a chronic or relapsing course into adulthood.

The morbidity of AN is minimised with early correction of the PCM (kwashiorkor). Ongoing effects to bone health and other organs have been demonstrated. There remains concern that the changes to brain structure and function, particularly in the more malnourished patients, do not fully recover even after nutritional rehabilitation. Protracted PCM certainly can result in organ failure

History	Clinical	Differential diagnosis	Investigations	Complications
Diet, eating or purging behaviour	Protein–calorie malnutrition	Hypothyroidism	Baseline investigations	Fluid and electrolytes (phosphate ↓)
Exercising	Mimics hypothyroidism	Diabetes mellitus	• ESR (low ESF typical)	Endocrine:
Perception of body shape, weight, health	Wasted	Addison's disease	• Evaluation of micronutrient deficiencies	• Delayed puberty
Menstrual history	Generalised pallor	Systemic lupus erythematosus	• Electrocardiogram (ECG)	• Amenorrhoea
Family history	Peripheral cyanosis	Inflammatory bowel disease	Imaging	Bone: osteopoenia
	Soft heart sounds	Brain tumour	• Dual energy X-ray absorptiometry (DEXA)	Haematology:
	Scaphoid abdomen		• Computed tomography (CT)	• Haemoglobin →
	Hepatomegaly			• Leucopenia, thrombocytopenia
	Pretibial/sacral oedema			• Iron deficiency anaemia
	Peripheral vascular insufficiency			Liver: non-alcoholic steatohepatitis (NASH)
				Heart: ventricular dysrhythmias; refeeding syndrome

FIGURE 25.1: Assessment of anorexia nervosa.

as illustrated by the diffuse glomerular sclerosis and renal failure seen in a small group of chronically malnourished patients.

In addition to this medical morbidity there is a substantial psychological morbidity. Patients have delayed growth and pubertal maturation. They become physically different, and socially isolated from peers around the time of diagnosis and during periods of hospitalisation.

The impact of AN has certainly been moderated with the development of multidisciplinary teams and the clinical collaboration of psychological and medical professionals.

SUMMARY

The overall (crude) mortality of this condition remains high. Despite the greater potential for medical complications because of the impact on growth and pubertal development, AN in children and adolescents carries a better prognosis. Early correction of protein calorie malnutrition increases the potential for recovery before chronic and irreversible organ changes occur. Early intervention and particularly early nutritional rehabilitation minimises the impact of AN on physical health. Weight restoration and nutritional rehabilitation remain the cornerstones of biological treatment with a two-track approach and appropriate psychosocial interventions to achieve recovery from this devastating illness (Figure 25.1).

FURTHER READING

Berkman ND, Lohr KN, Bulik CM. Outcomes of eating disorders: a systematic review of the literature. Int J Eat Disord 2007; 40:293–309.

Bulik CM, Berkman ND, Brownley KA, et al. Anorexia nervosa treatment: a systematic review of randomized controlled trials. Int J Eat Disord 2007; 40:310–20.

Herzog DB, Greenwood DN, Dorer DJ, et al. Mortality in eating disorders: a descriptive study. Int J Eat Disord 2000; 28:20–6.

Kohn MR, Golden NH, Shenker IR. Cardiac arrest and delirium: presentations of the refeeding syndrome in severely malnourished patients with anorexia nervosa. J Adolesc Health 1998; 22:239–43.

Chapter 26

PRACTICAL ISSUES IN NUTRITION AND SUPPLEMENTATION IN GASTROINTESTINAL DISEASE

KEY POINTS

- In upper gastrointestinal obstruction, endoscopic techniques facilitate access to the normal functional bowel distal to the obstruction, and thus restore normal digestion and absorption. It is imperative to simultaneously decompress the stomach proximal to the obstruction when feeding distally in order to avoid secretion build-up in the stomach.
- In lower gastrointestinal obstruction, the treatment is early surgery or total parenteral nutrition (TPN).
- Intestinal adaptation to intestinal loss may take up to 2 years. Thus, strong initial support is needed to optimise conditions for adaptation.
- The secret of adaptation is to make the remaining intestine work overtime.
- Tailoring TPN for the individual patient is essential.
- If less than 200 cm of small intestine without colon is present and IV supplementation becomes necessary, the condition is regarded as 'small bowel intestinal failure'. This is also the case if less than 50 cm of small intestine remains with colon, and TPN or home TPN becomes essential for survival.
- In intestinal fistulae the volume of output provides a good index of the site of the fistula.
- Treatment for low output fistulae is not TPN. Oral feeding should continue.
- Be wary of bowel rest in sick patients.

INTRODUCTION

The function of the bowel is to digest and absorb food. Consequently, it is no surprise that disorders of the gastrointestinal tract are associated with nutritional problems. In chronic gastrointestinal disorders, the situation becomes complicated by the secondary effects of malnutrition on digestive function. The mucosa has one of the highest protein turnover rates of any organ within the body, and the synthesis of pancreatic enzymes is directly dependent on an abundant supply of amino acids. Thus, in chronic malnutrition, digestive and absorptive function becomes impaired, leading to a vicious cycle of malabsorption, maldigestion, malabsorption, etc.

Equally important to realise is the tremendous depth of reserves in digestive and absorptive function. For example, we can survive following the loss of >90% of the small intestine if the colon remains intact. Similarly, maldigestion and fat malabsorption only occurs after we have lost >90% of our pancreatic enzyme secretion. However, it must be remembered that adaptation to loss takes time; in the situation of the small intestine up to 2 years. Consequently, strong initial support will be needed to optimise conditions for adaptation to occur.

NUTRITIONAL PROBLEMS

Management options for various nutritional problems are summarised in Figure 26.1.

Intestinal obstruction

In the days prior to total parenteral nutrition (TPN), intestinal obstruction was a fatal condition unless early surgery could correct the cause. In the 1970s and '80s, TPN was exclusively used to stabilise the patients before surgery could be performed. In the short term, this was usually successful, but when continued >2 weeks, complications began to outweigh benefits.

TPN therapy

- Benefits
  - Prevents fluid and electrolyte deficiencies
  - Maintains nitrogen balance
  - Prevents weight loss
  - Maintains life

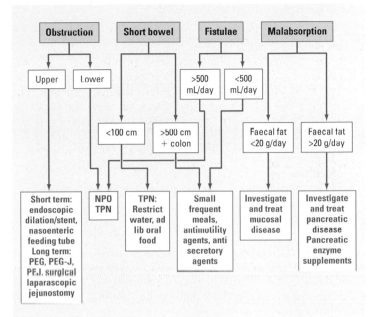

FIGURE 26.1: Nutritional problems.

NPO = non per os; PEG = percutaneous endoscopic gastrostomy;
PEG-J = percutaneous endoscopic gastrostomy with post-pyloric J extension;
PEJ = direct endoscopic jejunostomy; TPN = total parenteral nutrition.

- Risks:
  - It is unphysiological to feed directly into the right side of the heart
  - Catheter sepsis
  - Central vein thrombosis
  - Hyperglycaemia
  - Intestinal stasis:
    - Small intestine bacterial overgrowth
    - Mucosal atrophy and bacterial translocation
    - Endotoxaemia
    - Cholestasis
    - Pro-inflammatory cytokine over expression
  - Liver disease

Upper gastrointestinal obstruction

Because of concerns about TPN, endoscopic techniques have been developed to gain access to the normal functional intestine distal to the obstruction, and thus restore normal digestion and absorption.

- Oesophageal obstruction (e.g. cancer, stenosis, dysmotility):
  - Endoscopic dilation
  - Stenting
  - Percutaneous endoscopic gastrostomy (PEG).
- Gastric, duodenal and proximal jejunal obstruction:
  - Endoscopic dilation
  - Stenting
  - Percutaneous endoscopic gastrostomy with post-pyloric J extension (PEG-J)
  - Direct endoscopic jejunostomy (PEJ)
  - Double-lumen nasogastric decompression—jejunal feeding tube.

Note: It is imperative to simultaneously decompress the stomach proximal to the obstruction when feeding distally, as secretion will build up in the stomach leading to vomiting and possible aspiration.

Lower gastrointestinal obstruction

It is impossible to feed proximally with an intestinal obstruction because motility will be impaired and feed and secretions will build up without a chance for absorption to occur, producing vomiting. Consequently, the only alternatives are early surgery or TPN.

Short bowel

Short bowel syndrome results from surgical resection, congenital defect, or disease-associated loss of absorption and is characterised by the inability to maintain protein–energy, fluid, electrolyte or micronutrient balances when on a conventionally accepted, normal diet.

Traditionally, the short bowel syndrome has been defined by the loss of all but 200 cm of small intestine, bearing in mind that the average length of the small intestine is 4 metres. However, this is imprecise as function will be influenced by whether the colon is remaining or not, and whether the residual small intestine is healthy. It has been estimated that the colon represents another 100 cm of small intestine after adaptation (which can take up to 2 years), and colonic salvage of maldigested food can result in the absorption of a further 1000 kcal/day. Clearly, 200 cm of residual intestine with active Crohn's disease will not be equivalent to 200 cm of previously healthy mucosa. The most sensitive measure of remaining intestinal absorptive capacity is citrulline synthesis. Citrulline synthesis, and hence the functional bowel length, can be estimated from the fasting plasma citrulline concentration, which helps overcome errors in measurement of diseased bowel at surgery.

Management

The loss of small intestine, particularly the distal portion (which is usually the region removed, for example in Crohn's disease), results in a loss of the ability of the intestine to conserve fluids. The proximal small intestine characteristically has leaky junctions between the mucosal cells, which means that the presence of hypertonic or hypotonic fluid in the lumen results in the passive loss of either water or salt from the body. As there is no distal intestine to reabsorb this fluid or the intestinal and pancreatic secretions stimulated by eating, there is net loss of fluid and electrolytes from the body after eating. In order to maximise residual intestinal function it is important that patients:

- Avoid drinking water
- Increase the consumption of isotonic fluids containing a carbohydrate source and electrolytes; e.g. WHO solutions containing 100 g carbohydrates/litre and 70 mEq sodium
- Increase consumption of soups containing salt and carbohydrates
- Avoid large infrequent meals: 'nibble like a rabbit' all day long
- Consider nutritional supplementation with nutrient-dense liquid formula diets
- Supplement diet with nocturnal tube feeding 1000 kcal/8 h to make the gut work 24 hours a day.

Intestinal failure

Intestinal failure results from obstruction, dysmotility, surgical resection, congenital defect or disease-associated loss of absorption and is characterised by the inability to maintain protein–energy, fluid, electrolyte or micronutrient balance.

The first loss of function is the capacity to reabsorb secretions, resulting in fluid and electrolyte depletion, or 'dehydration'. It is only if <200 cm of small intestine and no colon remains that intravenous (IV) supplementation becomes necessary, and a state of 'small bowel intestinal failure' is said to exist. The same is true if <50 cm of small intestine remains with an intact colon, and TPN or home TPN then becomes essential for survival.

Measurement
The patient excretes less that 1000 mL urine and <5 mmol of sodium when on a normal diet.

Management: home TPN
It must be remembered that intestinal failure due to short bowel may recover through the process of adaptation. This process takes up to 2 years, and so intravenous (IV) nutritional requirements can be expected to decrease throughout this period. Adaptation occurs due to:
- Villous hyperplasia
- Dilation and hypertrophy of the residual bowel and slower motility
- Hypersecretion of digestive enzymes
- Hyperphagia
- Enhanced absorption
- Increased blood flow.

In order to maximise adaptation, food intake must be liberalised, as luminal nutrients are the chief stimulatory factors. Although this will increase stomal losses or diarrhoea, this must be accepted, as the quantity of absorbed nutrients will be maximised. The secret is to make the remaining bowel work overtime. Thus patients should be instructed to eat small frequent meals ('eat like rabbits'). In borderline patients, nocturnal tube feeding may well tip the balance in favour of nutritional autonomy. The longer food is in contact with the absorptive epithelium, the greater the chance for absorption, so the liberal use of antimotility drugs is encouraged, bearing in mind that much will be malabsorbed, so usual maximum doses can be exceeded (e.g. loperamide three tablets [6 mg] four times daily).

Tailoring TPN
1 Start with IV fluids and adjust to maintain a urine output of 1.5 L/day, and a sodium excretion of 20–80 mEq/d and potassium excretion 40–60 mEq/d.

2 Start with 80 g amino acids and 1000 kcal/day. Increase slowly to 1.5 g amino acids and 25 kcal/kg ideal body weight/day over 5 days.
3 Monitor urea and creatinine. If urea increases and creatinine stays stable, cut back on amino acids. If both increase, the patient is dehydrated and IV fluids need to be increased and urine volume monitored.
4 Long term, monitor body weight and adjust calories to maintain an ideal body weight, i.e. BMI of 23.5 kg/m².

Intestinal fistulae

Not all intestinal fistulae are treated the same. This stands to reason, as a fistula originating from the distal bowel will have little nutritional consequence, while a proximal fistula will result in major malabsorption of food, particularly if the leak is large. Consequently, it is important to first measure the fistula output. In an ideal world, the measurement of the contents of the fistulous fluid will provide even more specific guidelines for management, but this is costly and rarely done short of research studies. In general terms, the volume of output provides a good index of the site of the fistula: if output is >500 mL/day, it is likely to be proximal and associated with nutrient malabsorption, if it is <500 mL/day it is likely ileocolonic and therefore not associated with much malabsorption, as >90% of digestion and absorption occurs in the proximal gut. In a way, management is similar to that for short bowel syndrome discussed above, with the exception that high output fistulae may close spontaneously, and therefore TPN with bowel rest to reduce aggravating pancreaticobiliary secretions is recommended for up to 6 weeks. Low-output fistulae are *not* treated with TPN. Luminal nutrition helps the intestine recover, and oral feeding should continue in the form of small frequent meals, with IV supplementation of electrolytes and fluid as needed.

Malabsorption

Malabsorption is conventionally divided into conditions that interfere with:
- Mucosal absorption
- Food digestion.

Classic examples of diseases that interfere with mucosal function are coeliac disease and inflammatory and infiltrative disorders. Because such disorders are often patchy and because there is a redundancy of absorptive area, these diseases result in lower grades of malabsorption than diseases that impair digestive function, such as pancreatic diseases. It is therefore useful to measure the degree of fat malabsorption: in general mucosal disease results in fat malabsorption of <20 g/day, while pancreatic malabsorption usually causes losses >20 g/day. It is, however, extremely important to measure fat malabsorption accurately: it is amazing how frequently stool fats are measured in patients who are on restricted diets or even TPN, in which case such cut-off numbers are meaningless.

Measurement of fat malabsorption

- Patients *must* consume a 'normal' diet containing 100 g fat for 72 h.
- All stools must be collected from commencement of the diet after stools have been passed and discarded, to 72 h later when all stools must be collected, weighed and the fat content measured.

Management

Mucosal malabsorption can often be controlled by simply increasing the oral intake. Although this will inevitably increase stool losses initially, the proportion absorbed remains the same and so the *quantity* retained will increase. This is even true for vitamin B_{12} malabsorption in pernicious anaemia, as there is also a less efficient passive absorption mechanism. The ways of increasing nutrient intake is the same as those outlined above for the management of short bowel syndrome. For pancreatic malabsorption, commercial pancreatic enzyme supplements should be used. It must be remembered that the output of proteinaceous enzymes by the healthy pancreas is extremely large particularly during eating, approximately 20 g/day, and so enzyme supplementation has to follow a similar pattern and frequency (e.g. four capsules with meals and two with snacks). Much effort has been put into designing effective preparations that are not inactivated by gastric acid, that migrate with food through the pylorus and are only released on entering the duodenum. Despite this, it is rare to completely reverse steatorrhoea, but the improvement is usually sufficient to prevent further weight loss.

Bowel rest and pancreatic rest

Increasing knowledge about intestinal function and health has led to more cautious use of bowel rest, with or without TPN. This is because:

- the intestine depends upon luminal nutrients for the high turnover rate of mucosal proteins and maintenance of barrier function
- gut function and motility is stimulated by food
- the absence of feeding results in mucosal atrophy and disturbance of the bacterial flora with potential overgrowth with pathogens.

In contrast, bowel rest is advisable in the management of acute pancreatitis and in chronic pancreatic secretory disorders, such as fistulae and pseudocysts. If enteral feeding is delivered >40 cm past the ligament of Treitz, pancreatic stimulation is avoided, so that TPN is not the only way of feeding without stimulating the pancreas.

SUMMARY

There is a tremendous depth of reserves in digestive and absorptive function in the intestine. Adaptation is an important function but it can take up to 2 years, necessitating strong initial support.

TPN therapy is a vital component of the therapeutic armamentarium but it has both risks and benefits. Endoscopic techniques have facilitated access to the normal functional bowel distal to the obstruction. In lower gastrointestinal obstruction, the treatment is early surgery or TPN.

Short bowel syndrome is characterised by the inability to maintain protein–energy, fluid, electrolyte or micronutrient balances when on a conventionally accepted normal diet. The most sensitive measure of remaining bowel absorptive function is its citrulline synthesis capacity.

Intestinal failure is characterised by the inability to maintain protein–energy, fluid, electrolyte or micronutrient balance. Home TPN is an essential component of management but, in order to maximise adaptation, the remaining bowel should be made to 'work overtime' with oral intake. As part of the process, TPN should be tailored to the individual patient.

In the management of intestinal fistulae the volume of output provides a good index of the site of the fistulae. Treatment for low output fistulae (ileocolonic) is not TPN, as luminal nutrition helps the bowel to recover, and oral feeding should continue with IV supplementation.

Bowel rest is advisable in the management of acute pancreatitis and in chronic pancreatic secretory disorders, but, otherwise, caution is advised with regard to bowel rest.

FURTHER READING

Kaushik N, Pietraszewski M, Holst JJ, et al. Enteral feeding without pancreatic stimulation. Pancreas 2005; 31:353–9.

Matarese LE, O'Keefe SJ, Kandil HM, et al. Short bowel syndrome: clinical guidelines for nutrition management. Nutr Clin Pract 2005; 20:493–502.

Mullady DK, O'Keefe SJ. Treatment of intestinal failure: home parenteral nutrition. Nat Clin Pract Gastroenterol Hepatol 2006; 3:492–504.

O'Keefe SJ, Buchman AL, Fishbein TM, et al. Short bowel syndrome and intestinal failure: consensus definitions and overview. Clin Gastroenterol Hepatol 2006; 4:6–10.

Chapter 27

OBESITY SURGERY

DEFINITIONS OF OBESITY

The increasing prevalence of obesity is a worldwide phenomenon and it is a disease with protean adverse physical, social and psychological effects. The classification of obesity defines the relationship between a person's height and weight, the body mass index (BMI) to stratify patients according to their risk of obesity-related medical conditions (Table 27.1).

TABLE 27.1: Obesity definitions*		
	BMI (kg/m²)	Obesity class
Underweight	<18.5	–
Normal	18.5–24.9	–
Overweight	25.0–29.9	–
Obesity	30.0–34.9	I
	35.0–39.9	II
Extreme obesity	40.0+	III

*The term 'morbid obesity' relates to BMI 35.0–39.9 with medical comorbidities or BMI 40 and above.

TREATMENT OF OBESITY

There are many dietary, medical and therapeutic options available to clinicians treating patients with obesity and, in general, many of these treatments have been attempted by patients as they progress through various stages of their disease. Non-surgical treatments combining elements of diet, exercise and pharmacotherapy are demonstrated in the published literature to be effective in obtaining modest weight loss and perhaps allowing patients to 'hold' their weight, but have no long-term efficacy in those in whom massive sustained weight-loss is required. In general, weight-loss after surgical treatments is 5–10 times greater than that obtained by non-surgical methods, and the results in obesity comorbidity resolution, cost saving and mortality reduction cannot be matched by other methods.

Having surgery entails taking on some risks, so it is obvious that this is not a treatment that can be applied liberally. The effects of any operation, both positive and negative, may be permanent and some complications may develop insidiously many years later and, therefore, may not be related to the operation. Current, generally accepted criteria for selecting patients for surgery are listed in Table 27.2.

Weight-loss surgery

Obesity is a chronic, probably life-long disease and, therefore, the current surgical solutions are designed to cause permanent alterations to gastrointestinal physiology. These physiological

TABLE 27.2: Selection criteria for bariatric surgery	
Body weight	BMI >40 BMI 35–39.9 with medical comorbidities No endocrine cause
Resistant obesity	Obesity present >5 years Multiple failed non-surgical attempts
Psychological profile	No alcohol or drug use No or controlled psychiatric conditions Understanding of surgery and commitment to follow-up

alterations, while necessary for the maintenance of weight-loss, may become disordered and lead to the patient presenting for medical or surgical care. There are a range of bariatric surgical procedures currently undertaken, and a number of historical procedures that remain of interest due to the large number of patients who have undergone them in the past. Thankfully there is sufficient homology between all of the historic and current procedures to allow them to be grouped into categories when discussing them. Complications following surgery may be related to weight loss itself (e.g. gallstones), anatomic changes (e.g. vomiting, obstruction) or altered nutritional status (e.g. decreased intake, decreased absorption or gastrointestinal losses). Most of the subtle nutritional complications that can arise after this type of surgery are beyond the scope of this chapter and will not be discussed.

BARIATRIC OPERATIONS

Operations for morbid obesity are grouped into:
- 'Restrictive': vertical banded gastroplasty (VBG), fixed band and the laparoscopic adjustable gastric band (LAGB)
- 'Malabsorptive': jejunoileal bypass, biliopancreatic diversion, the Scopinaro procedure
- 'Combined': Roux-en-Y gastric bypass (RYGBP).

These terms are historically based and fail to take into account the often complex variations between individual operations; they also inadequately explain the mechanisms by which the procedures work.

Gastroplasty

Fixed gastroplasty

Stapled gastroplasty, of which the VBG has been the most frequently performed worldwide, has undergone multiple revisions in technique due to frequent staple-line disruption, stoma problems, reflux, vomiting and weight regain. Silent failure is common with loss of restriction and weight regain following staple line disruption, allowing patients to return to their asymptomatic, albeit obese, preoperative state. Surgeons practising during the 1980s and early 1990s will be familiar with the cruel paradox of the vomiting patient who still gains weight. This peculiarity shows how the term 'restrictive' is a misnomer, as an operation that restricts intake without offering satiety after limited solid food intake will enforce liquid calorie intake. Examination of adjustable gastric banding has shown that early satiety is a significant factor in the success of restrictive operations and that early satiety makes procedures that promote voluntary limitation of food intake (LAGB and RYGBP) tolerable to patients.

The main complications likely to cause presentation of VBG and the mechanistically similar fixed band patients relate to the stoma. The natural history of a fixed obstruction in any part of the gastrointestinal tract is proximal dilation, and if this occurs above an excessively tight or scarred stoma, patients experience increasing reflux and regurgitation with inability to tolerate solid food. Increasing the radius of the stomach 'pouch' above the obstruction increases the wall tension according to the law of Laplace, and leads to inability of the pouch to empty, which in turn leads to progressive dilation. Reflux, regurgitation and cough are common symptoms of this syndrome, and these symptoms are often associated with the presence of a hiatus hernia. If this complication cannot be controlled with proton pump inhibitors, surgical correction is mandated. Patients having re-operative surgery for complications resulting from an earlier operation should probably be seen by an experienced bariatric surgeon to help ensure a good outcome.

Adjustable gastroplasty

Laparoscopic adjustable gastric band (LAGB) is a procedure that has been responsible for the increase in uptake of bariatric surgery in many countries outside the USA. The band is placed just below the cardia, so that the volume of stomach above the band stoma is a couple of millilitres in size only (Figure 27.1).

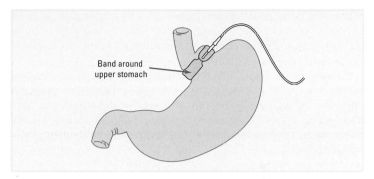

FIGURE 27.1: Laparoscopic adjustable gastric band (LAGB).

Bands placed lower on the stomach are often unstable and can 'slip' easily with prolapse of the stomach proximally, resulting in reflux and vomiting, which is reminiscent of VBG complications.

Severe perioperative problems after placement of a LAGB are rare, but operation-specific complications include injuries to vascular structures, the liver and spleen, as well as hollow viscus perforation. Early bolus obstruction after discharge, similar to that which occurs in some patients after Nissen fundoplication, may occur if solid food intake has been commenced too rapidly postoperatively, or if the patient has been vomiting with resulting stomal oedema. Perforation of the cardia or oesophagus at the time of surgery will often be missed by the surgeon as placement of the band involves blind dissection behind the stomach where it is bound to the crura of the diaphragm. A perforation at this location may cause significant intra-abdominal, retrogastric and mediastinal sepsis presenting several days after discharge. Any patient with significant pain and a fever following LAGB placement should be treated with extreme concern.

Late LAGB complications usually relate to stomal obstruction. If a band has been overfilled the stoma will be so tight that the patient may be unable to swallow saliva. This problem can invariably be fixed by accessing the port with a Huber (non-coring) needle and emptying the reservoir.

A more difficult cause of vomiting or reflux is stoma obstruction caused by pouch dilation and prolapse of stomach above the band. In extreme cases, this can cause strangulation and necrosis of the proximal stomach, so any LAGB patient in whom vomiting is not relieved by band deflation can be assumed to require an operation to remove or revise the band. Further contrast radiology may cause unnecessary delay and adversely affect the outcome, especially if the patient is unwell or in pain.

Erosion of the band into the stomach lumen is an uncommon occurrence and is usually asymptomatic except for patients complaining of weight regain, although abdominal pain may also be present due to localised sepsis. Eroded bands can usually be removed laparoscopically or endoscopically with surprisingly few sequelae.

Investigating patients after gastroplasty

The majority of patients will present with reflux and dysphagia symptoms, and in most of these cases the underlying pathology will be the result of an 'obstruction' with proximal dilation and/or a hiatus hernia. In many cases, the hiatus hernia will be small, and any barium studies will be misreported. In Figure 27.2 only the first barium swallow (left panel) was interpreted correctly as reflux and a small hiatus hernia, the second (second panel from the left) of a VBG with reflux and hiatus hernia and the third (second panel from the right) with reflux and a slipped gastric band were not. Note the transverse lie of the band on the AP radiograph, which is a finding that is always associated with anterior pouch prolapse. The correct orientation of the band is seen on the fourth image (right panel), with the lie of the band pointing at 2 o'clock on the anteroposterior film.

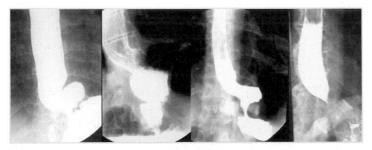

FIGURE 27.2: Barium studies post gastroplasty in four patients (three reflux patients, and one normal). The left panel shows a small hiatus hernia, second on the left shows a VBG and hiatus hernia. Second panel from the right shows a slipped gastric band and the right panel shows a normal barium swallow after successful gastroplasty.

At endoscopy there may or may not be evidence of oesophagitis, and care must be taken to look for a small hiatus hernia. Other studies, such as manometry or oesophageal pH studies are of no assistance and may give misleading results, especially as some gastroplasty patients can develop a 'pseudoachalasia' syndrome that cannot be properly characterised without removal of the obstructing lesion.

Acute post-gastric reduction surgery (APGARS) neuropathy
Any patient who suffers from intractable vomiting after an operation that has a gastroplasty component is at risk suffering a preventable and only variably reversible polyneuropathy—the acute post-gastric reduction surgery (APGARS) neuropathy. This is characterised by vomiting, significant and rapid weight loss and a constellation of symptoms that may include 'tingling', hyporeflexia, weakness and syndromes resembling Wernicke's or Korsakoff's psychosis. These patients typically have not been taking or absorbing mineral and vitamin supplements and may also be suffering from occult or suboptimally treated surgical complications. Admission to hospital, B_{12}, thiamine and multivitamin supplementation and search for and correction of surgical complications is recommended.

Malabsorptive operations
The pioneer bariatric operation was the jejunoileal bypass and, although the majority of patients undergoing this procedure lost a lot of weight, they did so at the expense of frequent and uncontrollable side effects including liver failure and profound malabsorption. Most of these patients have had the procedure reversed, but the legacy of procedures that work by inducing a malabsorption syndrome remains.

Of the current malabsorptive operations, the Scopinaro and biliopancreatic diversion (BPD) procedures are the most effective long-term operations available with regards to maintenance of weight loss, and they have unparalleled results in diabetes and hyperlipidaemia resolution. They involve a limited gastrectomy and subtotal small intestine bypass which is achieved by anastomosing the ileum to the stomach (or pylorus), and bypassing the entire jejunum which is then anastomosed to the terminal ileum. Typically patients will have a short 'enteric limb' in which carbohydrate is absorbed and a 'common channel' of 25–100 cm of terminal ileum where biliary and pancreatic juices are mixed with the food to allow limited fat absorption.

In essence, these operations convert patients with an uncontrolled obesity and metabolic disorder to patients with a controllable malabsorption and deficiency syndrome, but the margin for error is small and tolerance to the operation appears individually variable. Patients who have had these operations need strict lifelong supervision to avoid potentially dangerous and irreversible metabolic sequelae. Some patients require reversal or revision of the operation because of nutrition problems despite compliance, and those who stop taking supplements will develop marked osteopenia, fatigue, iron deficiency and fat soluble vitamin deficiency (A, D, E, K). Uncommonly, night blindness and other syndromes may develop. Complications resulting from stasis in the bypassed intestine are uncommon in modern forms of the operation but may present sporadically. A patient who is lost to follow-up after one of these operations who presents to another clinician should be treated with these deficiencies in mind and specialist help should be sought from either the operating surgeon or an endocrinologist. These patients have limited reserve and can become dehydrated and hypoalbuminaemic easily, so the patient should be admitted for all but the most trivial illnesses.

Gastric bypass

Gastric bypass is the most frequently performed bariatric procedure performed worldwide, and it may be performed via a laparoscopic or open approach. Gastric bypass is essentially just that, a bypass of the stomach, and gastroenterologists dealing with these patients can consider that they have had an operation analogous to a total gastrectomy (Figure 27.3).

Gastric bypass is essentially a 'restrictive' operation with strong satiety regulation mediated by early release of peptide YY and anorexic hormones after meals. This, and changes to small intestine motility, also leads to intolerance of high-density carbohydrate which will cause nausea and symptoms of 'early dumping'. The operation does not lead to protein or fat malabsorption as the length of the small intestine bypass is trivial. Bypassing the stomach will prevent acidification of the enteric stream and therefore cause potential but unpredictable and individually variable reductions in calcium, iron and B_{12} absorption.

Outside the early postoperative period where a therapeutic endoscopist may be asked to plug, glue or stent a leaking enteric anastomosis, potential complications revolve around the excluded stomach, the gastrojejunal anastomosis and bowel obstruction.

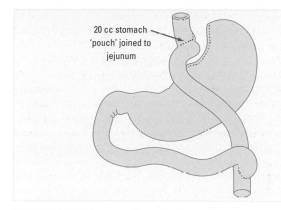

20 cc stomach 'pouch' joined to jejunum

FIGURE 27.3: Roux-en-Y gastric bypass.

The excluded stomach is surprisingly quiescent in these patients, and despite the obvious concerns regarding ulcer disease the reported rate of ulceration requiring treatment seems low. Long-term use of non-steroidal antiinflammatory drugs is not advised, and access to the stomach for endoscopy or endoscopic retrograde cholangiopancreatography (ERCP) will require additional laparoscopic or percutaneous techniques. The gastrojejunal anastomosis may become stenosed in about 5% of patients, and in the majority of cases this will be amenable to endoscopic balloon dilation; 12 mm dilation is usually sufficient to resolve symptoms.

The most significant complication following gastric bypass surgery is the risk of small bowel obstruction and internal herniation of bowel through mesenteric defects with volvulus or 'closed-loop' obstruction. This can present insidiously as recurrent abdominal pain, sometimes mimicking biliary colic, pancreatitis, or appendicitis. Vomiting and obstipation may occur very late in the clinical course of the illness as a prelude to or a result of intestinal infarction. Plain abdominal radiology is unreliable or misleading, but high-resolution computed tomography (CT) with oral and intravenous contrast will usually diagnose those with evolving obstruction, often only recognised as an abnormality in mesenteric vasculature. For patients with intermittent or recurrent symptoms, laparoscopy is the only diagnostic test with sufficient predictive value to either prove or disprove recurrent obstruction, and elective repair of any defects is usually straightforward.

SUMMARY

Bariatric surgery complications are common. Potential complications can be grouped into:

- Gastroplasty complications—vomiting, stomal obstruction, gastroenterostomy stricture and reflux (VBG, fixed and adjustable bands, gastric bypass)
- Excluded organ complications—bacterial overgrowth, peptic ulceration, occult bleeding (gastric bypass, intestinal bypass procedures)
- Intestinal obstruction and internal herniation (gastric bypass, intestinal bypass procedures)
- Gallstone disease (all)
- Malabsorption or decreased intake of, or abnormal loss of, protein, vitamins and minerals (all).

Most of these complications can be managed once a clear understanding of the underlying anatomy and, therefore, physiology has been obtained. Obtaining old records can be crucial in this regard. It should be recognised that many of these problems are complications rather than expected outcomes, and that anatomic defects underlying the complications may necessitate surgical correction.

FURTHER READING

Buchwald H, Buchwald J. Evolution of operative procedures for the management of morbid obesity 1950–2000. Obes Surg 2002; 12:705–17.

Buchwald H, Williams SE. Bariatric surgery worldwide 2003. Obes Surg 2004; 14:1157–64.

Colquitt J, Clegg A, Sidhu M, et al. Surgery for morbid obesity. Cochrane Database Syst Rev 2003; 2:CD003641.

Dixon AF, Dixon JB, O'Brien PE. Laparoscopic adjustable gastric banding induces prolonged satiety: a randomized blind crossover study. J Clin Endocrinol Metab 2005; 90:813–19.

Greenway SE, Greenway FL, Klein S. Effects of obesity surgery on non-insulin-dependent diabetes mellitus. Arch Surg 2002; 137:1109–17.

Livingston E. Obesity and its surgical management. Am J Surg 2002; 184:103–13.

Vage V, Solhaug JH, Berstad A, et al. Jejunoileal bypass in the treatment of morbid obesity: a 25-year follow-up study of 36 patients. Obes Surg 2002; 12:312–18.

Chapter 28

HOW TO PREPARE PATIENTS FOR ENDOSCOPIC PROCEDURES

KEY POINTS

Correct patient preparation involves:

- Informed consent—a discussion of the nature of the procedure as well as risks, benefits and alternatives.
- Assessment of patient fitness, which is generally dictated by the level of anaesthetic support available for the procedure.
- Patients should take their usual prescribed medications several hours prior to endoscopy with a sip of water.
- Patients with a coagulopathy or on warfarin require special consideration. Therapeutic endoscopy is safe with an INR <1.7.
- Special considerations for patients with diabetes. Instruct patients to halve the morning insulin dose and stop the morning oral hypoglycaemic agent. Schedule these patients early and monitor their blood glucose levels.
- Antibiotics to prevent endocarditis are no longer recommended for endoscopy procedures.
- Gastroscopy—ensure the patient is fasting (no solid food for at least 6 hours or clear liquids for at least 4 hours). In the emergency situation, airway protection via endotracheal tube should be considered.
- Acute gastrointestinal bleeding—intensive resuscitation is necessary.
- Endoscopic retrograde cholangiopancreatography (ERCP)— consent issues are very important because ERCP is potentially a dangerous procedure. Patients with biliary obstruction should receive prophylactic antibiotics.
- Colonoscopy—proper preparation is a prerequisite for adequate colonoscopic examination. Patients should fast prior to colonoscopy. Caution is advised with sodium phosphate purges in the elderly and in patients with renal impairment.
- Flexible sigmoidoscopy—enema just prior to procedure is usually sufficient preparation.

INTRODUCTION

Correct patient preparation is essential for safe and effective endoscopic procedures. These considerations can be divided into:

- Informed consent
- Assessment of patient fitness
- Procedure-specific issues (gastroscopy, endoscopic ultrasound, endoscopic retrograde cholangiopancreatography [ERCP] and colonoscopy)
- Patient-specific issues (underlying disease processes, medications and allergies).

INFORMED CONSENT

Informed consent is a process and *not* a signed piece of paper. Informed consent from a patient or their legal delegate is essential for all procedures, except for exceptional circumstances when the time to obtain valid consent would place the patient at risk. This decision must be made by the attending consultant. Informed consent involves a discussion of the nature of the procedure as well as risks, benefits and alternatives. Implicit in this is that the person obtaining the consent must understand the procedure and be able to answer the patient's questions. Patient information sheets are helpful, but do not replace the requirement to sit with the patient, explain the issues and provide an opportunity to answer questions. If language is a barrier to this discussion, the process should take place with a professional interpreter and not via a relative, who may not convey the message appropriately. In most institutions a signed consent form is necessary. Though not a legal requirement it does afford some protection should legal issues arise later, though it does *not* prove that the process was done properly. Ideally, the consent process should occur on a separate day to the procedure and not in the procedure room just prior to endoscopy, where the environment may be deemed to be coercive.

ASSESSMENT OF PATIENT FITNESS FOR PROCEDURE

Health professionals assessing patients for endoscopy should be aware of the American Society of Anesthesiologists (ASA) classification of patient risk (see Table 28.1). The degree of concern will be dictated somewhat by the level of anaesthetic support

TABLE 28.1: Definition of American Society for Anesthesiologists comorbidity status	
Class 1	Patient has no organic, physiologic, biochemical or psychiatric disturbance. The pathologic process for which the operation is to be performed is localised and does not entail systemic disturbance
Class 2	Mild to moderate systemic disturbance caused by either the condition to be treated surgically or by other pathophysiologic processes
Class 3	Severe systemic disturbance or disease from whatever cause, even though it may not be possible to define the degree of disability with finality
Class 4	Severe systemic disorders that are life-threatening, not always correctable by operation
Class 5	The moribund patient who has little chance of survival but is submitted to the operation in desperation

available for the procedure (which ranges between institutions from none to an anaesthesiologist, as well as varying for different types of procedures). In general, procedures on ASA class I and most class II patients can be safely performed in a well equipped endoscopy suite with appropriately trained staff. ASA class III patients might be better triaged to the operating room. This degree of patient risk must be identified prior to the endoscopy list so that appropriate patient assessment (and informed consent) can be undertaken as well as ensuring that the procedure is performed in the appropriate environment.

PROCEDURE-SPECIFIC ISSUES

Gastroscopy and endoscopic ultrasound

The main issue for gastroscopy (also known as oesophagogastro-duodenoscopy [EGD] or simply 'endoscopy') and endoscopic ultrasound (EUS) is safety to the patient through ensuring an empty stomach. Patients should not eat solid food for at least 6 hours or clear liquids for 4 hours prior to a gastroscopy. If the patient is known to have poor gastric emptying fasting for longer or dietary restriction to clear fluids for 24–48 hours prior to the procedure should be considered. In the emergency situation, airway protection via endotracheal tube should be considered.

Specific issues arise if the patient procedure involves irradiation of the abdomen, so a history of possible pregnancy should be elicited in young and middle-aged women. If the history suggests the possibility of pregnancy, this should be checked with a serum β-hCG (human chorionic gonadotrophin).

Contrast in the bowel lumen may prevent imaging of the relevant ducts with acute upper gastrointestinal bleeding.

Preparation for upper gastrointestinal bleeding

A period of intensive resuscitation is appropriate prior to undergoing upper endoscopy, which should be performed in the presence of a health professional trained in advanced life support and airway management. If there is a suspicion that there may be significant blood in the stomach it is reasonable to give the patient a prokinetic agent (such an intravenous erythromycin) 30 min prior to the procedure.

Endoscopic retrograde cholangiopancreatography

The same considerations regarding fasting and gastroscopy apply to endoscopic retrograde cholangiopancreatography (ERCP). In addition, because ERCP is potentially a very dangerous procedure, consent issues are especially important.

For this reason, patients who have had a recent barium enema, computed tomography (CT) scan with oral contrast or enteroclysis should have a plain abdominal X-ray to ensure that the region of interest is not obscured.

ERCP involves injection of iodinated contrast into the biliary and pancreatic duct systems. It is extremely unlikely that patients with iodine allergy would have an allergic reaction in this setting. Nonetheless, many radiologists recommend a regimen for these patients such as:

- Night before procedure: 50 mg prednisone
- Day of procedure: 25 mg prednisone; 150 mg ranitidine; 25 mg promethazine.

In addition, patients with uncontrolled hyperthyroidism should avoid an iodine load. This may involve delaying the procedure or using another contrast agent such as gadolinium.

Patients with biliary obstruction should receive prophylactic antibiotics prior to the commencement of the procedure (see below for a more detailed discussion of antibiotic prophylaxis). Endoscopic sphincterotomy (ES) of the ampulla of Vater is a common procedure during ERCP. Patients in whom ES is considered should have an international noramalised ratio (INR) <1.7 (ideally normalised) and should not take IIb/IIIa inhibitors such as clopidogrel for 7–10 days if the procedure is elective. Aspirin use does not preclude ES, but ideally should also be ceased 5 days before the procedure.

Colonoscopy

Proper preparation is a prerequisite for adequate colonoscopic examination. A poorly prepared colon may lead to missed pathology and often requires repeat examination.

Two colonic purges are commonly used: polyethylene-glycol (PEG)-based solutions and sodium phosphate-based solutions. Both are osmotic, though sodium phosphate is hypertonic whereas PEG-based solutions are essentially isotonic. Sodium phosphate purges have the advantage of requiring a smaller volume to be consumed (as they draw water into the bowel by osmotic pressure). This smaller ingested volume leads to better compliance. However, this may cause dangerous dehydration or electrolyte imbalances such as hyperphosphataemia. This is especially a concern in elderly patients or those with renal impairment. Furthermore, sodium phosphate purges may cause mild inflammation of the colonic mucosa and sometimes small aphthous ulcers. Therefore this type of purge is best avoided in patients undergoing colonoscopy to assess inflammatory bowel disease. PEG-based solutions cause less fluid and electrolyte disturbance, but may be difficult to ingest due to their large volume (3–4 litres). Only approximately 80% of patients complete a PEG-based purge.

Stimulant purgatives such as senna are not effective as sole agents and are rarely used. Fermentation of osmotic sugar purgatives such as mannitol, sorbitol and lactulose by gut bacteria may lead to high colonic concentrations of hydrogen gas. This can cause explosion if electrical current is used for polypectomy and, therefore, must not be used for colonoscopic preparation.

Patients should fast for at least 6 hours prior to colonoscopy since sedation associated with the procedure decreases protective reflexes and raises the possibility of aspiration of gastric contents.

Preparation for lower gastrointestinal bleeding

Acute massive haematochezia should be investigated with colonoscopy following a rapid purge. This usually involves at least 3–4 L PEG-based solution, until the effluent is pink. In patients unable to drink the solution, it may be administered using a nasogastric tube. A prokinetic agent may be helpful to speed this process. It should be noted that the passage of bright red blood per rectum in a haemodynamically unstable patient could be due to a duodenal source of bleeding, so these patients will often have an emergency upper endoscopy first.

Flexible sigmoidoscopy

One or two enemas are usually sufficient preparation just prior to flexible sigmoidoscopy. Often, no preparation is used if the procedure is performed for the investigation of acute diarrhoea. Fasting is not required unless the patient requires sedation (which is unusual).

PATIENT-SPECIFIC ISSUES

General considerations

Patients usually take their normal medications several hours prior to endoscopic procedures with a sip of water. Exceptions are drugs which are potentially harmful to the oesophagus if lodged there (such as bisphosphonates, potassium supplements, non-steroidal antiinflammatory drugs and tetracycline). Patients on bronchodilator therapy should be encouraged to bring their puffers to the hospital with them.

Diabetes mellitus

Medication for patients with diabetes requires special consideration. There are no controlled trials to guide management, but, generally, patients on oral hypoglycaemic agents omit their morning dose, while patients on insulin usually halve their morning dose. Close attention must be paid to the patient's blood glucose level during procedure preparation, before the procedure and after. Patients with diabetes should be first on the morning endoscopy list in order to minimise disturbance to their regimen and reduce fasting time.

Anticoagulant medications

The American Society for Gastrointestinal Endoscopy has published excellent guidelines for anticoagulant therapy. These are summarised in Table 28.2. In brief:

- Aspirin. There is no evidence that therapeutic endoscopic procedures (such as polypectomy and biliary sphincterotomy) cannot be performed on low-dose aspirin. Thus, use of aspirin in the preceding 5 days should not lead to cancelling the

procedure. Nonetheless, most practitioners would cease aspirin 5–7 days prior to an elective procedure.
- New antiplatelet agents. There is little data on which to base recommendations. In general, these drugs cause more profound platelet inhibition than aspirin and should be ceased 7–10 days prior to high-risk elective procedures (such as colonoscopy with polypectomy or biliary sphincterotomy, oesophageal dilation, etc). An important caveat is the patient on clopidogrel with

---

TABLE 28.2: The Amercian Society for Gastrointestinal Endoscopy guidelines on anticoagulants in patients undergoing endoscopic procedures

Acute gastrointestinal haemorrhage in the anticoagulated patient:
- The decision to reverse anticoagulation and the extent of anticoagulation reversal should be individualised, weighing the risk of thromboembolism against the risk of continued bleeding
- A supratherapeutic INR may be corrected with infusion of fresh frozen plasma
- Correction of the INR to 1.5–2.5 permits effective endoscopic diagnosis and therapy
- Reinstitution of anticoagulation should be individualised

Procedure risk	Condition risk for thromboembolism	
	High	Low
High	Discontinue warfarin 3–5 days before procedure	Discontinue warfarin 3–5 days before procedure
	Consider heparin while INR is below therapeutic level	Reinstitute warfarin after procedure
Low	No change in anticoagulation. Elective procedures should be delayed while INR is in supratherapeutic range	
	Aspirin and other non-steroidal antiinflammatory drug (NSAID) use	
	In the absence of a preexisting bleeding disorder, endoscopic procedures may be performed in patients taking aspirin or other NSAIDs	

From Gastrointest Endosc 1998;48:672–5, with permission.

INR = international normalised ratio.

a drug-eluting coronary stent. These patients are at risk of acute stent thrombosis, infarction and possibly death if their antiplatelet drugs are ceased. Management of these patients should be individualised in collaboration with their cardiologist.

- Warfarin. Safe therapeutic endoscopy can be performed with an INR <1.7. Diagnostic endoscopic procedures can be safely performed with a therapeutic INR. If a therapeutic procedure (polypectomy, biliary sphincterotomy, etc) is likely, the INR should be <1.7 prior to the procedure. The management of cessation of warfarin (i.e. whether the patient requires heparin cover and, if so, which type) depends upon the individual lesion and is best managed in collaboration with the patient's cardiologist.

- When to restart anticoagulation. There are few endoscopic data to guide practice and the decision depends partly upon the indication for anticoagulation (see Table 28.2). It is important to note that although most post-procedure bleeding occurs within 72 h of the procedure, delayed haemorrhage may occur up to 3 weeks after the procedure.

Antibiotic prophylaxis

There is very little scientific evidence to guide practice. Excellent guidelines are available from the American Society for Gastrointestinal Endoscopy, which are summarised in Table 28.3. In brief, endoscopic

TABLE 28.3: The American Society for Gastrointestinal Endoscopy guidelines on management of antibiotics in patients undergoing endoscopic procedures

Patient condition	Procedure contemplated	Antibiotic prophylaxis
High risk: • Prosthetic valve • History of endocarditis • Systemic pulmonary shunt • Synthetic vascular graft >1 year old • Complex cyanotic congenital heart disease	Stricture dilation Variceal sclerotherapy ERCP/obstructed biliary tree	Recommended
	Other endoscopic procedures, including EGD and colonoscopy (with or without biopsy/polypectomy), variceal ligation	Prophylaxis optional

TABLE 28.3: The American Society for Gastrointestinal Endoscopy guidelines on management of antibiotics in patients undergoing endoscopic procedures *(continued)*

Patient condition	Procedure contemplated	Antibiotic prophylaxis
• Moderate risk: • Most other congenital abnormalities • Acquired valvular dysfunction (e.g. rheumatic heart disease) • Hypertrophic cardiomyopathy • Mitral valve prolapse with regurgitation or thickened leaflets	Oesophageal stricture dilation Variceal sclerotherapy Other endoscopic procedures, including oesophagogastro-duodenoscopy and colonoscopy (with or without biopsy/polypectomy), variceal ligation	Prophylaxis optional Not recommended
Low risk: Other cardiac conditions (CABG, repaired septal defect or patent ductus, mitral valve prolapse without valvular regurgitation, isolated secundum atrial septal defect, physiologic/functional/innocent heart murmurs, rheumatic fever without valvular dysfunction, pacemakers, implantable defibrillators)	All endoscopic procedures	Not recommended
Obstructed bile duct	ERCP	Recommended
Pancreatic cystic lesion	ERCP, EUS-FNA	Recommended
Cirrhosis acute gastrointestinal bleed	All endoscopic procedures	Recommended
Ascites, immunocompromised patient	Stricture dilation Variceal sclerotherapy Other endoscopic procedures, including EGD and colonoscopy (with or without biopsy/polypectomy), variceal ligation	Not recommended Not recommended

TABLE 28.3: The American Society for Gastrointestinal Endoscopy guidelines on management of antibiotics in patients undergoing endoscopic procedures *(continued)*

Patient condition	Procedure contemplated	Antibiotic prophylaxis
All patients	Percutaneous endoscopic feeding tube placement	Recommended (parenteral cephalosporin or equivalent)
Prosthetic joints	All endoscopic procedures	Not recommended

Cardiac prophylaxis regimens (oral 1 h before, IM or IV 30 min before procedure)

Amoxycillin by mouth or ampicillin IV: adult 2.0 g, child 50 mg/kg

Penicillin allergic: clindamycin (adult 600 mg, child 20 mg/kg) or cephalexin or cefadroxil (adult 2.0 g, child 50 mg/kg), or azithromycin or clarithromycin (adult 500 mg, child 15 mg/kg), or cefazolin (adult 1.0 g, child 25 mg/kg IV or IM), or vancomycin (adult 1.0 g, child 10–20 mg/kg IV)

CABG = coronary artery bypass graft; ERCP = endoscopic retrograde cholangio-pancreatography; EUS-FNA = endoscopic ultrasound guided fine needle aspiration; IM = intramuscular; IV = intravenous.

From Hirota WK, Petersen K, Baron TH, et al. Guidelines for antibiotic prophylaxis for gastrointestinal endoscopy. Gastrointest Endosc 2003; 58:475–82, with permission.

procedures can be divided into high and low risk of significant bacteraemia and patient factors can similarly be classed in terms of risk from bacteremia. Low-risk procedures (such as gastroscopy and colonoscopy with or without polypectomy) never mandate the use of antibiotics, but they may be used at the clinician's discretion. High-risk patients (e.g. those with prosthetic heart valves, previous endocarditis, recent vascular graft) undergoing a high-risk procedure (such as oesophageal dilation or sclerosis of varices) used to require antibiotics but this is not longer recommended routinely. All other permutations of patient and procedure are guided by physician preference. When there is doubt, most clinicians take a pragmatic approach and give prophylactic antibiotics.

Due to the high risk of significant infective complications, prophylactic antibiotics are recommended for all patients undergoing some specific endoscopic procedures. These are:

- Percutaneous endoscopic gastrostomy (PEG) insertion
- Endoscopic pseudocyst drainage

- ERCP in the presence of biliary obstruction
- EUS-guided puncture of cystic lesions
- Any procedure in the bleeding patient with decompensated liver disease.

The choice of antibiotic should be dictated by protocols determined by the infectious diseases unit of the institution.

SUMMARY

Correct patient preparation is essential for safe and effective endoscopic procedures (Figure 28.1).

The issues that have to be considered are:

- Informed consent, which involves a discussion of the procedure as well as risks, benefits and alternatives. The person obtaining the consent must understand the procedure and be able to answer the patient's questions. Ideally the consent process should occur on a separate day to the procedure.
- Assessment of patient fitness for the procedure will be dictated somewhat by the level of anaesthetic support available for the procedure. The degree of patient risk must be identified prior to the endoscopy so that appropriate patient assessment and informed consent can be undertaken.

Informed consent	Assessment of patient fitness	Procedure-specific issues	Patient-specific issues
Discuss procedure and risks, benefits and alternatives Ideally, seek consent on a separate day to procedure	Correct patient preparation is essential Identify patient risk prior to endoscopy Level of anaesthetic support available important	• Gastroscopy: fasting. Airway protection in emergency. Resuscitation priority in upper gastrointestinal bleed • ERCP: consent issues important • Colonoscopy: proper preparation a prerequisite • Flexible sigmoidoscopy: enema just prior to procedure	Special considerations: • Diabetics on insulin • Anticoagulants • Antibiotics for high-risk patients undergoing high-risk procedures • No need for infective endocarditis prophylaxis

FIGURE 28.1: Preparation of patient for endoscopic procedures.

ERCP = endoscopic retrograde cholangiopancreatography.

- Procedure-specific issues. Ensure the patient has an empty stomach. In the emergency situation airway protection via endotracheal tube should be considered. Resuscitation is a priority in patients with upper gastrointestinal bleeding. Note that ERCP is potentially dangerous and consent issues are especially important. Also, because of radiation, enquire about possible pregnancy. If biliary obstruction is present, prophylactic antibiotics are required. Correct preparation is a prerequisite for adequate colonoscopic examination. Sodium phosphate purges can cause renal failure in the elderly. Preparation for flexible sigmoidoscopy usually requires one or two enemas just prior to the procedure.
- Patient-specific issues. Patients should take their usual medications several hours prior to the procedure. Special consideration should be given to patients with diabetes and patients on anticoagulants. Collaboration with the patient's cardiologist is advisable. Patients undergoing certain high-risk procedures require prophylactic antibiotics.

FURTHER READING

Barkun A, Chiba N, Enns R, et al. Commonly used preparations for colonoscopy: efficacy, tolerability, and safety – A Canadian Association of Gastroenterology position paper. Can J Gastroenterol 2006; 20:699–710.

Eisen GM, Baron TH, Domintz JA, et al. Guideline on the management of anti-coagulation and anti-platelet therapy for endoscopic procedures. Gastrointest Endosc 2002; 55:775–9.

Faigel DO, Eisen GM, Baron TH, et al. Preparation of patients for GI endoscopy. Gastrointest Endosc 2003; 57:446–50.

Hirota WK, Petersen K, Baron TH, et al. Guidelines for antibiotic prophylaxis for gastrointestinal endoscopy. Gastrointest Endosc 2003; 58:475–82.

Wexner SD, Beck DE, Baron TH, et al. A consensus document on bowel preparation before colonoscopy. Gastrointest Endosc 2006; 63:894–909.

Wilson W, Taubert KA, Gewitz M, et al. Prevention of infective endocarditis. Guidelines from the American Heart Association. Circulation 2007; April 19; [Epub ahead of print].

Zukerman MJ, Hirota WK, Adler DG, et al. The management of low-molecular weight heparin and nonaspirin antiplatelet agents for endoscopic procedures. Gastrointest Endosc 2005; 61:189–94.

Chapter **29**

ANAESTHESIA FOR ENDOSCOPY

KEY POINTS

- Patients do not need a deep level of anaesthesia, only moderate sedation—drug-induced depression of consciousness.
- A review of medications and results of investigations is necessary, in particular the presence of hepatic or renal impairment, which affects drug clearances and half-lives.
- All patients need reliable intravenous access, oxygen, pulse oximetry, accessible Ambu bag, emergency drugs, reversal drugs for benzodiazepines and narcotics and access to an electrocardiogram (ECG) and defibrillator.
- Sedation for endoscopy requires a combination of drugs. Midazolam, fentanyl and propofol are used in varying amounts to increase the comfort and tolerance of the patient to the procedure.

INTRODUCTION

In order to undertake upper or lower gastrointestinal endoscopy patients must be anaesthetised in some way. They do not need a deep level of anaesthesia, only moderate sedation—drug induced depression of consciousness. The purpose of this chapter is to give an outline of patient assessment (see Chapter 28 for more information), monitoring and drugs used in order to sedate patients undergoing procedures.

PATIENT ASSESSMENT

- Identification and introduction of anaesthetist to patient.
- Appropriate medical assessment of patient, especially cardiovascular and respiratory history (questionnaires are often helpful).
- Ask about previous sedation, anaesthetics, allergies, fasting and damaged or loose teeth (this is of particular interest for upper endoscopy).

- Clinical examination, review of medications and results of investigations. Hepatic and renal impairment are particularly relevant as they affect drug clearances and half-lives.

MONITORING CHECKLIST

- All patients need reliable intravenous access.
- All should have oxygen.
- All patients should have pulse oximetry.
- Pulse rate should be palpated and recorded.
- Blood pressure should be recorded.
- Electrocardiogram (ECG) and capnography may be required if cardiovascular or respiratory history.
- There should be an ambubag nearby (or means of inflating lungs).
- Emergency drugs.
- Reversal drugs for benzodiazepines and narcotics.
- Access to ECG and defibrillator.

ANAESTHESIA AND SEDATION

Anaesthesia should only be performed by medical practitioners with appropriate training in airway management and resuscitation.

Sedation for endoscopy requires a combination of drugs. Midazolam, fentanyl and propofol are used in varying amounts to increase patient comfort and tolerance of the procedure.

The use of narcotics and benzodiazepines avoids coughing in upper endoscopy and withdrawal response for colonoscopy.

Midazolam

Midazolam has anxiolytic, sedative-hypnotic and anticonvulsant activities. This is the benzodiazepine of choice because it has a rapid onset and ultra-short duration of action and has no active metabolites.

Midazolam is given intravenously with very rapid onset of action ranging from 15–20 seconds to a few minutes.

Midazolam is metabolised in the liver, thus there may be a need to decrease the dose if liver failure is present or expect a longer duration of action.

In the event of overdose, seen by respiratory depression, flumazenil, a specific benzodiazepine receptor antagonist, can be given. The plasma half-life of flumazenil is very short (2–5 min), so repeat doses may be required. The dosage is 0.1–0.2 mg boluses of up to 3 mg until reversal is seen.

Fentanyl

Fentanyl is a synthetic narcotic. It is eighty times more potent than morphine, yet has a much shorter duration of action. The plasma half-life of fentanyl is 20 minutes. It has a high hepatic extraction ratio (i.e. metabolism is dependent on liver blood flow). Fentanyl is haemodynamically stable, such that administration maintains blood pressure, and is generally safe to use in patients with impaired cardiovascular function.

Fentanyl dosages are individualised on a patient-to-patient basis. Doses may start with 10 µg boluses in older patients, and 25 µg boluses in young healthy people.

Overdose is often seen as a triad of coma, respiratory depression and pinpoint pupils. After establishing an airway, ventilation and administration of an opioid antagonist is required. Naloxone 0.01 mg/kg is the antagonist of choice. Patients may experience rebound sympathetic nervous system overdrive, which can result in dysrhythmias and pulmonary oedema. Naloxone's duration is very short so repeat doses or an infusion may be required.

Propofol

Propofol is an induction agent. It has a very short plasma half-life of 2–8 minutes. Its metabolism is also dependent on liver blood flow and it has inactive metabolites.

Propofol is less haemodynamically stable than fentanyl. It drops the blood pressure and can cause a reflex increase in heart rate and should be used with caution in patients with ischaemic heart disease. It can also lead to transient apnoea, and thus needs to be titrated slowly.

Propofol dosage is 10–20 mg boluses until its effect are seen. Propofol should not be used patients allergic to egg or soya bean. Thiopentone is a suitable alternative in this instance.

There is no reversal agent for propofol, but the effects are very short acting so maintain the airway, ventilation and blood pressure whilst needed and the patient will soon regain consciousness.

Thiopentone

Thiopentone is a barbiturate. It is used less and less these days because it has a longer duration of action than propofol (40 min).

It has much slower metabolism and 30% is excreted in the urine. Thus in endoscopy, which is done as a day surgery procedure, people awaken more slowly.

Thiopentone decreases blood pressure, increases heart rate and, thus, increases myocardial oxygen demand. Severe cardiovascular disease is a relative contraindication for thiopentone use.

SUMMARY

- Do a patient assessment—assess previous health, allergies, medications. Patient preparation is key.
- Check fasting status and provide informed consent (Figure 29.1).
- Examination—focus on the airway, and the respiratory and cardiovascular states.
- Monitoring—oxygen saturation, intravenous access, supplemental oxygen, pulse and blood pressure.
- Sedation—know your drugs: midazolam, fentanyl, propofol.

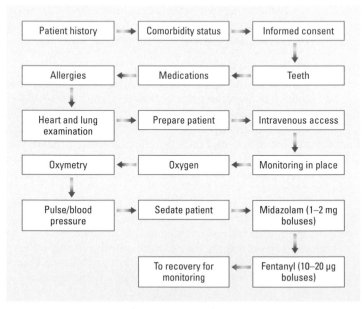

FIGURE 29.1: Preparing for conscious sedation.

FURTHER READING

Bailey PL, Zuccaro G Jr. Sedation for endoscopic procedures: Not as simple as it seems. Am J Gastroenterol 2006; 101:2008–10.

Rex DK. Review article: moderate sedation for endoscopy: sedation regimens for non-anesthesiologists. Aliment Pharmacol Ther 2006; 24:163–71.

Ristikankare M, Julkunen R, Heikkinen M, et al. Sedation, topical pharyngeal anesthesia and cardiorespiratory safety during gastroscopy. J Clin Gastroenterol 2006; 40:899–905.

Waring JP, Baron TH, Hirota WK, et al. Guidelines for conscious sedation and monitoring during gastrointestinal endoscopy. Gastrointest Endosc 2003; 58:317–22.

CHAPTER 30

EVALUATING ABNORMAL LIVER TESTS

KEY POINTS

- Liver enzyme abnormalities may be physiological or pathological.
- Any persistent elevation of liver function tests must be investigated.
- A detailed history and physical examination is mandatory.
- The degree and pattern of elevation of liver tests may provide clues to its aetiology.
- Upper abdominal ultrasonography is a useful non-invasive imaging procedure.

INTRODUCTION

Liver function tests (LFTs) are commonly performed as part of routine screening laboratory investigations. These include estimations of serum:

- alanine aminotransferase (ALT)
- aspartate aminotransferase (AST)
- alkaline phosphatase (ALP)
- gamma-glutamyltransferase (GGT)
- bilirubin (hepatic excretory function)
- albumin (hepatic synthetic function).

An elevated prothrombin time that is not corrected by the administration of vitamin K suggests reduced hepatic synthetic function.

Thrombocytopenia in the context of liver disease suggests hepatic fibrosis and impaired liver function with concomitant portal hypertension.

APPROACH TO THE PATIENT WITH ABNORMAL LFTs

The presence of any persistent abnormality of liver tests warrants further assessment. The initial step in evaluating a patient with raised liver enzymes is to undertake a thorough history and physical examination, with particular emphasis on risk factors for liver disease.

A detailed drug history is important including:

- prescribed medications in particular, antibiotics during the preceding 3 months
- alcohol intake
- ingestion of allopathic and traditional medications including vitamins and herbal preparations (CAM: complementary and alternatives medicines)
- recreational drugs.

Liver injury may manifest several weeks after drug cessation.

Risk factors for viral hepatitis must be elicited such as injecting drug use.

Sudden, marked elevations in transaminase levels necessitates exclusion of viral, drug-induced and ischaemic hepatitis.

INTERPRETING PATTERNS OF LIVER TEST ABNORMALITIES

The degree and pattern of liver tests' elevation may provide clues as to aetiology (Figure 30.1). A practically useful classification is provided below.

Liver test abnormalities are designated as:

1 'Hepatocellular' when there is an ALT increase of over twice the upper limit of normal or R $\geq$5, where R is the ratio of serum ALT/serum ALP in multiples of the upper limit of the normal range
2 'Cholestatic' if serum ALP is increased above twice the upper limit of the normal range or R $\leq$2
3 'Mixed' in pattern when both ALT and ALP are raised, and 2 $\leq$R $\leq$5. The ratio R may vary during the course of liver injury.

In the vast majority of patients with liver disease, the serum ALT exceeds the AST. Exceptions include those with alcoholic liver disease and those with cirrhosis from any aetiology.

The presence of liver test abnormalities in association with a low serum albumin or a prolonged prothrombin time infers significantly impaired hepatic synthetic function, while an elevated bilirubin reflects hepatic excretory dysfunction.

Disorders associated principally with elevations in aminotransferase levels

Aminotransferase levels are sensitive indicators of hepatic injury; ALT and AST are present normally in serum at low levels, usually less than 30–40 U/L.

AST is found in:

- liver
- cardiac muscle
- skeletal muscle
- kidneys
- brain
- pancreas
- lungs
- leucocytes and erythrocytes.

Because the highest levels of ALT are in the liver, an elevation of ALT is a more specific indicator of liver injury than the AST.

Common causes of liver enzyme abnormalities according to the pattern of enzyme elevation are presented in Table 30.1.

TABLE 30.1: Causes of elevated liver enzyme levels

Hepatocellular	Cholestatic

• Excessive alcohol consumption
• Drug-induced liver disease
  – Chronic hepatitis B and C
  – Non-alcoholic fatty liver disease
  – Haemochromatosis
• Autoimmune hepatitis
• Wilson's disease
• Alpha$_1$-antitrypsin deficiency
	• Drug-induced liver injury
	• Choledocholithiasis
	• Primary biliary cirrhosis
	• Primary sclerosing cholangitis
	• Pancreatic carcinoma
	• Neoplastic infiltration
	• Sarcoidosis

Additional laboratory tests useful in identifying specific disorders are listed in Table 30.2.

TABLE 30.2: Laboratory tests to clarify the cause of liver test abnormalities

Laboratory test	Diagnosis
• Hepatitis C antibody	• Positive test suggests chronic hepatitis C infection
• Hepatitis B surface antigen	• Positive test suggests chronic hepatitis B infection
• Hepatitis B e antigen	• Positive test suggests active viral replication
• Serum ferritin, transferrin saturation	• Iron overload suggests haemochromatosis
• Antimitochondrial antibodies	• Detected in primary biliary cirrhosis
• Antinuclear antibodies, anti-smooth muscle antibodies	• Detected in autoimmune hepatitis
• Serum caeruloplasmin	• Reduced in Wilson's disease
• Serum alpha$_1$-antitrypsin	• Decreased in alpha$_1$-antitrypsin deficiency

Causes of elevated aminotransferase levels

Alcohol-related liver disease (ALD)

- The diagnosis of alcohol-related liver disease is supported by the finding of a ratio of AST to ALT of at least 2:1.
- The degree of elevation of aminotransferase levels may provide further evidence for a diagnosis of ALD. It is rare for AST levels to be greater than 8 times the normal value in patients with alcohol abuse, and even less common for ALT levels to exceed 5 times the normal value. ALT levels may be normal in patients with severe ALD.
- ALT levels >300 U/L in those with significant alcohol intake usually indicates the presence of another cause for the liver test elevation (e.g. coincident drug toxicity or viral hepatitis).
- A GGT level that is twice normal in patients with an AST:ALT ratio of at least 2:1 strongly implicates alcohol as the likely cause for the liver enzyme abnormalities. However, the lack of specificity of GGT precludes its use as a single test to diagnose alcohol abuse.

Laboratory features suggestive of alcohol abuse are:
- AST:ALT >2
- ALT <300 U/L
- Elevated GGT

- Raised MCV (mean corpuscular volume)
- Thrombocytopenia which corrects following abstinence from alcohol.

Drug-induced liver disease

- Almost any medication, herbal preparation or illicit substance can cause abnormal liver tests. Meticulous history taking is critical. Changes in liver tests may persist long after cessation of the offending agent. Prevention and treatment of drug-induced liver disease is predicated on awareness and early cessation of the suspected offending agent. Commonly implicated drugs are listed in Table 30.3.

TABLE 30.3: Commonly prescribed medications causing abnormal liver tests

Class of medication	Examples
• Antibiotics	• Flucloxacillin, minocycline
• Antiepileptics	• Carbamazepine, phenytoin
• Antipsychotics	• Chlorpromazine
• Antituberculotics	• Isoniazid, rifampicin
• Lipid-lowering medications	• HMG-CoA reductase inhibitors (statins)
• Non-steroidal antiinflammatory drugs	• Ketoprofen, naproxen
• Oestrogens	• Oral contraceptive pill

Chronic viral hepatitis

Chronic hepatitis C: afflicts up to 1% of Australians, with 85% of incident cases related to injecting drug use. All patients with chronic HCV infection should be considered for antiviral therapy, which demonstrates excellent cost effectiveness.

- Risk factors for acquiring hepatitis C infection include:
  - Having received blood transfusions prior to February 1990
  - Injecting drug use
  - Exposure to non-sterile instruments including acupuncture needles, needle stick injury, tattooing, body piercing
  - Snorting cocaine
  - Country of birth (South East Asia, Mediterranean region, Middle East, Africa, South America): probably relates to use of non-sterile medical equipment
  - Infants born to hepatitis C virus (HCV)-infected mothers.

- In a patient with risk factors, a diagnosis of chronic hepatitis C infection is suggested by the presence of a positive hepatitis C antibody test with or without a raised ALT.
- Up to 30% of patients with a positive antibody result have no ongoing HCV viraemia, particularly if the ALT is persistently normal. The positive antibody result in this instance reflects prior exposure to the virus.
- Confirmation of hepatitis C infection can be sought by the detection of hepatitis C virus RNA in serum (polymerase chain reaction [PCR] test).
- A liver biopsy should be considered to assess the severity of liver damage in any viraemic patient with chronic hepatitis C and an elevated ALT.
- Individuals who are viraemic with persistently normal ALTs are currently not eligible for treatment but should be monitored.

Chronic hepatitis B: results when immune elimination does not occur following acute infection and the hepatitis B virus (HBV) continues to replicate (see Chapter 36).

- At risk populations include:
  - those from countries with high hepatitis B endemicity (e.g. South East Asia)
  - indigenous Australians
  - individuals with a history of injecting drug use.
- Serologic testing for hepatitis B infection includes tests for hepatitis B surface antigen, hepatitis B surface antibody and core antibody. A positive test for hepatitis B surface antibody and core antibody indicates the presence of immunity to hepatitis B.
- A positive hepatitis B surface antigen is indicative of hepatitis B infection. Viral replication can be assessed by determining hepatitis B e antigen status:
  - Patients who are hepatitis B e antigen positive have high levels of replicating virus.
  - When hepatitis B e antigen is negative but ALT levels are paradoxically raised, individuals may be infected with a mutant form of hepatitis B virus or have another cause for liver injury.
- The presence of mutant HBV can be confirmed by determining serum HBV DNA levels. Those infected with mutant HBV often run a more aggressive course.

- Patients with chronic hepatitis B have an approximately 30% lifetime risk of developing hepatitis B-related complications including hepatocellular carcinoma and liver failure.
- Any patient who is surface antigen and e antigen positive with an elevated ALT (especially if >100 U/L) or with precore mutant hepatitis B and elevated ALT should be considered for specialist assessment, liver biopsy and treatment with potent antiviral drugs, such as lamivudine.

Non-alcoholic fatty liver disease (NAFLD)

- Non-alcoholic fatty liver disease is the most common cause for liver test abnormalities in Western countries, affecting 20% of obese and 3% of lean individuals (see Chapter 39).
- Hepatic steatosis and non-alcoholic steatohepatitis (NASH) can manifest as mild elevations in serum aminotransferase levels ($<4 \times$ normal value). Patients with NASH usually have an AST:ALT ratio less than 1:1, unless cirrhosis intervenes which can reverse this ratio.
- Hepatic steatosis and NASH are found in association with disorders of insulin resistance:
  - Type 2 diabetes
  - Obesity (central)
  - Hyperlipidaemia (hypertriglyceridaemia, low HDL).
- Ultrasonography is useful in the assessment of a patient with suspected NASH. Fatty involvement of the liver appears on ultrasonography as a hyperechoic liver but such an appearance is non-specific, and indistinguishable from that due to hepatic iron deposition or fibrosis.
- Steatosis and NASH can be distinguished on liver biopsy, with the former showing bland fatty infiltration (steatosis), while NASH is characterised by steatosis as well as inflammation and variable fibrosis.
- Steatosis is a benign, non-progressive or slowly progressive condition. In contrast, a proportion of patients with NASH can progress to cirrhosis and liver failure. Serious consideration has to be made in implementing lifestyle modifications early in this group of patients including regular exercise, a low-fat weight-reduction diet, as well as careful monitoring and control of underlying disorders of insulin resistance.

Haemochromatosis

- Hereditary haemochromatosis is a common genetic disorder (1 in 200) that can present with abnormal liver tests (see Chapters 37 and 42).
- A transferrin saturation value (serum iron divided by total iron binding capacity) >45% is suggestive of haemochromatosis.
- Serum ferritin provides less specific information as it is an acute phase reactant and is often raised in conditions such as alcoholic liver disease and NAFLD.
- Genetic testing can now be performed to identify the mutations (C282Y and H63D) in the haemochromatosis (*HFE*) gene.
- A liver biopsy is necessary to assess the degree of fibrosis if:
  - iron overload is present on iron studies but no *HFE* mutation is found on genetic testing, or
  - a patient with the *HFE* mutation is older than 40 years of age, has a serum ferritin >1000 μg/L, abuses alcohol or has hepatomegaly or an abnormal AST.
- If the individual has an elevated transferrin saturation and is a C282Y homozygote, or a compound heterozygote C282Y/H63D, then a liver biopsy can be avoided if the patient is under the age of 40 years and the serum aminotransferase levels are normal.
- Family screening is *mandatory* in all first-degree relatives of patients with hereditary haemochromatosis.

Autoimmune hepatitis

- Typically, this condition affects young women who present with a hepatocellular pattern of elevation of liver enzymes and raised serum globulins (predominantly IgG) (see Chapter 38).
- Autoimmune markers for this condition include antinuclear antibodies and antibodies against smooth muscle and liver-kidney microsomes. A liver biopsy is essential in confirming the diagnosis.
- Untreated, autoimmune hepatitis can rapidly progress to cirrhosis and liver failure. Patients must be referred early for assessment and immunosuppressive therapy.

Wilson's disease

- Wilson's disease is a rare genetic disorder in which copper accumulates in the liver and brain in excess of normal metabolic needs. The underlying defect in copper homeostasis is a reduction in the biliary excretion of copper (see Chapter 42).

- All young patients (<40 years) with new onset liver test abnormalities should be screened for Wilson's disease by way of a serum caeruloplasmin level. Serum caeruloplasmin levels are reduced in 85% of affected individuals. Ophthalmological assessment looking for Kayser-Fleischer rings is recommended.
- A 24-hour urine collection to quantify copper excretion may be useful, particularly if a clinician is strongly suspicious of the diagnosis of Wilson's disease in a patient with absent Kayser-Fleischer rings and a normal serum caeruloplasmin level.
- Liver biopsy is recommended to measure hepatic copper levels and ascertain the degree of hepatic fibrosis.

Alpha$_1$-antitrypsin deficiency

- This is an uncommon cause for abnormal liver tests in adults. Decreased levels of alpha$_1$-antitrypsin can be detected by direct measurement of serum levels. The diagnosis is established by determination of the genotype of the affected individual.

Other liver test abnormalities

Alkaline phosphatase levels

- Liver and bone are two sources of ALP.
- Benign causes of elevated ALP levels:
    - Third trimester of pregnancy (passage of placental ALP into the maternal circulation)
    - Adolescents (leakage of bone ALP into blood)
    - Serum ALP gradually increases from the age of 40 up to the age of 65, especially in women.
- The initial step in evaluating an elevated ALP level is to consider it in tandem with a serum GGT. A raised ALP in the presence of an elevated GGT suggests that the ALP is of liver origin.
- If liver enzymes demonstrate a 'cholestatic' pattern, chronic cholestatic and infiltrative liver disorders should be considered (Table 30.1).

Gamma-glutamyltransferase levels

- GGT is found in hepatocytes and biliary epithelial cells.
- Raised levels of GGT can be found in a wide variety of clinical conditions including:
    - pancreatic disease
    - myocardial infarction
    - renal failure

  – chronic obstructive pulmonary disease
  – diabetes.
- Patients taking phenytoin and barbiturates commonly have an elevated GGT.
- The sensitivity of an elevated GGT for detecting alcohol ingestion ranges from 52% to 94%. Its lack of specificity makes it unreliable for this purpose. Measurement of serum GGT is best used as an adjunct in interpreting the pattern of elevations of the other liver tests.

Hyperbilirubinaemia

- Hyperbilirubinaemia may be present in association with both hepatocellular (e.g. viral hepatitis) and cholestatic (e.g. bile duct obstruction) patterns of liver test abnormalities.
- Familial abnormalities of bilirubin metabolism should be entertained once haemolytic or overt liver diseases have been excluded.
- The most common abnormality is Gilbert's syndrome, which is a benign, mild, unconjugated hyperbilirubinaemia (not due to haemolysis), in the setting of normal synthetic liver function and histology. It affects up to 5% of the population and is inherited as an autosomal dominant condition. Jaundice is mild and intermittent, with exacerbations following infection or fasting and may be associated with malaise, nausea and right upper quadrant discomfort. Gilbert's syndrome has an excellent prognosis, with normal lifetime expectancy (see Chapter 42).

Assessment of a patient with 'cholestatic' liver tests

- In the assessment of cholestatic liver tests not considered to be drug related, ultrasonography is recommended to assess the hepatic parenchyma and bile ducts.
- If biliary dilatation or choledocholithiasis is found, then diagnostic and therapeutic endoscopic retrograde cholangiopancreatography should be undertaken.
- If no obstructive lesion is identified on ultrasonography then the patient will require referral to exclude rare conditions such as primary biliary cirrhosis, primary sclerosing cholangitis or granulomatous hepatitis. Serologic testing for antimitochondrial antibodies is used to screen for primary biliary cirrhosis. If a patient tests positive, the diagnosis is confirmed by liver biopsy.

SUMMARY

Liver enzyme abnormalities may be physiological or pathological. Persistent elevation of liver tests must be investigated. Eliciting a detailed history and performing a thorough physical examination is mandatory (Figure 30.1).

Assess the degree and pattern of elevation of liver tests. Serologic testing for common causes of liver dysfunction should be undertaken. Upper abdominal ultrasonography is a useful non-invasive imaging procedure. Liver biopsy should be considered in consultation with a gastroenterologist.

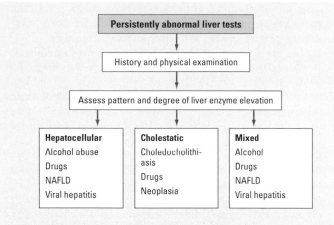

NAFLD = non-alcoholic fatty liver disease.

FIGURE 30.1: Evaluating liver function test abnormalities.

FURTHER READING

Dunn W, Angulo P, Sanderson S, et al. Utility of a new model to diagnose an alcohol basis for steatohepatitis. Gastroenterology 2006; 131:1057–63.

Keegan A. Abnormal liver function test results. In: Talley NJ, Martin CJ. Clinical gastroenterology: a practical problem-based approach. 2nd edn. Sydney: Elsevier; 2006:373–423.

Sherlock S, Dooley J. Diseases of the liver and biliary system. 11th edn. Oxford: Blackwell Science; 2002.

CHAPTER 31

ASCITES

KEY POINTS

- Portal hypertension due to cirrhosis is the most common cause of ascites in Western countries, accounting for approximately 80% of cases.
- Peritoneal malignancies and right heart failure account for most of the remaining cases.
- The serum-to-ascites albumin gradient (SAAG) correctly differentiates patients with ascites related to portal hypertension (gradient ≥11 g/L) from those with non-portal hypertension-related aetiologies (gradient <11 g/L) in over 97% of instances.
- The ascitic white cell count (WCC) is usually normal (total count <500/μL, neutrophil count <250/μL) in patients with uncomplicated portal hypertension-related ascites and raised in those with non portal hypertensive aetiologies, with the exception of hypoproteinaemic states and disorders associated with increased vascular permeability, such as the ovarian hyperstimulation syndrome.
- A simple initial algorithm based on the patient's medical history, physical examination, the SAAG and ascitic WCC allows a focused approach to further investigation aimed at determining the precise cause of ascites, upon which effective management relies.

INTRODUCTION

Ascites is excessive fluid in the peritoneal space. It is suggested clinically by the finding of shifting dullness and confirmed by imaging such as ultrasonography. Causes can be broadly categorised as portal hypertension-related or non-portal hypertension-related (Table 31.1). The latter include reduced plasma oncotic pressure, peritoneal inflammation, disruption to lymphatic drainage and increased vascular permeability. Despite this diversity in possible cause and mechanism, portal hypertension due to cirrhosis accounts for approximately 80% of cases in Western countries. Peritoneal malignancies and right heart failure account for

TABLE 31.1: Causes of ascites

Portal hypertention-related	Non-portal hypertention-related
Primary liver disease	*Peritoneal inflammation*
• Cirrhosis ± complicating portal vein obstruction or spontaneous bacterial peritonitis	• Bacterial peritonitis (spontaneous or due to perforated gut or intra-abdominal abscess)
• Pre-sinusoidal pathology:	• Tuberculosis
– Nodular regenerative hyperplasia	• Pancreatic enzymes
– Schistosomiasis	• Bile
• Acute liver failure	• Pelvic inflammatory disease
• Alcoholic hepatitis	• Connective tissue disorders
• Diffuse liver infiltration	*Reduced plasma oncotic pressure*
Primary venous pathology	• Nephrotic syndrome
• Hepatic veno-occlusive disease	• Protein-losing enteropathy
• Budd-Chiari syndrome	• Malnutrition
• Hypercoagulable state	*Impaired lymphatic drainage*
• Tumours:	• Lymphatic obstruction
– Hepatocellular carcinoma	– Lymphoproliferative disorders
– Renal cell carcinoma	– Peritoneal malignancies
– Adrenal carcinoma	– Tuberculosis
• Membranous webs	• Lymphatic tear
• Acute portal vein obstruction	– Trauma
• Trauma:	– Cirrhosis
– Acute pancreatitis	*Increased vascular permeability*
– Intra-abdominal sepsis	• Peritoneal malignancies
– Hypercoagulable state	• Ovarian hyperstimulation syndrome
Right heart failure	

most of the remaining cases. Tuberculosis is a common cause in patients from endemic areas. Although acute portal vein thrombosis commonly results in transient ascites, chronic portal vein obstruction does not usually cause ascites in the absence of underlying liver disease.

Spontaneous bacterial peritonitis (SBP), an infection of ascitic fluid with a single bacterial species in the absence of any primary intra-abdominal source, may complicate the clinical course of patients with preexisting ascites, often resulting in an exacerbation of peritoneal fluid accumulation. Less commonly, ascites develops de novo as a consequence of SBP. Most instances of SBP occur in cirrhotic patients and clinical studies have identified several subgroups at particularly high risk (Table 31.2). Overall, SBP is present in up to 20% of all cirrhotic patients undergoing paracentesis, although the incidence is notably lower in recent outpatient-based series. SBP is also well recognised to occur in patients with acute liver failure and those with nephrotic syndrome and other hypoproteinaemic states.

TABLE 31.2: Proven risk factors for the development of spontaneous bacterial peritonitis in patients with cirrhosis

- Decompensated hepatic function
- Small intestinal bacterial overgrowth
- Gastrointestinal haemorrhage
- Ascitic fluid protein concentration ≤10 g/L

The initial approach to the investigation of patients with ascites is based on four key components, namely the history, physical examination, the serum-to-ascites albumin gradient (SAAG) and the ascitic white cell count (WCC). Such a schema, which reliably allows categorisation into portal hypertension-related and other aetiologies in most cases, allows a focused approach to further investigation so that the precise cause of ascites in an individual patient can be ascertained. Given the wide range of possible causes of ascites and their differing treatments, this is mandatory if appropriate management is to be implemented.

INITIAL INVESTIGATION

History taking and physical examination are directed towards the range of possible aetiologies listed in Table 31.1, with particular emphasis on the more common possibilities, such as liver disease, right heart failure, peritoneal malignancies and, depending on patient demographics, tuberculosis. The possibility of underlying cirrhosis should not be dismissed in patients without peripheral stigmata of chronic liver disease, such as palmar erythema and spider naevi, as these are often absent, especially in those with non-alcoholic aetiologies.

Calculation of the SAAG complements the clinical assessment in correctly differentiating patients with ascites related to portal hypertension (gradient ≥11 g/L) from those with non-portal hypertension-related aetiologies (gradient <11 g/L) in over 97% of instances. The accuracy of this ratio obviates the need in routine practice for more invasive investigations for portal hypertension, such as measurement of the hepatic venous pressure gradient.

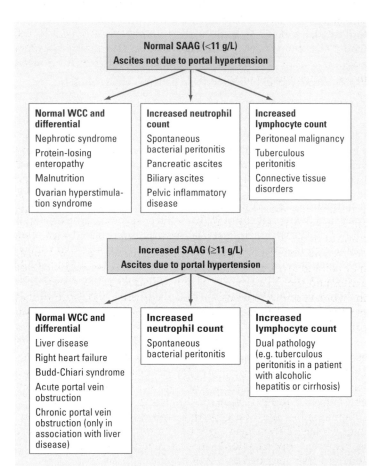

FIGURE 31.1: Initial diagnostic algorithm based on consideration of the serum-to-ascites albumin gradient (SAAG) and ascitic white cell count (WCC) patterns.*

* Normal ascitic WCC <500/μL with neutrophil count <250/μL

Further investigation is mandatory to determine the actual cause of ascites within the two broad categories of portal hypertension-related and other aetiologies. Consideration of the ascitic WCC and differential in combination with the SAAG is of particular value (Figure 31.1). The ascitic WCC is usually normal (total count <500/μL; neutrophil count <250/μL) in patients with uncomplicated portal hypertension-related ascites, such as due to cirrhosis, and raised in all non-portal hypertensive aetiologies, with the exception of hypoalbuminaemic states and disorders associated with increased vascular permeability, such as the ovarian hyperstimulation syndrome.

FURTHER INVESTIGATION

Portal hypertension-related ascites (SAAG ≥11 g/L)

The possibilities of intrinsic liver disease, right heart failure and venous obstruction must be addressed in patients with portal hypertension-related ascites. Standard liver function tests are important but may be entirely normal. Abdominal imaging, generally with ultrasound in the first instance, may demonstrate features of cirrhosis or extensive infiltration, along with other features of associated portal hypertension, such as splenomegaly and venous collaterals. Evidence of cytopenia on full blood count may point to hypersplenism. A clinical association between cirrhotic ascites and the development of hepatorenal syndrome, especially in hyponatraemic patients, is well recognised and, accordingly, markers of renal function and the serum sodium concentration can be important clues pointing to otherwise clinically inapparent (silent) liver disease with portal hypertension as the cause of ascites. Liver biopsy may be required. To minimise the risk of haemoperitoneum, this should be performed only after ascites has been effectively treated. The transjugular biopsy route is an alternative to the percutaneous approach if this is problematic. Coagulopathy must be reversed with clotting factor support and/or platelet transfusion prior to biopsy. If right heart failure is suspected, investigations such as echocardiography and lung function tests may be needed to establish the cause.

Patency of the portal and hepatic veins is usually adequately assessed by Doppler-ultrasound or dynamic computed tomography (CT). A high index of clinical suspicion is important for diagnosing hepatic veno-occlusive disease and Budd-Chiari syndrome, the latter resulting from hepatic venous outflow block. Tender, non-pulsatile hepatomegaly is a clinical hallmark of these disorders, although can be difficult to detect when ascites is tense. An underlying hypercoagulable state, most commonly related to a myeloproliferative disorder, is present in approximately 75% of patients with Budd-Chiari syndrome and should be sought. The possibility of an underlying malignancy should also be excluded. Associated thromboses in the inferior vena cava and/or portal vein are present in up to 20% of cases.

Ascites due to causes other than portal hypertension (SAAG <11 g/L)

Cytological examination of ascitic fluid remains the gold standard test for ascites due to peritoneal malignancy, although sensitivity is as low as 40%–60% in some series, even when up to 500 mL of fluid is analysed. Ascitic fluid fibronectin levels have been reported to have high diagnostic accuracy in discriminating between malignant and non-malignant causes of ascites. Laparoscopy-guided peritoneal biopsy may be required. The latter is the most reliable test for tuberculous peritonitis. A raised adenosine deaminase level in ascitic fluid has a specificity >90%, although reported sensitivities are widely variable. Mycobacteria are identified on culture of ascitic fluid in fewer than 20% of cases. Molecular diagnosis by polymerase chain reaction techniques is becoming more routinely available. Over 70% of patients with tuberculous peritonitis have no evidence of pulmonary disease. A raised ascitic amylase level, generally in the order of 2,000 IU/L, is typical of pancreatic ascites, while an ascitic bilirubin value in excess of that in serum is compatible with a biliary aetiology. Further imaging of the pancreas and biliary tree, respectively, should be undertaken in these latter circumstances.

Spontaneous bacterial peritonitis

The spectrum of clinical features of spontaneous bacterial peritonitis (SBP) extends from a fulminant presentation with peritonism and shock to an asymptomatic state manifest only by deterioration in laboratory variables. Abdominal pain with fever or hypothermia, often with an increased volume of ascites which may become refractory to diuretic therapy, are characteristic features. However, the majority of patients present with such non-specific symptoms as general malaise, anorexia, nausea or vomiting. Presentation with deterioration in mental status due to precipitation or exacerbation of hepatic encephalopathy is well recognised. Consequently, a high index of suspicion is mandatory if patients with SBP are to be identified and this diagnosis should be sought in any patient with ascites whose clinical status deteriorates.

An ascitic fluid neutrophil count ≥250/µL is the single most reliable test for SBP, with sensitivity approaching 90%. Other causes of neutrocytic ascites (as listed in Figure 31.1) must be excluded but, due to the relative frequencies with which these occur in cirrhotic patients, most instances of a raised ascitic neutrophil count in patients with cirrhosis are due to SBP. The sensitivity of traditional ascitic fluid culture is only 33%. This is improved to around 75% by the bedside inoculation of ascitic fluid into blood culture bottles. Gram stain of ascitic fluid is usually negative, as the concentration of infecting bacteria is generally only very low. Since neither the ascitic fluid neutrophil count nor ascitic culture has 100% sensitivity for SBP, even in combination, it is appropriate to make a clinical diagnosis of this disorder in patients with a suggestive clinical picture, even when these standard tests are negative. Assessment for the presence of bacterial DNA in ascites may be helpful in this latter circumstance, but is not yet widely available in clinical practice. The SAAG has no value in identifying patients with SBP. This gradient remains ≥11 g/L in patients with underlying portal hypertension-related ascites and <11 g/L in those with SBP complicating ascites of another aetiology, such as nephrotic syndrome.

SBP must be differentiated from secondary bacterial peritonitis due to perforation of the gut or an intra-abdominal abscess. A polymicrobial ascitic culture, especially in association with a raised ascitic neutrophil count, is an important clue to these latter possibilities. Gram stain may be positive for multiple organisms, especially in the case of secondary bacterial peritonitis related to gut perforation. A polymicrobial culture in association with a neutrophil count <250/µL suggests needle perforation of the gut during diagnostic or therapeutic paracentesis.

Chylous ascites
When ascites appears milky, the triglyceride content should be measured in order to differentiate between true chylous and pseudochylous ascites, the latter due to scattering of

light by aggregates of cholesterol, phospholipid and protein derived from degenerating malignant or inflammatory cells. Lymphatic obstruction in association with lymphoproliferative disorders or tuberculosis is a common cause of chylous ascites. This may also occur in patients with nephrotic syndrome and those with uncomplicated cirrhosis, due to rupture of overloaded lymphatics.

TREATMENT

Portal hypertension-related ascites

As sodium retention is a key feature in the pathogenesis of ascites related to portal hypertension, the goal of medical therapy is to induce a negative sodium balance by use of diuretics in combination with dietary sodium restriction, aiming for loss of body weight in the order of 0.5–1.0 kg/24 h, without precipitating hyponatraemia or azotaemia (Table 31.3). Refractory ascites, defined by lack of response to a sodium-restricted diet and high-dose diuretic therapy, occurs in a minority of patients. Second-line options for this group are listed in Table 31.3. Specific interventions may be necessary in carefully selected patients with ascites due to Budd-Chiari syndrome or veno-occlusive disease. These include thrombolytic therapy, angioplasty with or without venous stenting, transjugular intrahepatic portosystemic shunt (TIPS), surgical portacaval or mesoatrial shunt and orthotopic liver transplantation (OLT).

TABLE 31.3: Treatment options for ascites related to portal hypertension

Treatment	Example
First-line	Dietary sodium restriction (80 mmol/day)
	Diuretics: spironolactone ± frusemide
	Fluid restriction only if hyponatraemic
Second-line	Therapeutic paracentesis
	Peritoneovenous shunt
	Transjugular intrahepatic portosystemic shunt (TIPS)
	Orthotopic liver transplantation (OLT)

Treatment of any underlying hypercoagulable state is mandatory in those with Budd-Chiari syndrome.

Ascites due to causes other than portal hypertension

The primary focus of treatment in patients with non-portal hypertension-related ascites is on the underlying cause, such as antituberculous chemotherapy in those with tuberculous peritonitis or endoscopic or percutaneous stenting of a biliary leak in cases of biliary peritonitis. Therapeutic paracentesis may be required. The intraperitoneal installation of cytotoxic agents may provide effective palliation in selected patients with chemotherapy-sensitive tumours.

Spontaneous bacterial peritonitis (SBP)

Empiric antibiotic treatment should be commenced immediately after diagnostic paracentesis in patients in whom SBP is clinically suspected or after the demonstration of neutrocytic ascites in other patients. It is inappropriate to wait for the result of ascitic culture in view not only of the suboptimal sensitivity of this test but also of the risk of rapid clinical deterioration. The antibiotic of choice is generally a third-generation cephalosporin. The quinolones, ofloxacin or ciprofloxacin, are also efficacious. The appropriateness of the chosen antibiotic regimen may be reviewed when ascitic fluid culture and sensitivity results eventually become available. Granulocyte-macrophage colony stimulating factor has been shown in vitro to reverse defects in neutrophil phagocytosis and chemotaxis in cirrhotic patients and may have a role in the management of SBP in selected patients, such as those with severe infection and an incomplete initial response to antibiotics.

Although resolution of SBP is usually achieved with the use of appropriate antibiotics and despite improvements in the general medical care of cirrhotic patients, the in-hospital mortality rate remains 20%–40%. This is largely related to underlying hepatic decompensation and a high prevalence of hepatorenal syndrome. The latter occurs in approximately 30% of patients with SBP, predominantly in those with pre-existing renal impairment, and is progressive despite cure of infection in half of these cases. The development of renal failure is the most important predictor of in-hospital mortality associated with SBP. Survivors of an episode of SBP should be evaluated for orthotopic liver transplanation in view of the high risk of recurrence and poor overall prognosis.

SUMMARY

Despite the many possible causes of ascites, broad categorisation into portal hypertension-related and non-portal hypertension-related processes is usually possible based on a relatively simple algorithm based on the history, physical examination and determination of the serum-to-ascites albumin gradient and ascitic white cell count. Such a schema allows a focused approach to further investigation in order to ascertain the precise cause in an individual patient. This is vital if appropriate management is to be implemented.

FURTHER READING

Aslam N, Marino CR. Malignant ascites. Arch Intern Med 2001; 161:2733–7.

Navasa M, Rodes J. Bacterial infections in cirrhosis. Liv Int 2004; 24:277–80.

Riordan SM, Williams R. Infection and the intestinal flora in cirrhosis. J Hepatol 2006; 45:744–57.

Romney R, Mathurin P, Ganne-Carrie N, et al. Usefulness of routine analysis of ascitic fluid at the time of therapeutic paracentesis in asymptomatic outpatients. Gastroenterol Clin Biol 2005; 29:275–9.

Runyon BA, Montano AA, Akriviadis EA, et al. The serum-ascites albumin gradient in the differential diagnosis of ascites is superior to the exudates/transudate concept. Ann Intern Med 1992; 117:215–20.

Such J, Frances R, Munoz C, et al. Detection and identification of bacterial DNA in patients with cirrhosis and culture-negative, nonneutrocytic ascites. Hepatology 2002; 36:135–41.

Chapter 32

CHOLESTASIS AND JAUNDICE

KEY POINTS

- Biliary, hepatocellular and systemic conditions may all cause cholestasis and jaundice.
- Elevated bilirubin and cholestatic enzymes (ALP and GGT) suggest a biliary cause. Elevated bilirubin and transaminases (ALT and AST) suggest a hepatocellular cause.
- Imaging with abdominal ultrasound is essential to evaluate for the presence of biliary obstruction and parenchymal liver disease, giving useful information about both the underlying cause for cholestasis and any complications of liver disease.
- A liver screen should be performed to narrow the differential diagnosis for cholestasis.
- Treatment of cholestasis is primarily aimed at treating the underlying cause.
- Pruritis is a troublesome symptom of cholestasis, and can occur with elevated bile acids, even when the bilirubin is within normal range. There is a range of specific treatments available.
- Cholestatic disorders contribute to mortality and morbidity and are, in some settings, an important indication for liver transplantation.

INTRODUCTION

Cholestasis and jaundice are common clinical occurrences which flag the presence of an underlying disease process. Diseases of the liver and biliary tree are a significant cause of morbidity and mortality and an important indication for liver transplantation in certain settings. This chapter outlines an approach to dealing with this common problem.

Definitions

Cholestasis can be defined as 'the excess of biliary substances in the blood'. Cholestasis may be accompanied by jaundice and/or deranged liver biochemistry. Although cholestasis commonly occurs in the context of biliary obstruction, it may occur without evidence of biliary pathology.

CAUSES OF CHOLESTASIS

Cholestasis can broadly be divided into that caused by mechanical obstruction, and that caused by non-obstructive or hepatocellular causes. Table 32.1 lists the causes of cholestasis. Mechanical obstruction may develop in either the extrahepatic biliary tree or the smaller intrahepatic bile ducts. Non-obstructive intrahepatic cholestasis may arise from parenchymal disease affecting the small bile ducts and canaliculi or conditions affecting the hepatocytes directly (causing an excess of bile products to be formed). Considering the possible underlying causes of cholestasis will guide the history, examination and investigation of a patient with cholestasis. Important causes to consider include the following.

1 Cholelithiasis and choledocholithiasis: cholelithiasis (stones in gall bladder) is common, occurring in up to 25% of Caucasian population, and more in certain ethnic groups. Choledocholithiasis (stone in bile duct) complicates 15%–20% of patients with cholelithiasis. Major risk factors for cholelithiasis include age, female gender, family history, obesity, diabetes and hyperlipidaemia. States with elevated oestrogen and progesterone (pregnancy, oral contraceptives and hormone therapy) are also lithogenic.

2 Malignancy: malignancies (primary and secondary) can cause cholestasis both by mechanical obstruction (e.g. large intrahepatic tumours, cholangiocarcinomas or pancreatic tumours) or by disruption of normal hepatocyte function (hepatocyte destruction).

3 Primary sclerosing cholangitis (PSC): an idiopathic inflammatory disorder of bile ducts characterised by small and large bile duct strictures, portal fibrosis and cirrhosis. Patients have abnormal liver function tests at diagnosis, but only approximately half of the patients are symptomatic at this time. Coexisting inflammatory bowel disease is found in 62% of the patients. High-dose ursodeoxycholic acid has been used to manage cholestasis and endoscopic therapy for dominant bile duct strictures, however the role of these therapies requires further investigation. The risk of developing cholangiocarcinoma is high.

4 Primary biliary cirrhosis (PBC): an autoimmune disease of the bile ducts, occurring predominantly in women, which if untreated can progress to fibrosis and cirrhosis.

TABLE 32.1: Causes of cholestasis

Mechanical obstruction		Non-obstructive intrahepatic cholestasis		Systemic illness
Extrahepatic	*Intrahepatic*	*Small bile ducts/canalicular*	*Hepatocellular*	
Malignant	Malignant	• Primary biliary cirrhosis	• Viral	• Right heart failure
• Cholangiocarcinoma	• Metastatic malignancy	• Primary sclerosing cholangitis	• Alcoholic hepatitis	• Haemolysis
• Pancreatic carcinoma		• Vanishing bile duct syndrome	• Drug induced	
• Ampullary carcinoma		– Chronic rejection in liver transplants	• Autoimmune	
• Gall bladder carcinoma		– Sarcoidosis	• Malignant infiltration	
• Metastases to lymph nodes in porta hepatis	Benign	– Drugs	• Vascular occlusion	
	• Abscess	• Inherited	– Budd-Chiari syndrome	
Benign	• Primary sclerosing cholangitis	– Benign recurrent cholestasis	– Portal vein thrombosis	
• Choledocholithiasis	• Suppurative cholangitis	– Progressive familial intrahepatic cholestasis	• Metabolic/Hereditary	
• Primary sclerosing cholangitis	• Congenital fibrosis	– Gilbert's syndrome	– NAFLD/NASH	
• Chronic pancreatitis		– Crigler-Najjar syndrome	– Iron overload	
• AIDS cholangiopathy		– Dubin-Johnson syndrome	– Wilson's disease	
• Congenital		– Rotor syndrome	– Alpha₁-antitrypsin deficiency	
– Choledochocele		• Cholestasis of pregnancy	– Galactosaemia	
			– Tyrosinaemia	
			– Cystic fibrosis	

AIDS = acquired immunodeficiency syndrome; NAFLD = non-alcoholic fatty liver disease; NASH = non-alcoholic steatohepatitis.

Antimitochondrial antibodies are found in 95% of patients with PBC. Ursodeoxycholic acid is the only treatment established to modify disease progression in PBC.

5 Drug-induced cholestasis: this can occur with a number of pharmacological agents and may be associated with variable degrees of hepatitis. The offending drug should be promptly discontinued. In some circumstances, drug induced cholestasis may progress to vanishing bile duct syndrome, veno-occlusive disease or liver failure.

6 Hepatocellular causes: any acute or chronic hepatocellular injury can cause cholestasis (e.g. viral or alcoholic hepatitis). This is characterised by a predominant elevation in the serum transaminases and the cholestasis usually resolves sometime after the resolution of the underlying acute hepatocellular injury.

7 Congenital: a choledochocele is a cystic dilatation of the common bile duct, which may cause intermittent biliary obstruction. It is rare, occurring in approximately 1:100,000–150,000 live births. About 80% are diagnosed before 10 years of age, classically presenting as a triad of right upper quadrant pain, a mass and jaundice. In adults this is a rare presentation with abdominal pain and tenderness being the most common features. Endoscopic and surgical therapies are possible.

8 Inherited defects of bilirubin uptake, glucuronidation and transport:

a Unconjugated hyperbilirubinaemia:

  i Gilbert's syndrome: the most common inherited disorder of bilirubin glucuronidation. Diagnosed in young adults who present with mild icterus or isolated hyperbilirubinaemia. Impaired conjugation of bilirubin is due to reduced bilirubin UDP glucuronosyl transferase activity.

  ii Crigler-Najjar syndrome (Type I & II): congenital non-haemolytic jaundice with glucuronosyltransferase deficiency. A rare, autosomal recessive disorder of bilirubin metabolism presenting as neonatal jaundice (kernicterus).

b Conjugated hyperbilirubinaemia: characterised clinically by mild icterus presenting in the second decade of life.

  i Dubin-Johnson syndrome: rare condition except in Sephardic Jews (incidence is 1:3000) due to altered excretion of bilirubin into the bile ducts.

  ii Rotor syndrome: due to defective hepatic storage of bilirubin.

c Defects in canalicular transport: a range of molecular defects can result in impaired transport of bile acids, phospholipids and ions that express as progressive familial forms of cholestasis.

9 Haemolysis: although haemolysis due to any cause leads to an excess of biliary substances in the blood (unconjugated hyperbilirubinaemia) and may cause clinically evident jaundice, it is not usually associated with cholestatic symptoms. An exception to this is haemolytic disease of the newborn which causes kernicterus, a condition with significant risks to the neonate.

ASSESSMENT

History

Fatigue is the most common symptom of chronic cholestasis. Other symptoms include jaundice, pruritis and steatorrhoea. There may be a history of haemorrhage due to poor vitamin K absorption or bone pain and fractures due to poor vitamin D and calcium absorption (in cases of chronic cholestasis resulting in hepatic osteodystrophy or osteoporosis).

Specific questioning will help determine the underlying aetiology of the cholestasis.

- Enquire about the presence, site and character of abdominal pain. The absence of pain is also relevant. Ask about associated nausea, vomiting and the timing of these symptoms.
- Fevers, chills and rigors suggest hepatobiliary obstruction or an infectious aetiology.
- Enquire about constitutional symptoms suggestive of underlying malignancy (weight loss, appetite change) and perform a specific systems review for other symptoms of malignancy.
- Ask about intercurrent conditions, especially:
  - Pregnancy
  - Metabolic disorders
  - Autoimmune disorders
  - Malignancy
  - Inflammatory bowel disease
  - Cardiac disease
  - Haematological conditions.

- Take a family history with particular focus on liver disease, autoimmune diseases, malignancies, neonatal jaundice or cholestasis of pregnancy.
- A thorough drug history (including complementary and over-the-counter drugs) is essential to evaluate for the possibility of a drug-induced cholestasis.
- Ask about the level of alcohol consumption (in grams per day) and illicit or recreational drug use. Risk factors for viral hepatitis and human immunodeficiency virus (HIV) should be elicited (intravenous drug use, tattoos, blood product transfusions, foreign travel, infectious contacts, occupation, sexual history).

Physical examination

Start with general inspection. Scleral icterus is first visible when the serum bilirubin is greater than twice the upper limit of normal. There may also be generalised jaundice (yellowing of the skin). Check for scratch marks (suggesting pruritis), bruising (vitamin K deficiency) and muscle wasting (malabsorption, malignancy).

Then check the nursing observations. Check for fever, hypotension and tachycardia which suggest sepsis/infection. Assess if the patient is orientated to time, person and place. Examine for asterixis (hepatic flap) and fetor, which suggest hepatic encephalopathy. Check for signs of chronic liver disease (palmar erythema, spider naevae, gynaecomastia, dilated abdominal wall veins). Examine for lymphadenopathy in all lymph node groups.

Examine the abdomen for organomegaly and masses. A small shrunken liver with splenomegaly suggests chronic liver disease. An enlarged liver suggests acute hepatitis, hepatic congestion, primary biliary cirrhosis or an infiltrating process (malignant or non malignant). A nodular liver suggests malignancy, cystic disease or cirrhosis.

The presence of a palpable gall bladder in a patient with painless jaundice is worrying (Courvoisier's sign)—this suggests compression of both the cystic duct and bile duct, usually due to malignancy of the head of the pancreas. A tender gall bladder suggests cholecystitis—if there is associated jaundice, a gallstone in the common bile duct (choledocholithiasis) is likely. Choledocholithiasis alone causes abdominal pain, but rarely tenderness on examination unless there is associated pancreatitis or cholecystitis.

Check for shifting dullness (ascites), which, if present, suggests hepatic decompensation.

Investigations

Basic laboratory tests: biochemistry (liver function tests, electrolytes and creatinine), full blood count and coagulation profile. Note the degree of hyperbilirubinaemia and the presence of hypoalbuminaemia and coagulopathy (which together suggest hepatic decompensation). Disorders of the bile ducts predominantly cause elevation in gamma glutamyltransferase (GGT) and alkaline phosphates (ALP). In disorders affecting hepatocytes, the serum transaminases (alanine aminotransferase [ALT] and aspartate aminotransferase [AST]) predominantly may be elevated. There is often mixed liver function test derangement, in which case further investigations may be necessary to narrow the differential diagnosis (see Chapter 30).

Non-invasive imaging modalities

Ultrasound is an essential basic imaging modality to investigate for biliary and hepatic parenchymal pathology. The size and echogenicity of the liver, the presence of biliary duct dilatation, cholelithiasis/choledocholithiasis and the gall bladder may all be assessed. The pancreas and spleen should also be assessed for size and space occupying lesions, and Doppler flow studies of the hepatic and portal veins performed to check for thrombosis or other impedance to blood flow. The presence and volume of ascites should also be noted.

Computed tomography (CT) scans or magnetic resonance cholangiopancreatography (MRCP) may be needed to further characterise abnormal findings.

Invasive imaging modalities (with therapeutic capability)

Endoscopic retrograde cholangiopancreatography (ERCP): ERCP allows imaging of both the pancreatobiliary tree as well as therapeutic intervention with sphincterotomy, biliary dilatation, biliary duct balloon trawl, lithotripsy and stenting. The complications of pancreatitis, cholangitis, bleeding and perforation should be weighed against benefits of the procedure.

Percutaneous transhepatic cholangiography (PTC): this ultrasound-guided procedure is an alternative or adjunct in patients who will not tolerate ERCP, or in those patients in whom ERCP is technically difficult (e.g. in cases of non-dilated biliary system or abnormal anatomy). Biliary stenting and percutaneous biliary drainage is also possible with this method.

Endoscopic ultrasound (EUS): EUS has been used to image the hepatobiliary tree, pancreas and adjacent structures. Its precise role in the investigation and management of cholestatic disorders is under evaluation.

Table 32.2 summarises the sensitivity and specificity of the range of imaging modalities available for detecting choledocholithiasis.

Liver screen

If basic investigations exclude obstructive causes for cholestasis, investigations for parenchymal or intrahepatic causes may be needed. The following liver screen should be considered.

- Viral causes:
  - Hepatitis A IgM, HBsAg (hepatitis B surface antigen), HBcAb (hepatitis B core antibody), HBeAg (hepatitis B e antigen) and HBeAb (hepatitis B e antibody)
  - Hepatitis B DNA PCR (polymerase chain reaction) and/or hepatitis C RNA PCR and genotype if serology positive
  - Epstein-Barr virus (EBV) IgG and IgM, cytomegalovirus (CMV) IgG and IgM.

TABLE 32.2: Sensitivities and specificities of imaging modalities used to detect cholelithiasis, choledocholithiasis and biliary obstruction

Modality	Cholelithiasis		Choledocholithiasis		Biliary obstruction	
	Sensitivity	*Specificity*	*Sensitivity*	*Specificity*	*Sensitivity*	*Specificity*
Ultrasound (US)	84%	99%	50%–75%	–	55%–91%	–
Computed tomography (CT)	Poor	Poor	50%–75%	–	–	–
Magnetic resonance cholangiopan-creatography (MRCP)	Similar to US	Similar to US	80%–100%	85%–100%	95%	97%
Endoscopic ultrasound (EUS)	100%	85%	88%–97%	96%–100%	–	–

- Autoimmune causes:
  - Antimitochondrial antibody (AMA), antineutrophil cytoplasmic antibody (ANCA), anti-liver/kidney microsomal antibody (Anti-LKM Ab), anti-smooth muscle antibody
  - Gamma globulin level.
- Malignant causes:
  - Alpha-fetoprotein (AFP), human chorionic gonadotrophin (β-hCG), electrophoresis (EPG), immunoelectrophoresis (IEPG), carbohydrate antigen (CA 19-9).
- Metabolic causes:
  - Fasting glucose, insulin, C-peptide
  - Fasting cholesterol and triglycerides
  - Thyroid function tests
  - Copper and caeruloplasmin
  - Iron studies
  - Alpha$_1$-antitrypsin level (and genotype if level reduced).
- Haemolysis
  - Blood film, lactate dehydrogenase (LDH), reticulocytes, haptoglobins, Coombs test.

Liver biopsy

Percutaneous liver biopsy is considered the gold standard for diagnosis of liver disease. A liver biopsy may be necessary before committing a patient to specific treatments with significant adverse effects or toxicity. Liver biopsy is also useful to determine disease severity and prognosis by evaluating extent of fibrosis or cirrhosis. Specialty consultation should be considered before a liver biopsy because of the risks associated with the procedure (see Chapter 33).

MANAGEMENT

1 Treat underlying cause:
   - In cases of mechanical obstruction, consider endoscopic retrograde cholangiopancreatography (ERCP) to relieve dominant strictures, malignant obstruction or choledocholithiasis
   - Surgery
   - Systemic conditions: treat heart failure, malignancies, etc
   - See chapters on treating specific underlying disorders.
2 Remove exacerbating/precipitating factors:
   - Hepatotoxic drugs
   - Alcohol.

3 Treat complications of chronic cholestasis:
   - Treat cholangitis with antibiotics
   - Correct nutritional/vitamin deficiencies
   - Treat any manifestations of hepatic decompensation (see Chapter 47).
4 Symptomatic treatment (see Table 32.3):
   a For mild cholestatic pruritus—nonspecific measures:
      - Warm baths
      - Antihistamines: promethazine 10–20 mg b.d. and 25–75 mg nocte (sedating), or loratadine or cetirizine 10 mg daily (non-sedating).
   b For moderate to severe pruritus, or mild pruritus that does not respond to simple measures:
      - Cholestyramine (4 g daily) or
      - Colestipol (15–30 g daily in 2–4 divided doses) or
      - Ursodeoxycholic acid (15 mg/kg daily in two divided doses).
      If these fail, consider:
      - Rifampicin 150 mg b.d. (monitor liver function tests for drug induced/idiosyncratic liver derangement)
      - Phenobarbitone 90 mg q.i.d. (alternative to rifampicin—has the disadvantage of somnolence during the first few weeks of use).
   c Refractory pruritis: these patients may need an acute pain team consultation or consideration for use of investigational techniques:
      - Opioid antagonists, e.g. naloxone
      - Plasmapheresis
      - Phototherapy
      - Extracorporeal albumin dialysis
      - Emerging therapies – pharmacologic modulation of xenobiotic/nuclear receptors.
      Liver transplantation should also be considered in refractory cholestatic pruritis.
5 Consider:
   a Biliary reconstruction
      - High mortality from surgery, especially if cirrhotic.
   b Liver transplantation—85% five-year survival. Indications include:
      - Haemorrhage due to oesophageal varices or portal gastropathy
      - Intractable ascites

- Recurrent bacterial cholangitis
- Progressive muscle wasting
- Hepatic encephalopathy
- Refractory cholestatic pruritis.
c Pregnant women: obstetric liaison is essential (see Chapter 48).
  - Pregnant women are susceptible to all the usual causes of cholestasis as listed above.
  - Cholestasis of pregnancy: severe cholestasis with significant symptoms may occur from 20 weeks gestation. The cholestasis resolves following delivery of the baby. Ursodeoxycholic acid may improve symptoms and may also improve fetal outcome especially if serum bile acids exceed 40 µg/mL:
    - Ursodeoxycholic acid 15 mg/kg orally, daily in two divided doses, or
    - Cholestyramine 4 g daily.

TABLE 32.3: Mechanism of action of drugs to manage cholestasis

Cholestyramine	Cholestyramine resin combines with bile acids forming a complex that is excreted in the faeces. This non-systemic action results in a partial removal of the bile acids from the enterohepatic circulation, preventing their reabsorption
Colestipol	An oral hypolipidaemic that binds bile acids in the intestine, i.e. works like cholestyramine
Ursodeoxycholic acid (UDCA)	A hydrophilic bile acid. The assumption is that replacing the bile acid pool UDCA may reduce hepatocyte damage
Rifampicin	May decrease pruritus by competing with bile acids for hepatic uptake, thereby minimising bile acid toxicity to the hepatocyte. May also induce microsomal enzymes that promote 6-alpha-hydroxylation and subsequent glucuronidation of toxic bile salts
Phenobarbitone	Sedative properties
Opioid antagonists	Opiate receptors may be implicated in pathogenesis of pruritis therefore blocking these receptors theoretically may improve symptoms

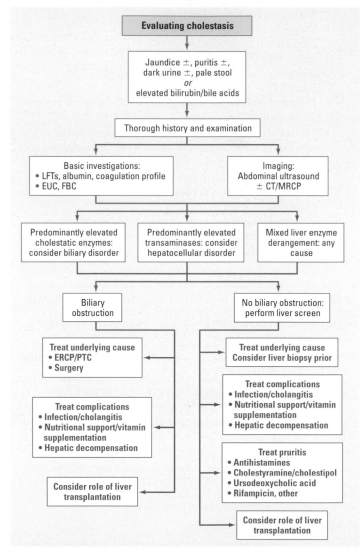

FIGURE 32.1: The evaluation of cholestasis.

CT = computed tomography; ERCP = endoscopic cholangiopancreatography;
EUC = electrolytes, urea, creatinine; FBC = full blood count; LFTs = liver function
tests; MRCP = magnetic resonance cholangiopancreatography; PTC = percutaneous
transhepatic cholangiography.

SUMMARY

Both cholestasis and jaundice can arise due to biliary, hepatocellular and systemic conditions. Biochemical clues may suggest the underlying mechanism for the cholestasis: elevated bilirubin and cholestatic enzymes (ALP and GGT) suggest a biliary cause; elevated bilirubin and transaminases (ALT and AST) suggest a hepatocellular cause (Figure 32.1). Imaging with abdominal ultrasound gives useful information about both the underlying cause for cholestasis and any complications of liver disease. A full liver screen will narrow the differential diagnosis for cholestasis. Treatment of cholestasis is primarily aimed at treating the underlying cause, but a range of symptomatic treatments is available. In particular, pruritus is a troublesome symptom of cholestasis, and can occur with elevated bile acids, even when the bilirubin is within normal range.

One must appreciate that cholestatic disorders contribute to mortality and morbidity and, in some settings, these disorders are an important indication for liver transplantation.

FURTHER READING

Balistreri WF, Bezerra JA, Jansen P, et al. Intrahepatic cholestasis: summary of an American Association for the Study of Liver Diseases single-topic conference. Hepatology 2005, 42:222–35.

Demery PA, Seidman DS, Stevenson DK. Neonatal hyperbilirubinaemia. N Engl J Med 2001; 344:581–90.

Glantz A, Marschall HU, Mattsson LA. Intrahepatic cholestasis of pregnancy: relationships between bile acid levels and fetal complication rates. Hepatology 2006; 40:467–74.

Glasova H, Beuers U. Extrahepatic manifestations of cholestasis. J Gastroenterol Hepatol 2002; 17:938–48.

Kaplan MM, Gershwin ME. Primary biliary cirrhosis. N Eng J Med 2005; 353:1261–73.

Levy C, Lindor KD. Drug-induced cholestasis. Clin Liver Dis 2003; 7:311–30.

LIVER BIOPSY

INTRODUCTION

Liver biopsy remains an important tool in the investigation of hepatic dysfunction. It can obtain qualitative information regarding liver architecture, as well as type and degree of acute hepatic injury, and can both identify and qualify degree of fibrosis. A biopsy is usually performed after numerous non-invasive liver tests have been obtained.

It is also useful in evaluating and monitoring treatment of hepatic abnormalities and diseases, including post-transplant, and in guiding future management.

BIOPSY METHODS

Percutaneous: most commonly used method, and safe when performed by an experienced operator. Use of ultrasound as a marker for needle entry improves safety.

Transjugular: a more invasive method, and most commonly used in patients with bleeding diatheses, or those with other conditions that would make percutaneous approach unsafe, such as morbid obesity or massive ascites, or after a failed attempt at percutaneous biopsy.

Laparoscopic: invasive, and requires a surgical approach, and therefore general anaesthetic. Often performed in conjunction with another surgical procedure (e.g. cholecystectomy). Has an advantage over percutaneous biopsy in malignant hepatic lesions and in cirrhosis, and provides a higher diagnostic yield.

Ultrasound or CT-guided fine needle aspiration: obtains only a small number of cells, and is used mainly to target specific liver lesions, rather than sample a homogeneous liver.

Indications

- Grading and staging of chronic hepatitis B.
- Grading and staging of chronic hepatitis C in genotype 1, or hepatitis B and C coinfection.
- Diagnosis of abnormal liver tests, usually after at least 6 months of inconclusive serological tests.
- Diagnosis of non-alcoholic steatohepatitis (NASH), autoimmune hepatitis and alcoholic liver disease.
- Diagnosis of haemochromatosis with ferritin >1000 µg/L and Wilson's disease.
- Primary biliary cirrhosis and sclerosing cholangitis.
- Evaluation of liver function post-transplant, and to assess potential donor.
- Assessment of drug effects on the liver (e.g. long-term methotrexate therapy).
- Diagnosis of a liver lesion.
- Pyrexia of unknown origin.

Histology is not needed prior to therapy for hepatitis C in some centres, therefore biopsy is not always necessary. Biopsy may stage the disease satisfactorily, but is not good for predicting clinical response to treatment.

Percutaneous biopsy of a neoplastic lesion has the small potential for seeding, and is therefore not usually performed. A lesion >2 cm with a high alpha-fetoprotein (AFP) in serum is highly sensitive for malignancy.

Biopsy is the only method of assessing fibrosis in NASH (see Chapter 39). Patients with a BMI >30 kg/m^2, diabetes or age >45 years should be biopsied. Up to 20% of NASH patients will have severe fibrosis.

Diagnosis of viral hepatitis or NAFLD does not require biopsy.

At least six portal tracts are needed for accurate diagnosis. Specimen should be at least 2 cm in length.

Contraindications

Absolute

- Previous unexplained bleeding.
- Uncooperative patient.
- Suspected vascular lesion or echinococcal disease.
- Poor resuscitation facilities.
- Accurate biopsy site not identified by percussion or ultrasound.

Relative

- Non-steroidal antiinflammatory drug (NSAID) use in last 7 days.
- Platelets <60,000/mL.
- Prothrombin time >4 seconds.
- Prolonged bleeding time (>10 minutes).
- Haemophilia.
- Ascites.
- Obesity.
- Right-sided pleural or diaphragmatic infections.
- Acute renal failure.
- Skin infection at the potential biopsy site.

} May be corrected by appropriate methods prior to biopsy

PATIENT PREPARATION

- Thorough history and examination.
- Fully informed consent, including:
  - Indication for biopsy
  - Alternatives
  - Limitation of biopsy
  - A full understanding of the risks and complications.

Check:

- Patient is fasted or has had a light breakfast prior to biopsy.
- Patient uses the bathroom prior to biopsy, and understands they need to lie still post procedure.

- Patient should be resting and feel comfortable. Low-dose benzodiazepine premedication is sometimes useful.
- An ultrasound has been performed, if required, to mark the biopsy site.
- Patient has not inadvertently used aspirin, NSAIDs, warfarin or other anticoagulant medications, including many herbal preparations e.g. *Ginkgo biloba*, fish oil.
- Administration of relevant factors that decrease risk of post-procedure bleeding, e.g. fresh frozen plasma (FFP), desmopressin acetate, platelets.
- Patient should be close to hospital in case of delayed complication.

EQUIPMENT

- Suction needle: more likely to cause fragmentation of specimen, which reduces accuracy and therefore avoided in suspected cirrhosis.
- Cutting needle: more likely to cause bleeding due to longer time within the liver.
- Spring-loaded cutting needle: most commonly used.

COMPLICATIONS

- Up to 96% occur within 24 hours.
- Up to 60% occur within 2 hours.
- Complications are more likely to occur:
  - In patients over 50 years
  - In patients with minor coagulopathy
  - When two or more passes are made.
- Mortality varies in series from 0.01% to 0.25%.
- Pre-biopsy ultrasound reduces complication rate.
- Needle gauge should not change complication rate.

Major complications (1%) include:
- Bleeding 0.1%–0.5%
- Haemobilia up to one week post-procedure
- Jaundice and pain—rare.

Minor complications (6%–13%) include:
- Pain at biopsy site—most common
- Vasovagal episode
- Vomiting.

POST PROCEDURE

- Right lateral position for up to 2 hours.
- Supine for a further 1 hour.
- Monitor blood pressure and pulse every 15 minutes for first hour, then every 30 minutes until discharge.
- Patients should have a realistic expectation of post-procedure recovery. In surveys, 30% of patients would refuse a future repeat biopsy.

SUMMARY

Liver biopsy is a relatively safe investigation in experienced hands, and remains the gold standard for investigation of hepatic dysfunction or architectural abnormality. The percutaneous method is most commonly used, and can be done as an outpatient. Indications for biopsy include investigation of abnormal liver function tests, grading and staging of chronic hepatitis B or C, and monitoring treatment post liver transplant. Non-invasive serological and liver function tests should be obtained prior to biopsy. Major contraindications to percutaneous biopsy include bleeding tendencies, morbid obesity and ascites. Alternative methods of biopsy include laparoscopic or transjugular techniques. Informed consent is vital, with a full explanation of risks, possible complications and alternative investigations. Most patients will experience a small amount of pain at the biopsy site.

FURTHER READING

Bravo AA, Sheth SG, Chopra S. Liver biopsy. N Engl J Med 2001; 344:495–500.

Campbell MS, Reddy KR. Review article: the evolving role of liver biopsy. Aliment Pharmacol Ther 2004; 20:249–59.

de Ledinghen V, Combes M, Trouette H, et al. Should a liver biopsy be done in patients with subclinical chronically elevated transaminases? Eur J Gastroenterol Hepatol 2004; 16:879–83.

Firpi RJ, Soldevila-Pico C, Abdelmalek MF, et al. Short recovery time after percutaneous liver biopsy: Should we change our current practices? Clin Gastroenterol Hepatol 2005; 3:926–9.

van der Poorten D, Kwok A, Lam T, et al. Twenty-year audit of percutaneous liver biopsy in a major Australian teaching hospital. Int Med J 2006; 36:692–9.

Chapter 34

ACUTE HEPATITIS

KEY POINTS

- Acute hepatitis generally denotes conditions of self-limiting hepatic injury.
- The majority are caused by viral hepatitis with variable geographic prevalence.
- History of travel, family contacts, immunocompetency, blood transfusions, intravenous (IV) drug usage, sexual practice, tattoos, body piercing, birthplace and prior vaccination can provide useful information for differential diagnosis.
- Drug-induced hepatitis is an important consideration as it can lead to fulminant hepatitis unless it is reversed early by removal of the offending agent and, if available, treatment with antidote.
- Most cases of acute hepatitis are expected to resolve in weeks with supportive therapy although some might represent the early phase of a chronic process.

GENERAL CONSIDERATIONS

The term acute hepatitis is not well defined. It generally denotes conditions of self-limiting hepatic injury, although, in many instances, it also encompasses the early phase of chronic liver diseases such as hepatitis B and C. Implicit in the definition, liver histology at the time of presentation should have no evidence of chronicity, such as fibrosis.

Most cases of acute hepatitis are caused by viral hepatitis. Systemic infections such as pneumonia are also commonly associated with non-specific and reactive hepatitis. A smaller cohort is associated with drugs, vascular abnormalities, metabolic disturbance, autoimmunity, pregnancy and systemic illness, such as cardiogenic shock and metabolic disturbance (Table 34.1). However, in fulminant hepatic failure or subfulminant hepatic failure, drugs can become a dominant cause of acute hepatitis. The scope of this chapter will focus primarily on acute viral hepatitis.

TABLE 34.1: Differential diagnoses of acute hepatitis

Viral hepatitis	*Systemic infections*
• Hepatitis A–E • Epstein-Barr Virus (EBV) • Cytomegalovirus (CMV)	• Bacterial infections • Tuberculosis
Drugs	*Metabolic*
• Paracetamol (acetaminophen) • Flucloxacillin • Amoxycillin plus clavulanic acid • Isoniazid • Sulfonamides • Phenytoin • Ketoconazole • Over-the-counter medications	• Hyperglycaemia • Hyperthyroidism • Wilson's disease
	Autoimmunity • Autoimmune hepatitis
Vascular	*Pregnancy associated conditions*
• Ischaemic hepatitis • Budd-Chiari syndrome	• Cholestasis of pregnancy • Haemolysis, elevated liver enzymes and low platelets (HELLP) syndrome • Acute fatty liver of pregnancy (AFLP)

CLINICAL PRESENTATION

The clinical spectrum of acute hepatitis may range from mild symptoms and signs (Table 34.2) associated with recent onset of liver enzyme abnormalities to fulminant hepatic failure. Most symptoms and signs are non-specific (Table 34.2) though there are some manifestations associated with specific conditions, and if present, are helpful in differential diagnosis (Table 34.3).

TABLE 34.2: Non-specific symptoms and signs of acute hepatitis

• Malaise	• Myalgia
• Flu-like symptoms	• Jaundice
• Weight Loss	• Pruritis
• Anorexia	• Dark urine
• Nausea	• Hepatomegaly
• Vomiting	• Ascites
• Diarrhoea	• Encephalopathy
• Arthralgia	• Fever

TABLE 34.3: Diagnostically helpful associations of acute hepatitis	
Infectious mononucleosis Lymphadenopathy Pharyngitis Splenomegaly Thrombocytopenia Haemolytic anaemia	*Hepatitis C* Cryoglobulinaemia *Metabolic disturbance* Hyperthyroidism Kayser-Fleischer rings
Hepatitis B Polyarteritis nodosum	*Drugs* Desquamating dermatitis Eosinophilia

DIFFERENTIAL DIAGNOSES

A diagnostic algorithm is suggested for assessing a patient presenting with acute hepatitis (Figure 34.1). There may be obvious clues at the outset such as pregnancy, history of paracetamol overdose or recent drug use. Serology for common causes of viral hepatitis and paracetamol level should be requested as initial investigations. Failing to identify an obvious cause, other less common causes would need to be considered and liver biopsy may be necessary.

Acute viral hepatitis

The most common cause of acute hepatitis found on audits of consecutive presentations to the emergency department is hepatitis B, followed by hepatitis A and C (Table 34.4). History of travel, family contacts, immunocompetency, blood transfusions, intravenous (IV) drug usage, sexual practice, tattoos, body piercing, birthplace and prior vaccination can provide useful information for differential diagnosis.

The geographic differences in the prevalence of acute viral hepatitis also need to be borne in mind in differential diagnosis. In Western countries, most cases of hepatitis B and C are acquired as an adult through sexual transmission or drug use. Hepatitis E is unusual in Western countries but common in the Indian subcontinent (Table 34.4). On the other hand, in Asian countries, notably Taiwan, almost half the cases are represented by hepatitis B carriers presenting either with an exacerbation of hepatitis B infection or with superimposed non-B hepatotropic viral infections (Table 34.4).

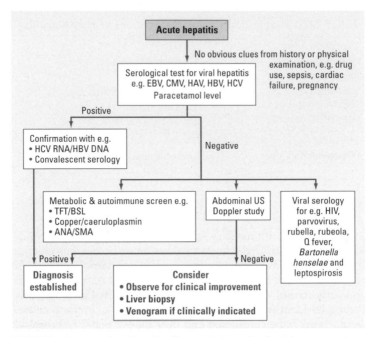

FIGURE 34.1: An algorithm for diagnostic investigations for acute hepatitis.

ANA = antinuclear antibody; BSL = blood sugar level; CMV = cytomegalovirus; EBV = Epstein-Barr virus; HAV = hepatitis A virus; HBV = hepatitis B virus; HCV = hepatitis C virus; HIV = human immunodeficiency virus; SMA = anti-smooth muscle antibody; TFT = thyroid function tests; US = ultrasound.

TABLE 34.4: Prevalence of acute viral hepatitis	
Western countries	
Acute hepatitis B	30%–60%
Hepatitis A	25%–50%
Acute hepatitis C	15%–20%
EBV hepatitis	2%–10%
Hepatitis G	1%
CMV hepatitis	1%

TABLE 34.4: Prevalence of acute viral hepatitis *(continued)*	
Asian countries	
Acute hepatitis B	5%–13%
Acute exacerbation of chronic hepatitis B	15%–40%
Acute hepatitis C	21%
Acute hepatitis C in hepatitis B carriers	12%
Hepatitis A	3%–4%
Hepatitis E	2%–70%*
Hepatitis A, D, E in hepatitis B carriers	20%
Non A–E hepatitis	16%
Superimposed non A–E hepatitis in hepatitis B carriers	15%
* There is significant geographical variability with the higher proportion of hepatitis E virus accounting for presentation of acute hepatitis reported in India. CMV = cytomegalovirus; EBV = Epstein-Barr virus.	

The incubation interval ranging from 2 to 7 weeks for hepatitis A and E, up to 26 weeks for hepatitis B and C, is often helpful in assessing for potential source of contacts. Serological testing is generally adequate in confirming the aetiology of acute viral hepatitis. Histology is rarely required and often unhelpful for distinguishing one condition from another.

Epstein-Barr virus hepatitis

Epstein-Barr virus (EBV) infection is transmitted via oral contact. While infection is typically subclinical, it can manifest the clinical syndrome of infectious mononucleosis in a small subset of patients, with fever, exudative pharyngitis, lymphadenopathy, hepatosplenomegaly and atypical lymphocytosis. The illness is more likely to develop in a younger patient as most individuals over the age of 40 have had past contact with EBV and therefore immune to subsequent re-infection. In older patients, the diagnosis may not be immediately apparent as they are less likely than younger patients to have lymphadenopathy and pharyngitis.

Of patients with EBV infection, 80%–90% have mild hepatic parenchymal injury with most expected to resolve spontaneously. Rarely, it could manifest as cholestatic hepatitis, progress to chronic hepatitis or fulminant hepatic failure. Most cases of fatality are associated with immunodeficiency. Hence, depending on the age of the patient, testing for human immunodeficiency virus (HIV) status, X-linked lymphoproliferative disease and complement deficiency should be considered in those presenting with fulminant hepatitis.

Laboratory investigations

Atypical lymphocytes	Not pathognomonic
	May be found in toxoplasmosis, rubella, roseola and CMV
Lymphocytosis	Usually 12–18 × 10⁹/L
Heterophile antibody	Detectable within 1 week of symptoms Sensitivity 70%–92% and specificity 96%–100%
EBV IgM	Directed at the viral capsid antigen, early antigen and anti-EBV nuclear antigen

Cytomegalovirus infection

Clinical manifestations of cytomegalovirus (CMV) infection are similar to EBV but cervical lymphadenopathy is more frequent in EBV than CMV. It may occur as a result of primary infection or reactivation of a latent viral infection. The infection is transmitted by direct contact. CMV infection is rarely symptomatic in previously healthy adults. It is the most prevalent cause of acute hepatitis in young infants. In such cases, a subgroup may develop massive hepatocellular necrosis, giant cell hepatitis, cholestasis, cirrhosis or hepatic failure associated with poor prognosis and increased mortality.

Laboratory Investigations

Atypical lymphocytosis	Not pathognomonic
CMV IgM	False positive may be associated with pregnancy, rheumatoid arthritis, Sjögren's syndrome and antinuclear antibody (ANA)-positive patients

Hepatitis A

Hepatitis A virus (HAV) infection is transmitted via the faecal–oral route. It is the most common cause of viral hepatitis, accounting for a quarter of acute hepatitis in some regions. Seroprevalence varies, ranging from 13% in Sweden, 60% in Australia, to 100% in highly endemic areas such as Africa, Asia and South America. HAV is notable for its relative resistance to degradation, which permits transmission within the population leading to a high attack rate of 70%–90% and secondary attack rate of 15%–20%.

Hepatitis A infection is often self-limiting. Fulminant hepatitis is rare. Infrequently, it may develop a cholestasis variant, relapse after recovery or lead to autoimmune diseases.

Laboratory investigations

HAV IgM	Confirms acute HAV infection
	Peak during the acute phase of infection
	Undetectable after 3–4 months although 25% may have IgM persistence up to 6 months or more
HAV IgG	Indicates previous exposure and immunity to hepatitis A
	Rising HAV IgG levels is indicative of recent exposure
HAV RNA	Not clinically useful as the virus is usually undetectable at the time of clinical manifestation

Hepatitis B

This infection is discussed in more detail in Chapter 36. Acute infection in immunocompetent adults is often self-limiting. Fulminant hepatitis is rare but associated with a poor prognosis. Individuals at risk of chronicity include those who acquired hepatitis perinatally or those with HIV coinfection. Acute hepatitis B infection may be associated with a number of extrahepatic manifestations including polyarteritis nodosa, vasculitis-induced neuropathy, renal disease, rash, arthritis and Raynaud's phenomenon.

Laboratory investigations

Hepatitis B surface antigen	Marker of hepatitis B infection
Hepatitis B surface antibody	Detection in the presence of hepatitis B core IgG indicates resolution of hepatitis B infection and immunity
	Detection in the absence of hepatitis B core IgG indicates immunity from past vaccination
Hepatitis B core IgM	Detectable with the onset of symptoms during acute infection for up to 6 months
	Not able to distinguish between acute infection and a flare as it may also reappear in chronic carriers during a severe flare
Hepatitis B core IgG	Often persists for a lifetime and therefore the best marker of exposure to hepatitis B
Hepatitis B e antigen	Marker of viral replication of wild type hepatitis B
HBV DNA	Marker of viral replication
	Threshold of detection varies with different assays, being the most sensitive with Taqman fluorescent-probe real time PCR at 10 copies/mL

Hepatitis D

The hepatitis D virus (HDV) is transmitted most efficiently among hepatitis B-infected patients through injection. It is therefore most prevalent among injecting drug users coinfected with hepatitis B, from 31% in Ireland to 91% in Taiwan. Perinatal transmission of hepatitis D is rare and vertical transmission of the virus has not been reported. Infection is most prevalent in Italy, Eastern Europe, Central America, Western Asia and some Pacific Islands.

Coinfection of hepatitis D and B is often self-limiting, characterised by a biphasic increase in alanine aminotransferase (ALT), and associated with higher risk of severe or fulminant hepatitis than hepatitis B infection alone. Acute superinfection of hepatitis D in established hepatitis B-infected patients may lead to a flare, which results in clearance of both infections. Chronic superinfection of hepatitis D is thought to hasten disease progression in a subgroup of hepatitis B-infected patients.

Laboratory investigations

HDV IgM	Associated with detectable hepatitis B core IgM in coinfected patients and the absence of hepatitis B core IgM in superinfection
HDV antigen	Often transiently detectable in low titres during late incubation phase and therefore of little clinical utility
IIDV RNA	Not routinely available

Hepatitis E

The hepatitis E virus (HEV) is transmitted via the faecal–oral route. Epidemics of hepatitis E infection occur with ingestion of faecally contaminated water supply. Hepatitis E is the most common cause of enterically transmitted hepatitis being endemic in subcontinental India, Asia, Southeast Pacific, the Middle East, Africa and Central America. Most sporadic cases in non-endemic areas occur primarily in travellers returning from endemic countries. The incidence of infection through household contact is low (0.7%–2.2%). Clinical presentation is usually seen among individuals 15–40 years of age. Most cases are self-limited infections, which resolve in 6 weeks, but fatality can be associated with fulminant hepatitis, of which pregnant women are at higher risk.

Laboratory investigations

HEV IgM	Enzyme immunoassay directed at the structural regions ORF2 and ORF3
	Sensitivity 80%–100%
HEV antigen	Usually undetectable by the time ALT levels peak
	Can be detected in liver tissue and stool
HEV RNA	Not routinely available

Drug-induced hepatitis

Drug-induced liver injury accounts for less than 5% cases of acute hepatitis. Most cases are self-limiting upon withdrawal of the offending drug. However, rarely, some may develop chronicity associated with cirrhosis or vascular complications. Other cases progress to fulminant hepatitis with hepatic failure. Some agents may present with a hepatocellular pattern while others may become predominantly cholestatic.

The most crucial clinical approach to the diagnosis is to ascertain the chronological relationship between the onset of acute hepatitis and commencement of the drug as well as the response upon withdrawal. However, some forms of injury are idiosyncratic and there may be a lag period between the development of hepatitis and time of commencing the drug.

MANAGEMENT

Most cases of acute hepatitis often only require symptomatic relief with intravenous fluids and antiemetics. In the case of paracetamol overdose, N-acetylcysteine should be instigated as soon as possible. Rarely, fulminant hepatic failure develops requiring intensive care unit support and possible assessment for liver transplant.

The majority are expected to resolve in weeks. In some, the course of the illness may become chronic when symptoms are less prominent but progressive hepatic injury occurs. Specific intervention would depend on the aetiology concerned.

SUMMARY

Most cases of acute hepatitis are viral in aetiology and expected to resolve in weeks with supportive therapy. Drug-induced hepatitis constitutes a minority of cases but needs to be considered at the outset as the condition is usually reversible upon removal of the offending agent and instigation of antidote.

FURTHER READING

Ater MJ, Gallagher M, Morris TT, et al. Acute non A-E hepatitis in the United States and the role of hepatitis G virus infection. Sentinel Counties Viral Hepatitis Study Team. N Engl J Med 1997; 336:741–6.

Crum N. Epstein Barr virus hepatitis: case series and review. South Med J 2006; 99:544–7.

Watanabe S, Arima K, Nishioka M, et al. Comparison between sporadic cytomegalovirus hepatitis and Epstein-Barr virus hepatitis in previously healthy adults. Liver 1997; 17:63–9.

Chapter 35

THE HEPATITIS C-POSITIVE PATIENT

KEY POINTS

- Hepatitis C is the leading cause for liver transplantation.
- Specific viral nucleic acid testing is available to confirm the diagnosis of acute and chronic hepatitis C virus (HCV) infection.
- Antiviral therapy should be considered for every patient with acute or chronic HCV infection with provision of counselling and support services.
- Hepatitis C genotype and viral load are useful in predicting a response to therapy; liver biopsy may be useful in providing a long-term prognosis.
- The combination of pegylated interferon and ribavirin is the international standard of therapy for patients with chronic HCV infection.
- Individualisation of antiviral therapy is possible based on genotype and virological response in the first weeks of treatment.

EPIDEMIOLOGY

Prevalence and natural history

The prevalence of hepatitis C virus (HCV) infection varies worldwide with relatively low prevalence in North America and Europe compared with higher prevalence in Asia and southern Europe. The prevalence in Australia is approximately 0.1%, making HCV infection a common cause of chronic liver disease. Recent estimates from the Hepatitis C Projections Working Group 2006 suggest that around 200,000 people were chronically infected with the virus at the end of 2005 in Australia and that the prevalence will triple over the next 20 years. Of chronically infected individuals, 10%–15% will develop liver cirrhosis over a 20-year period. Once cirrhosis is established, hepatocellular carcinoma (HCC) develops at an annual incidence of 2%. In most countries where data are available, HCV infection is the leading cause of liver transplantation. The Hepatitis C Projections

Working Group concluded that the current number of people receiving treatment would need to be increased three-fold to reduce the proportion of patients living with advanced liver disease due to HCV infection.

Risk factors for acquiring HCV infection

HCV is a blood-borne virus and, therefore, a history of blood exposure can be elicited in many patients. The introduction of routine antibody screening of blood products substantially reduced the risk of transmission from blood transfusion to less than 1 in 200,000 units transfused. The implementation of nucleic acid testing has further reduced the risk to around 1 in 1,000,000 donations. There is a high prevalence of HCV infection in injecting drug users and, in Australia, the majority of patients acquired the infection through the sharing of infected needles or equipment during injecting drug use. Other less common routes of exposure include skin or mucosal penetration from tattooing or contaminated medical instruments. Sexual transmission and vertical transmission from mother to child is uncommon. Transmission following needlestick injury in a healthcare setting is also uncommon; estimates range from 0% to 6%. Post-exposure prophylaxis is not recommended.

VIROLOGY

HCV is a small, enveloped, single-stranded RNA virus of 9.5 kb that encodes a single polyprotein that is cleaved into structural and regulatory proteins. The structural region contains the core and two envelope proteins (E1 and E2). The non-structural proteins function as proteases (NS3/4) and polymerases (NS5B) and provide important targets for a new class of small molecules undergoing early phase trials for the treatment of HCV infection. Error-prone replication results in the rapid evolution of diverse quasispecies within an infected individual. It is estimated that more than 10 trillion virion particles are produced daily in both acute and chronic phases of infection.

HCV is classified on the basis of similarity of nucleotide sequence into major genetic groups designated genotypes. A recent reclassification has resulted in six major genotypes with a number of subtypes that vary geographically. Genotypes 1, 2 and 3 are common in North America, Europe, Japan and Australia; genotype

4 is common in the Middle East including Egypt, genotype 5 in South Africa and genotypes 6 and its subtypes in Asia. All major genotypes have been identified in Australia, although genotypes 1 and 3 are more common.

DIAGNOSTIC TESTING

Diagnosis of HCV exposure relies on serological assays. HCV infection is confirmed through nucleic acid testing for viral genomes (HCV RNA). Serological assays are based on the detection of specific antibodies to HCV recombinant antigens by enzyme immunoassays. The widely used second- and third-generation immunoassays can detect antibodies within 4–10 weeks after infection. False positives are common when screening low-risk populations and false negatives can occur in immunocompromised individuals, for example in HIV/HCV coinfection.

Detection of HCV RNA distinguishes previous exposure from current infection. Qualitative HCV RNA tests, based on the polymerase chain reaction (PCR), have a lower detection limit than quantitative viral load tests. Commercial tests used to quantitate HCV viraemia include a branched DNA assay (Versant™ HCV RNA 3.0, Bayer) and PCR-based assays such as the Cobas Monitor Amplicor® HCV 2.0 and the HCV TaqMan™ (Roche Diagnostics). All systems deliver reliable, but not always directly comparable, results. While a standardised practice of expressing viral load in international units (IU/mL) has been proposed to allow comparison of different assay results, it is prudent to monitor an individual patient during treatment using only one assay to avoid inter assay variability that may affect management decisions.

CLINICAL COURSE OF HCV INFECTION

Acute HCV infection

Acute HCV infection is commonly asymptomatic and thus infrequently recognised clinically. Systematic reviews suggest that approximately 25% of patients may spontaneously clear acute HCV infection although the exact proportion is unclear. Acute HCV may be associated with a clinical syndrome of fatigue, lethargy, low-grade fever and right upper quadrant discomfort. Serum HCV RNA typically becomes detectable 7–21 days after exposure and specific antibodies appear subsequently. Jaundice occurs in less than 20% of acute infections. Interestingly, the patients who develop clinically apparent acute hepatitis clear the virus and avoid chronic disease with greater frequency than those who have clinically silent disease (see *Treatment* section). The host and viral factors that influence resolution of HCV infection remain unclear.

Chronic HCV infection

The majority of persons exposed to HCV will develop chronic infection with persistence of detectable serum HCV RNA for more than 6 months. A certain proportion of these patients will have persistently normal liver function tests; in these patients the risk of progression to advanced liver diseases is low. In patients with abnormal alanine aminotransferase (ALT), the overall fibrosis progression rates are higher and some will progress through increasing stages of fibrosis to cirrhosis (Figure 35.1).

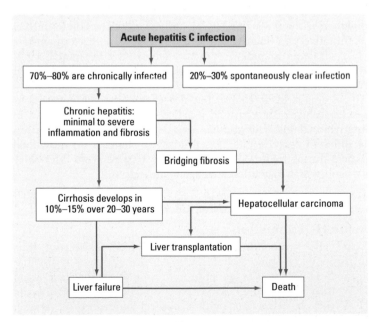

FIGURE 35.1: Hepatitis C natural history.

Complications of chronic HCV infection

Progression to cirrhosis

The primary concern for patients with chronic HCV infection is the evolution from chronic hepatitis to advanced fibrosis and cirrhosis. Estimates of progression to cirrhosis have been examined in different populations of HCV-infected patients. In studies involving liver clinic populations, rates of progression to cirrhosis have been estimated at 20%–35% at 20–30 years, which may reflect referral and selection bias. Progression to cirrhosis in community based groups, such as blood donors newly diagnosed with HCV infection, is generally lower, approximately 2%–5% after 10–20 years of infection. In the majority of community-based studies, subjects tend to be younger and a larger proportion will have normal liver function tests, which may be associated with milder disease.

Factors that affect progression to cirrhosis could be related to the virus or to the host. Interestingly, viral factors appear to play the least important role and there are no convincing data to link either HCV genotype or viral load with liver injury, although both of these factors are critical in predicting treatment outcome. Several host factors significantly influence the likelihood of progression to cirrhosis; these include age at infection (cirrhosis occurs more frequently in older compared with younger patients), gender (progression is lower among women than men) and lifetime alcohol intake. Insulin resistance (obesity, diabetes and steatohepatitis) and genetic polymorphisms in inflammatory mediators are likely to be associated with fibrosis progression.

Progression to hepatocellular carcinoma

The risk of HCC is increased 25-fold in HCV-infected patients compared with HCV-negative controls. Virtually all HCV-related HCC cases occur among patients with advanced fibrosis or cirrhosis. The annual risk of HCC development in patients with HCV cirrhosis is 1%–4% in Western populations and higher in Asian populations (up to 7%). Factors affecting progression to HCC include male gender, older age, duration of HCV infection (most cases occur after 25–30 years of chronic infection), daily alcohol intake >60 g (>6 standard alcoholic drinks/day) and coinfection with HBV.

ASSESSING LIVER INJURY

Liver function tests

Traditional 'liver function tests' such as serum alanine aminotransferase (ALT) and aspartate aminotransferase (AST) provide a relatively insensitive indication of the degree of hepatic inflammation. These enzymes do not correlate well with either the extent of liver injury or the risk of disease progression. Serum ALT can be used to monitor treatment efficacy in addition to viral testing. However, serum ALT may be elevated even when HCV RNA is not detected because of other factors such as hepatic steatosis and hepatic iron content. Other markers such as a low albumin, elevated bilirubin and prolonged coagulation tests more accurately indicate impairment of liver function.

Histology

Histological staging provides the most reliable estimate of hepatic fibrosis and likelihood of disease progression, although it is subject to sampling error and variability in interpretation. Liver biopsy is an invasive procedure and major complications occur in 0.06%–0.3% of biopsies; however death as a direct result of liver biopsy is extremely rare. In the future, it is possible that indirect markers of fibrosis may obviate the need for a liver biopsy. Liver biopsy can provide an assessment of disease progression rate if the date of onset of infection is known; this may be helpful in counselling patients about treatment. Liver biopsy in patients with chronic hepatitis C can indicate prognosis, exclude other forms of liver disease, predict the likelihood of responding to antiviral therapy and provide baseline histology that can be factored into future management decisions.

TREATMENT

Interferon and ribavirin

Interferons are naturally occurring antiviral proteins that produce an 'antiviral state' to promote elimination of virally infected cells. Jay Hoofnagle and colleagues first reported using recombinant alpha interferon to treat non-A, non-B hepatitis in 1986. John McHutchison and colleagues showed in 1998 that the addition of ribavirin, a guanosine analogue, in combination with interferon reduced the relapse rate following the end of therapy, and thus improved the overall sustained response rate. The precise mechanism of ribavirin's antiviral activity is unknown; it is ineffective against HCV when given alone. Currently the combination of pegylated interferon and ribavirin is the international standard of therapy for patients with chronic HCV infection. Addition of polyethylene glycol (pegylation) to the interferon molecule allows for weekly administration; ribavirin tablets are taken daily in divided doses.

Treatment regimens

The outcome of antiviral therapy can be defined biochemically by serum ALT normalisation and virologically by the lack of serum HCV RNA detection using a sensitive method such as PCR. A response at the completion of a treatment course is defined as an end-of-treatment response (ETR) but the desirable goal is a sustained response. A sustained virological response (SVR) is defined as undetectable HCV RNA 6 months following the completion of treatment. Non-responding patients include those who relapse (achieve an ETR but re-develop detectable serum HCV RNA) and patients with persistently detectable serum HCV RNA after adequate treatment durations.

Treatment of patients with acute symptomatic HCV infection with pegylated interferon alone may be effective in preventing chronic HCV infection in up to 90% of cases. Most studies have shown that the addition of ribavirin is not required for successful treatment. The timing of treatment remains controversial, but many studies have treated after 12 weeks' observation in order to allow for spontaneous resolution.

For patients with chronic HCV infection, the recommended treatment duration with pegylated interferon and ribavirin varies by genotype. Patients with genotype 1 should receive treatment with either peginterferon alfa-2a (180 μg weekly) or peginterferon alfa-2b (1.5 μg/kg weekly) plus weight-based ribavirin daily for 12 months. Patients with genotypes 2 and 3 should receive the same interferon dosages plus ribavirin for 6 months; recent data suggest that a ribavirin dose of 800 mg/day is sufficient for these patients. Unfortunately, there are few data to guide therapy for patients with genotypes 4, 5 and 6, although it is generally thought that patients with genotype 4 require therapy for 12 months and patients with genotype 6 may only require treatment for 6 months. The overall SVR rate following therapy with pegylated interferon and ribavirin is approximately 55%; patients with genotype 1 have lower response rates than patients with non-1 genotypes. There is currently no consensus on the most effective treatment for patients who have either relapsed or failed to respond to pegylated interferon plus ribavirin.

Treatment with interferon may be individualised by considering genotype and, more recently, viral kinetics during therapy (see Table 35.1). Patients with genotype 1 who achieve an early virological response (EVR), generally defined as ≥2 log reduction in HCV RNA by week 12, are more likely to achieve an SVR

TABLE 35.1: Virological testing during HCV antiviral therapy	
Genotype 1	
Week 12	Quantitative HCV RNA ≤2 log reduction → Discontinue therapy
	Quantitative HCV RNA ≥2 log reduction → Continue therapy to week 24
Week 24	Qualitative HCV RNA detectable → Discontinue therapy
	Qualitative HCV RNA undetectable → Continue therapy to week 48
Week 48	End of therapy—check HCV RNA by qualitative PCR
Week 72	End of follow-up—check HCV RNA by qualitative PCR (this determines sustained virological response or relapse)

Recent developments:
- Genotype 1 patients with low viral load may only require 24 weeks total therapy if HCV RNA is undetectable by week 4
- Genotype 1 patients who achieve undetectable HCV RNA between weeks 12 and 24 may benefit from extended therapy for 72 weeks to increase the duration of HCV RNA negativity

Genotypes 2 and 3

There are no recommendations for HCV RNA testing between commencement and end of treatment

Recent developments:

Patients who achieve undetectable HCV RNA by week 4 may only require 12–16 weeks total therapy to achieve a SVR

HCV = hepatitis C virus; PCR = polymerase chain reaction; RNA = ribonucleic acid; SVR = sustained virological response.

compared with patients who do not reach this threshold. Those patients who achieve a 2 log reduction by week 12 should continue therapy until week 24; if they have undetectable HCV RNA by qualitative PCR at that time, then they should continue therapy until week 48. Patients who fail to achieve an EVR or who have detectable HCV RNA at week 24 should stop treatment, since the likelihood of achieving a SVR is less than 2%. Recent studies have looked at shortening treatment duration in genotype 1 patients with low pretreatment viral loads (Table 35.1) and prolonging treatment duration in genotype 1 patients with high viral loads.

Patients with HCV genotype 2 and 3 infection are currently treated for 24 weeks with pegylated interferon and ribavirin and achieve SVR rates of 80%. Recent studies have questioned whether treatment duration could be shortened by individualising treatment based on rapid or early virological responses. Shorter treatment duration with equivalent SVR rates seems feasible only in patients who are HCV RNA negative by week 4 and some patients, for example those with genotype 3 and a high viral load, may require longer treatment durations.

Adverse events associated with treatment

Interferon

Common side effects with interferon therapy include a 'flu-like' syndrome of myalgias, lethargy and fatigue during the first few weeks of therapy although tachyphylaxis to these symptoms is the rule. Interferons also affect mood, and irritability and depression are common, sometimes treatment-limiting, side effects. Neutropenia and thrombocytopenia are also common but reversible events that mandate close monitoring of patients during treatment.

Ribavirin

A dose dependent haemolytic anaemia, leading to a 20–40 g/L fall in serum haemoglobin, is common in patients treated with ribavirin. Less common side effects include upper respiratory tract symptoms and skin rashes. Ribavirin is a known teratogen and both patients and their partners must undertake adequate contraception during, and for 6 months following, treatment.

Prior to commencing therapy patients should have a baseline full blood examination, urea, electrolytes, creatinine, thyroid function tests and pregnancy testing. Patients with diabetes or hypertension should have an ophthalmological examination. Counselling prior to treatment and ongoing support during treatment are important in helping patients adhere to a difficult treatment regimen; those patients who complete a course of treatment have the best chance of eradicating HCV.

Long-term benefits of antiviral therapy

The most important goal of therapy is improved survival and there are now data indicating that hepatic fibrosis may regress and that HCC may occur less often in treated patients. Histological improvement, measured as a reduction in fibrosis stage, has been noted even in patients with cirrhosis prior to treatment. Other studies have shown a significant risk reduction for developing HCC in treated patients compared with untreated patients. Generally, patients who achieve a sustained virological response show the greatest benefit, but some improvement can be seen even in patients who remain viraemic. On the basis on these observations, several, prospective, large international trials are underway examining the role of maintenance interferon therapy in viraemic, non-responding patients.

Future therapy for HCV infection

New antiviral therapy for chronic HCV infection includes modified interferons, such as albumin bound to interferon (Albuferon), which provides a longer half-life compared with pegylated interferons. A number of specifically targeted antiviral therapies have been developed against essential HCV proteins, such as the viral polymerase and protease. Phase II trials are underway with these direct small molecule inhibitors, which will likely be combined with interferon and/or ribavirin. Immune-based therapies involve stimulation of innate immunity through activation of toll-like receptors and through the development of therapeutic vaccination to stimulate adaptive immunity.

SUMMARY

The pandemic of hepatitis C remains an important public health issue and a major challenge to individual patients in regard to understanding the impact of this chronic viral infection on their health and in making a decision whether to undertake a demanding treatment regimen. The international standard therapy is a combination of pegylated interferon and ribavirin, which achieves viral eradication in 55% of patients overall, although this proportion varies with genotype and viral load. Individualisation of treatment is possible based on virological responses during therapy in different genotype groups. Treatment is associated with significant adverse effects so that ongoing medical and nursing support is required. A number of new treatment approaches, based on direct antiviral agents and immune manipulation, are likely to improve patient outcomes in the future.

FURTHER READING

De Francesco R, Migliaccio G. Challenges and successes in developing new therapies for hepatitis C. Nature 2005; 436:953–60.

Halfon P, Penaranda G, Bourliere M, et al. Assessment of early virological response to antiviral therapy by comparing four assays for HCR RNA quantitation using the international unit standard: implications for clinical management of patients with chronic hepatitis C virus infection. J Med Virol 2006: 78:208–15.

Hoofnagle JH, Mullen KD, Jones DB, et al. Treatment of chronic non-A, non-B hepatitis with recombinant human alpha interferon. A preliminary report. N Engl J Med 1986; 315:1575–8.

Manns M, Wedemeyer H, Cornberg M. Treating viral hepatitis C: efficacy, side effects and complications. Gut 2006; 55:1350–9.

McCaughan G, George J. Fibrosis progression in chronic hepatitis C virus infection. Gut 2004; 53:318–21.

McHutchison JG, Gordon SC, Schif ER, et al. Interferon alfa-2b alone or in combination with ribavirin as initial treatment for chronic hepatitis C. Hepatitis Interventional Therapy Group. N Engl J Med 1998; 339:1485–92.

Micallef J, Kaldor J, Dore G. Spontaneous viral clearance following acute hepatitis C infection: a systematic review of longitudinal studies. J Viral Hep 2006; 13:34–41.

Prati D. Transmission of hepatitis C virus by blood transfusions and other medical procedures: a global review. J Hepatol 2006; 45:607–16.

Chapter **36**

THE HEPATITIS B-POSITIVE PATIENT

KEY POINTS

- Chronic hepatitis B virus (HBV) infection is common, affecting approximately 3.5 million people worldwide.
- There are three antigens and each has corresponding antibodies:
  - Surface antigen (HBsAg) indicates current infection, and surface antibody (HBsAb) indicates immunity
  - E antigen (HBeAg) indicates active viral replication and high infectivity. E antibody (HBeAb) indicates clearance of HBe antigen
  - Core antigen is never found in the serum. HBV core antibody (HBcAb IgM) generally indicates infection within the previous 10 months. HBcAb IgG indicates past infection.
- HBV-DNA is the best test for viral replication.
- There are two main settings for HBV transmission:
  - Transmission in early life in a highly endemic area (mother to baby or infection by other members of the extended family within the first year of life)
  - Transmission in adolescence or adult life by injecting drug use and sexual contact.
- The natural history of chronic HBV can be divided into three phases:
  - Immunotolerant replicative phase. High viral replication but transaminases and histology virtually normal
  - E antigen clearance phase. May be rapid with development of e antibody and minimal hepatitis or prolonged with cycles of regeneration and repair. Mutations in the precore or the basal core promoter regions may develop
  - Residual integrative phase. Regard people in this phase as potentially having cirrhosis.
- Three common scenarios:
  - The 'healthy' or asymptomatic chronic carrier
  - The chronic carrier with liver disease
  - Acute hepatitis B.
- Antiviral treatment. A number of drugs have been approved for treatment of chronic HBV infection, including interferon alfa-2b, lamivudine, adefovir dipivoxil, entecavir, peginterferon alfa-2a and telbivudine.

- Transplantation may be appropriate in highly selected patients.
- Screening for hepatocellular carcinoma (HCC). The most common program is ultrasound and alpha-fetoprotein at 6-monthly intervals.

INTRODUCTION

At least 350 million people worldwide are chronically infected with hepatitis B virus (HBV).

Acute hepatitis B is subclinical in young children, and only 50% of adults are likely to be symptomatic. Acutely infected adults have a 90% chance of clearing the surface antigen within 6 months, whereas young babies and children have a <10% chance of clearing HBV.

This chapter focuses mainly on the chronic carrier.

THE ANTIGENS AND THEIR ANTIBODIES

Table 36.1 and Figure 36.1 summarise the tests available for HBV and their clinical relevance. There are three antigens, and each has corresponding antibodies:

- Surface antigen (HBsAg) indicates current infection, and surface antibody (HBsAb) indicates immunity (either from vaccination, or from past infection)
- E antigen (HBeAg) indicates active viral replication and high infectivity. HBeAg is highly immunogenic, and much of the host immune response is directed against this antigen rather than against HBsAg. E antibody (HBeAb) has no protective role—its presence simply indicates clearance of HBeAg
- Core antigen is never found in serum. However core antibodies are detectable as a marker of past infection. As a general rule, HBcAb IgM indicates infection within the previous 10 months, and so can be used as a marker of recent infection (occasionally it can also re-appear in the serum of chronic carriers during a severe flare). HBcAb IgG indicates past infection, duration undefined
- HBV DNA is the best test for active viral replication. It is always positive if HBeAg is present, and may be positive when HBeAb is positive, in the case of precore mutant infection.

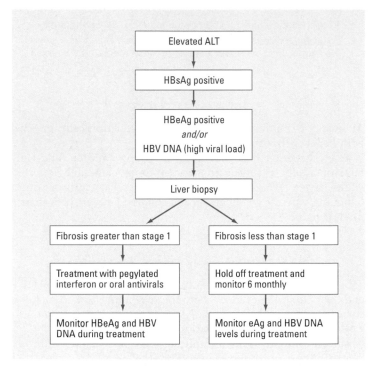

FIGURE 36.1: Indications for biopsy and treatment.

ALT = alanine aminotransferase; HBeAg = hepatitis B e antigen; HBsAg = hepatitis B surface antigen; HBV = hepatitis B virus.

TRANSMISSION OF HBV

HBV is highly infectious in someone who has replicating virus—the virus will be present in all body fluids at high concentration. There are two main settings for HBV transmission. The most common global setting is transmission in early life in a highly endemic area (i.e. most parts of the world except the highly Westernised countries of Western Europe, USA, Canada and Australia). Transmission can occur from mother to baby (95% likelihood in mother with replicating HBV). Babies who do not acquire it from their mothers in these areas have a high chance of being infected by other members of the extended family within the first year of life. Such young children do not develop symptoms,

TABLE 36.1: Clinical investigations in chronic hepatitis B

Clinical situation	HBsAg	HBsAb	HBeAg	HBeAb	HBV DNA	HBcAb IgM	HBcAb IgG	Liver function test
Immunity post vaccine	Neg	Pos	Neg	Neg	Neg	Neg	Neg	Normal
Acute HBV	Pos	Neg	Pos (briefly)	Neg	Pos (briefly)	Pos	Neg	Abn
Chronic infection, minimal activity (phase 3)	Pos	Neg	Neg	Pos	Low level pos	Neg	Pos	Normal
Resolved infection (phase 4)	Neg	Pos (may be very low titre)	Neg	Pos	Neg	Neg	Pos	Normal
Phase 2 (suitable for treatment)	Pos	Neg	Pos	Neg	Pos	Pos/Neg	Pos	Abn
Phase 1	Pos	Neg	Pos	Neg	Pos	Pos	Pos	Abn

Abn = abnormal; HBcAb = hepatitis B core antibody; HBcAg = hepatitis B core antigen; HBeAb = hepatitis B e antibody; HBeAg = hepatitis B e antigen; HBsAb = hepatitis B surface antibody; HBsAg = hepatitis B surface antigen; Neg = negative; Pos = positive.

but remain subclinical for the first few decades of life (Figures 36.2 and 36.3). Most people in these endemic regions are either carriers or immune by adult life. Such transmission is responsible for most of the world's burden of HBV-related disease.

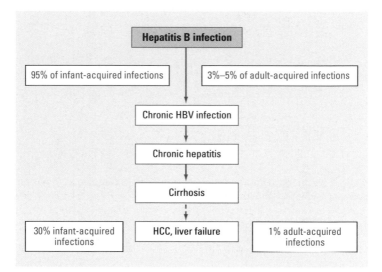

FIGURE 36.2: The outcome of HBV depends upon age of acquisition.
HBV = hepatitis B virus; HCC = hepatocellular carcinoma.

The second setting is transmission in adolescence or adult life by more 'Western' practices, such as injecting drug use, and sexual contact. Other risk factors are listed in Table 36.2.

TABLE 36.2: Some risk factors for acquisition of hepatitis B virus

- Perinatal
- Sexual contact (especially male–male)
- Close family/domestic contact
- Injecting drug use
- Blood transfusion
- Non-sterile medical injections
- Tattoos
- Living or working in crowded condition (e.g. prisons)
- Living or working in institutions for the intellectually disabled
- Contact with renal dialysis
- Folk/cultural practices involving skin penetration

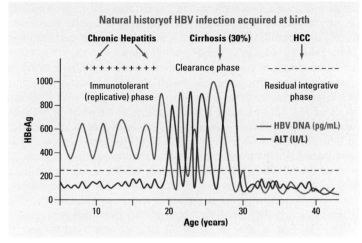

FIGURE 36.3: The natural history of hepatitis B virus acquired at birth, showing: phase 1—the immunotolerant replicative phase; phase 2—the e antigen clearance phase; phase 3—the residual integrative phase.

From Digestive Health Foundation 2000, with permission.

ALT = alanine aminotransferase; HBeAg = hepatitis B e antigen; HBV = hepatitis B virus; HCC = hepatocellular carcinoma.

NATURAL HISTORY OF HEPATITIS B

The outcome of hepatitis B depends almost entirely on the age of infection: young babies and children have a 90% chance of becoming a chronic carrier, but adults have less than 10% chance (Figure 36.2). The individual infected as a baby has an eventual 30% chance of dying from the consequences of hepatitis B (females 15%; males 45%), whereas the person who has acquired the infection in adult life has <1% chance. The reasons for this difference are the duration of the replicative or 'highly infectious' phase of the infection: this is related, in turn, to the level of immunological maturity of the host.

Infection acquired in early life: the three phases

Infection acquired early in life is the most common setting worldwide. The HBV is not recognised as a foreign protein until immunological maturity, generally between 15 and 40 years. Consequently, during the first two, three or four decades of life the virus continues to replicate, but there is no immune response i.e. transaminases are normal, and histology virtually normal—this is the immunotolerant replicative phase. At a variable age, often around 20 years, 'hepatitis' develops for the first time (i.e. transaminases rise). This is the beginning of the 'e antigen clearance phase'. This phase can be quick, with rapid development of e antibody and minimal hepatitis, or prolonged, with ongoing cycles of regeneration and repair, leading to cirrhosis in 30% of cases. During these flares, alanine aminotransferase (ALT) will rise and the DNA will temporarily fall, only to rise again with the next flare. Eventually the third phase, the residual integrative phase, will be reached. By this stage 30% of people will have significant liver injury, but this is usually not clinically apparent for some time. Thus, people in this phase must be regarded as potentially having cirrhosis, which may be detectable only on liver biopsy.

The DNA level at a single point in time has been shown to predict later complications. However, there is not proof that lowering DNA prevents complications (except in the case of decompensation). Though it has become a widely accepted premise that lowering DNA below 4 logs (10^4 copies/mL) will improve outcome.

On occasion, the e antigen clearance phase will be partially resolved by development of a mutant strain, selected out under immunological pressure—pressure which has suppressed the wild-type virus, but allowed mutations to replicate. The most common mutations are known as the precore mutant, relating to specific mutations in the precore region of the genome, and the basal core promoter mutations. These strains are more likely to develop with certain genotypes (strains) of HBV, which have geographical variation. The precore and basal core promoter mutations are unable to produce e antigen (Table 36.3) although they continue to replicate and cause significant liver damage.

Diagnosis and clinical significance of the three phases

The phase of infection in a chronic HBV carrier can be identified by ordering three blood tests. Generally, in this situation, the surface antigen has already come back positive, and long-standing infection is suspected because of the clinical setting (e.g. born in highly endemic region). The blood tests to order are ALT, HBV DNA and HBe antigen/antibody. The phases of infection (Figure 36.3) are detailed below.

TABLE 36.3: The diagnosis of wild type and precore mutant HBV

	Wild type	**Precore**
HBsAg	Positive	Positive
HBeAg	Positive	Negative
Anti-e	Negative	Positive
DNA	Positive	Positive
ALT	Elevated	Elevated

- Immunotolerant replicative phase: highly infectious, subclinical, antiviral treatment will not be effective, person should be monitored for beginning of clearance phase (ALT normal, eAg positive, DNA levels high).
- E antigen clearance phase: highly infectious often in flares, antiviral treatment indicated, may be clinical, occasionally severe hepatitis (ALT high, DNA high, eAg positive, eAb negative).
- Residual integrative phase: less infectious, too late for antiviral treatment, person may develop decompensated chronic liver disease or hepatocellular carcinoma (HCC), may be appropriate for transplantation (ALT normal, DNA low, eAg negative, eAb positive).
- Precore mutant: less infectious, but likely to develop liver disease and HCC. A limited response to antiviral therapy is expected and patients may be suitable for transplantation (ALT high, DNA high, eAg negative, eAb positive).

Hepatitis B acquired in adolescence or adult life: resolved infection

In this setting, characteristic of infection in the 'Western' world, the host has reached immunological maturity, there is no immunotolerant replicative phase, and he/she and enters the 'clearance phase' immediately. Thus, there is a high chance of clearing hepatitis B surface antigen within 6 months (Figure 36.1; Table 36.1). Following this most individuals will have markers of the resolution phase only and, in general, the chance of liver disease or HCC is very low.

HEPATITIS B IN PRACTICE

Three common scenarios are usually encountered, and each scenario prompts specific questions.

Scenario 1: The 'healthy' or asymptomatic chronic carrier

Is this person a chronic carrier? (>6 months HBsAg)

Where the person comes from provides a clue. If the person was born in a highly endemic region, it is often taken for granted that he/she is a chronic carrier. Sometimes, a previous sAg result will be available or there may be documentation of sAg present for more than 6 months. In any case, the IgM core Ab will be negative. If acute/recent infection is suspected, go to Scenario 3.

Do they have clinical liver disease?

Symptoms: jaundice, bruising, bleeding, oedema, ascites, muscle wasting, tiredness, drowsiness, gastrointestinal bleeding.

Examination: stigmata of chronic liver disease, signs of portal hypertension (ascites, splenomegaly) or decompensation (jaundice, bruising, muscle wasting, drowsiness, flap, fetor).

If yes, go to Scenario 2.

What phase of infection are they in?

Order ALT, HBV-DNA, HBeAg/eAb.

1 Replicative phase: If <15 years old, assess every 5 years with blood tests, if >15 years, assess every 6 months with blood tests to identify clearance phase, then refer for antiviral treatment (see below).
2 eAg clearance phase: refer for treatment (see below).
3 Residual phase: can offer liver biopsy; see 6 or 12 monthly for blood tests, consider screening for HCC (see below).
4 Precore mutant: refer for possible treatment.

Interrupting further transmission

Does the patient and family understand the following:
- Need for testing and vaccination of all close and family contacts?
- Potential for blood spread?
- Potential for sexual and close contact spread?

Scenario 2: the chronic carrier with liver disease

All of the above questions are relevant as well as the following.

Does this patient have clinical chronic liver disease?

Symptoms: jaundice, bruising, bleeding, oedema, ascites, muscle wasting, tiredness, drowsiness, gastrointestinal bleeding

Examination: stigmata of chronic liver disease (spider naevi, gynaecomastia, hepatomegaly), signs of portal hypertension (ascites, splenomegaly) and decompensation (jaundice, bruising, muscle wasting, drowsiness, flap, fetor).

Has anything precipitated the decompensation?

Look for sepsis (including spontaneous bacterial peritonitis), hypovolaemia, electrolyte imbalance, gastrointestinal bleeding, protein load and sedative use.

Management

- Manage the decompensation and precipitants appropriately.
- Investigate for possible HCC.
- Antiviral treatment indicated in compensated or decompensated with replicating or precore mutant disease (see below).
- Consider referral for liver transplantation.

Scenario 3: acute hepatitis B

When to suspect?

Usually adult/adolescent with potential risk factors (e.g. injecting drug use, imprisonment, sexual contacts), no remote risk factors, usually with acute illness. May be icteric.

Examination: jaundice, may have spider naevi, hepatosplenomegaly, can develop hepatic failure.

Investigation: ALT high, DNA often low by the time symptoms develop, eAg often negative by the time of presentation, HBsAb may be already positive, and so the only way to be reasonably certain of recent acquisition of HBV is to order HBcAb IgM.

Remember that there may be alternative or additional causes for jaundice in a chronic HBV carrier—in other words, this current episode may not be acute HBV. Thus, investigations should include a detailed drug history (prescribed and non-prescribed), testing for hepatitis C (by serology and polymerase chain reaction [PCR]), testing for hepatitis D (which can coinfect or superinfect those people with HBV), testing for hepatitis A and E, Epstein-Barr virus and cytomegalovirus. Also test for Wilson's disease, iron studies and autoimmune hepatitis.

Management
Watch and wait, as adults have 90% chance of clearing HBsAg spontaneously.

Interruption of further transmission
See above for counselling information.

ANTIVIRAL TREATMENT

A number of drugs have been approved for treatment of chronic HBV infection. They are interferon alfa-2b, lamivudine, adefovir dipivoxil, entecavir, peginterferon alfa-2a and telbivudine. The adverse side effects of interferon alfa-2b has resulted in peginterferon alfa-2a superseding it.

Table 36.4 compares interferon and nucleoside analogue therapy. Interferon affords a chance of long-term remission to selected patients, at the cost of side effects. Antiviral therapy is often beset by frequent resistance with need to change antivirals. Thus these patients need to be monitored every 3 months with HBV DNA and liver function tests and future trials may indicate a benefit from combination antiviral treatment in preventing resistance.

TABLE 36.4: Pros and cons—interferon alfa and antivirals

	Interferon	Antivirals
Route	Subcutaneous	Oral
Duration of treatment	24 weeks	Open-ended
Side effects	Marked	Minimal
Risk of resistance	No	Yes
Effectiveness in selected patients	30%	30% at 2 years
Precore mutant disease	Minimal effectiveness	Requires long-term treatment, risk of resistance
Can be used sequentially	Yes, prior to antivirals	Yes, prior to other antivirals as resistance develops

TRANSPLANTATION

Liver transplantation can be successfully accomplished in highly selected individuals. Patients must fulfill all other criteria for transplantation, and preferably not have mutant virus. Patients are treated with antivirals and large doses of hyperimmune immunoglobulin. Infection of the donor liver with host HBV is universal, but the aim of the antiviral treatments is to prevent severe disease post transplantation. With these regimens, survival can be equivalent to other indications for transplantation.

SCREENING FOR HEPATOCELLULAR CARCINOMA

There is no evidence that screening for HCC in patients with chronic hepatitis B infection prolongs survival. Nevertheless, most liver clinics recommend HCC screening to patients with chronic HBV. The highest risk groups are those with long duration of infection (i.e. perinatally acquired), and those with cirrhosis, particularly males, a family history of HCC and those with high HBV DNA levels and/or active hepatic inflammatory activity. The most common program is ultrasound and alpha-fetoprotein every 6 months. A suspicious lesion on ultrasound should be followed up with a triple-phase computed tomography (CT) scan, and possibly further investigations after that.

SUMMARY

On a global scale, chronic hepatitis B infection is common, affecting approximately 3.5 million people. The are two main settings for HBV transmission: transmission in early life in a highly endemic area (mother to baby or infection by other members of the extended family within the first year of life) or transmission in adolescence or adult life by injecting drug use and sexual contact. The presence of HBsAg indicates current infection, whereas the presence of HBsAb indicates immunity. The presence of HBeAg indicates active viral replication. HBV DNA measurements provide a viral load and are a useful means of monitoring the adequacy of response to therapy. While most infected individuals develop adequate immunity, a smaller proportion become 'carriers' and an even smaller number develop chronic active hepatitis. The latter may lead to the development of cirrhosis and HCC. Patients with chronic active hepatitis need to be assessed for treatment. Such therapies include peginterferon alpha-2a and oral nucleoside/

nucleotide analogues. They not only require long-term ongoing treatment, but are associated with the development of viral resistance. Patients are at risk of progressing to cirrhosis and HCC. Those with progressive cirrhosis may benefit from liver transplantation. Six-monthly HCC monitoring is best targeted at patients with cirrhosis. Vaccination is the best strategy for preventing this infection.

FURTHER READING

Hoofnagle JH. Hepatitis B-preventable and now treatable. N Engl J Med 2006; 354:1074–6.

Jacobson IM. Therapeutic options for chronic hepatitis B: considerations and controversies. Am J Gastroenterol 2006; 101 Suppl 1:S13–18.

McMahon BJ. Selecting appropriate management strategies for chronic hepatitis B: who to treat. Am J Gastroenterol 2006; 101 Suppl 1:S7–12.

Perrillo RP, Gish RG, Peters M, et al. Chronic hepatitis B: a critical appraisal of current approaches to therapy. Clin Gastroenterol Hepatol 2006; 4:233–48.

Chapter 37

SUSPECTED IRON OVERLOAD OR HIGH SERUM FERRITIN

KEY POINTS

- Iron is a component of a number of essential proteins.
- Iron surplus to body needs is stored in ferritin, while iron is transported in serum bound to transferrin. Transferrin saturation and serum ferritin increase with increasing iron stores.
- Transferrin saturation is affected by dietary iron intake. A raised random transferrin saturation should be repeated fasting. Serum ferritin is increased in inflammation and by liver disease.
- Increased body iron stores are seen in hereditary haemochromatosis, a group of diseases caused by mutations in proteins involved in iron regulation. HFE1 is the most prevalent of these disorders and is caused by mutations of *HFE*, particularly homozygosity for the C282Y mutation.
- Secondary iron overload occurs with repeated blood transfusion or iron infusion, chronic anaemia, chronic liver disease and inflammatory states.
- In subjects with an appropriate ancestry, *HFE* genotyping should be performed if fasting transferrin saturation is ≥45%. When serum ferritin is >1000 µg/L, liver biopsy should be considered.
- Treatment options rely on deceasing iron stores. This can usually be achieved by phlebotomy.

INTRODUCTION

High serum ferritin is usually detected during screening studies for causes of chronic liver disease or where iron overload is suspected, as in patients requiring repeated transfusions for thalassaemia or other causes of inadequate red cell production.

It is important to note that serum ferritin is influenced by liver injury and inflammation, so an elevated serum ferritin does not necessarily indicate increased body iron stores.

IRON METABOLISM

Iron is present at about 35–45 mg/kg body weight in men and women respectively (typically 2–3 g). Iron uptake in the gut is the key step regulating iron stores and is stimulated by iron deficiency and chronic anaemia. Approximately 10%–20% of dietary iron (1–2 mg/day) is absorbed in the proximal small intestine. Once in enterocytes, iron needs to be released into the circulation, where it complexes with transferrin to be transported around the body. Iron is used in a variety of essential proteins including haemoglobin (60%–70% of body stores); and myoglobin, cytochromes and other cellular enzymes (10% of body stores). The liver is the principal storage site for iron (typically 20%–30% of body stores), in protein, ferritin; and in haemosiderin, where it can be detected histologically with Perl's stain. Iron is lost from the body (about 1 mg/day) in bile and urine, and with the shedding of enterocytes and skin. In women, iron is also lost with menses and pregnancy. In pathological states, iron can be depleted by gastrointestinal blood loss and excessive menstrual losses.

Serum iron studies

A request for serum iron studies usually results in measurement of serum ferritin, iron and transferrin. Ferritin is the storage protein for iron in reticuloendothelial cells and hepatocytes. The serum concentration of ferritin represents the balance between secretion/leakage from cells and hepatic clearance. It provides an indirect guide to iron stores. However, serum ferritin is an acute phase reactant and its concentration increases with inflammation, and also as a consequence of hepatocyte injury.

Serum iron is included on some routine blood tests of electrolytes and liver enzymes. It is affected by dietary intake, shows diurnal variation, and is not a reliable indicator of iron stores. Transferrin is the major iron transporting protein in the body. Transferrin saturation reflects iron stores and is usually elevated (>50%) before the serum ferritin increases. Transferrin is calculated from the serum iron and total iron binding capacity, which depends on serum transferrin concentration. Measuring fasting transferrin saturations decreases the effects of diet and diurnal variation, and a value of >45% is suggestive of iron overload.

Consequences of iron overload

Iron surplus to body needs is stored in the liver. Iron overload can result in liver injury and hepatic fibrosis that can progress to cirrhosis, which in turn can be associated with liver failure and hepatocellular carcinoma. Cirrhosis typically occurs when body iron stores are >5 g. The risk of developing cirrhosis is increased in the presence of a cofactor for liver injury, such as alcohol or non-alcoholic fatty liver disease. Iron can also accumulate in the heart, resulting in cardiomyopathy and conduction defects; the pancreas, leading to diabetes; the pituitary gland, leading to hypogonadotrophic hypogonadism; joints, causing arthritis; and skin, resulting in bronze pigmentation.

Causes of high serum ferritin

Serum ferritin is increased in iron overload, liver injury and in inflammatory states. Iron overload can occur with inherited abnormalities of iron metabolism, particularly hereditary haemochromatosis (HFE), repeated blood transfusion and dietary iron overload (including hazardous alcohol consumption). The most common cause of iron overload in Western countries is haemochromatosis. There are a number of different types of haemochromatosis. HFE1 is the most common type of haemochromatosis and is an autosomal recessive condition caused by mutation of the *HFE* gene, in particular a cysteine to tyrosine mutation at amino acid 282, designated Cys282Tyr or C282Y. This mutation interferes with the regulated movement of iron from enterocytes into the body, so that iron accumulation can occur despite adequate iron stores. This depends on factors like dietary iron intake, and iron depletion through blood loss or pregnancy. The C282Y mutation appears confined to populations with Northern European ancestry and in these groups the prevalence of C282Y homozygotes is about 1 in 200 to 1 in 400. Approximately 50% of C282Y homozygotes will develop significant iron overload, depending on diet, blood loss and other genetic factors. Another *HFE* mutation that appears to play a role in HFE1 is the H63D mutation, which seems to only be associated with iron overload in combination with C282Y. Other genes implicated in haemochromatosis include transferrin receptor 2, ferritin heavy chain, ferroportin 1, hepcidin and hemojuvelin.

ASSESSMENT

Assessment relies on history and physical examination for inflammatory conditions or liver disease; and serological studies of iron markers, liver enzymes and screening for liver disease, and inflammatory state; and *HFE* gene testing. In haemochromatosis, the earliest phenotypic change is in transferrin saturation, with 45% generally being considered the upper limit of normal. This occurs prior to elevation of serum ferritin. If iron overload is suspected, transferrin saturation should be repeated after an overnight fast to avoid the diurnal and postprandial changes in this measurement. A fasting transferrin saturation of >45% will detect most patients with HFE1 and is the recommended threshold for *HFE* genotyping. Cirrhosis is usually associated with ferritin >1000 µg/L and this is often taken as a cutoff value for liver biopsy. Confirmation of increased iron stores relies on measurement of hepatic iron. This has usually been done on liver biopsy material, but new magnetic resonance imaging (MRI) modalities have been shown to accurately measure hepatic iron stores. Liver biopsies are also undertaken to determine if cirrhosis is present as this has prognostic significance and may lead to screening for oesophageal varices and hepatocellular carcinoma.

Causes of hyperferritinaemia and iron overload include:

- Inflammatory states—including the metabolic syndrome, and chronic rheumatologic conditions
- Chronic anaemia—conditions associated with chronic anaemia, such as haemolytic anaemia, hereditary sideroblastic anaemia and thalassaemia, that stimulate erythropoiesis can also stimulate increased iron uptake
- Transfusional iron overload—these include conditions where there is a need for repeated transfusions such as thalassaemia, bone marrow failure and sickle cell disease. Iron accumulation may also occur with parenteral iron administration
- Chronic liver disease—serum ferritin is increased with liver cell damage and release of ferritin into the circulation. This can be dramatic (ferritin in the thousands) in acute liver injury. Iron overload also occurs with chronic liver disease and cirrhosis, where it is seen more commonly as hepatocellular rather than biliary injury. It is particularly associated with non-alcoholic fatty liver disease, alcoholic liver disease, chronic viral hepatitis and porphyria cutanea tarda.

- Haemochromatosis—HFE1 is an autosomal recessive condition caused by *HFE* mutations, particularly homozygosity of the C282Y mutation. A small proportion (several per cent) of C282Y/H63D compound heterozygotes develop mild iron overload. Other *HFE* genotypes are not associated with significant iron loading. HFE2 and 3 are rare, autosomal conditions associated with raised transferrin saturation. They have been identified in people from southern Europe (Italy and Portugal). HFE2 is juvenile haemochromatosis (onset of clinical manifestations <30 years). HFE2A is an autosomal recessive condition caused by mutations in hemojuvelin (*HJV*). *HJV* mutations have also been identified in Japanese populations. HFE2B is caused by mutations in hepcidin (*HAMP*). HFE3 is clinically similar to HFE1 and is caused by mutations in the transferrin receptor 2 (*TFR2*), which is present on hepatocytes. HFE4 is autosomal dominant, caused by mutations in ferroportin 1 (*SLC11A3*). It is associated with normal or slightly raised transferrin saturation. HFE5 occurs with ferritin heavy chain mutations (*FTH1*). Routine genetic testing is only available for *HFE* mutations.
- Other hereditary hyperferritinaemias—hereditary hyperferritinaemia cataract syndrome is an autosomal dominant disease caused by mutation in the ferritin light chain (*FTL*) that can be associated with congenital cataracts. Transferrin saturation is normal and iron overload does not occur. Hereditary acaeruloplasminaemia is a rare autosomal recessive condition associated with absence of serum caeruloplasmin that can result in hepatic iron overload. It can be associated with neurological disorders due to cerebral iron deposition.

MANAGEMENT OF IRON OVERLOAD

Patients with iron overload who can tolerate phlebotomy should undergo weekly or biweekly venesection of a unit of blood (500 mL) until serum ferritin is <50 μg/L. The haemoglobin should be checked prior to each venesection to ensure it has not fallen by ≥20% from the previous value. Once 'de-ironing' has been achieved, the frequency of venesection can be reduced to 3–4 times per year. In patients who are unable to tolerate phlebotomy (including patients with anaemia), de-ironing can be achieved by chelation. A number of chelating agents are available including desferrioxamine at a dose of 40 mg/kg body weight/day. This is expensive and cumbersome to administer, requiring infusion over 8–12 hours. Recently oral chelating agents (deferiprone) have entered clinical practice. Their role in relation to desferrioxamine is being determined.

Phlebotomy is so successful there is no need to modify intake of foods containing iron. Vitamin C increases iron absorption and should be avoided. Alcohol also appears to increase iron uptake. There are few data supporting phlebotomy for iron overload associated with chronic liver disease.

PROGNOSIS

The prognosis of hyperferritinaemia depends on the underlying condition. In transfusion-dependent patients prognosis depends on cumulative iron load and adequacy of chelation therapy. In HFE, prognosis depends on recognition and adequate de-ironing. If patients are not cirrhotic, survival is similar to patients without HFE. However, once cirrhosis has occurred, there is increased risk of cirrhosis-related complications, particularly hepatocellular carcinoma.

SUMMARY

Iron is a component of a number of important proteins including haemoglobin, myoglobin, cytochromes and other key enzymes. Body iron stores are controlled by regulating uptake from the gut. Iron surplus to body needs is stored in hepatocytes and the reticuloendothelial systems as ferritin.

Iron is transported in blood bound to the protein transferrin. Serum ferritin and the saturation of transferrin with iron both increase with increasing iron stores. However, transferrin saturation shows diurnal variation related to dietary iron intake. As a consequence, an elevated random transferrin saturation should be repeated with a fasting sample to confirm body stores are increased. Serum ferritin is an acute phase reactant, and so is increased in inflammation. It is also elevated by liver diseases and leakage from damaged hepatocytes.

Increased body iron stores are seen in hereditary haemochromatosis, a group of diseases caused by mutations in proteins involved in iron regulation. HFE1 is the most prevalent of these disorders in populations with northern European ancestry, affecting 1 in 200–400 people. It is caused by mutations in *HFE*, almost exclusively homozygosity for the C282Y mutation. Other genes implicated in hereditary haemochromatosis include hepcidin, hemojuvelin, transferrin receptor 2, ferroportin and the ferritin light chain. There are other rare genetic causes of hyperferritinaemia. Secondary iron overload occurs with repeated blood transfusion or iron infusion, chronic anaemia, chronic liver disease and inflammatory states.

Evaluation of suspected iron overload requires history taking, physical examination and appropriate laboratory investigations to rule out chronic inflammation or liver disease and determine if there is secondary iron overload (Figure 37.1). In subjects with an appropriate ancestry, *HFE* genotyping should be performed if fasting transferrin saturation is ≥45%. When serum ferritin is >1000 µg/L, liver biopsy should be considered.

Treatment options rely on decreasing iron stores. This can be achieved by phlebotomy or chelation therapy, if phlebotomy is not possible.

FURTHER READING

Aguilar-Martinez P, Schved J-F, Brissot P. The evaluation of hyperferritinemia: an updated strategy based on advances in detecting genetic abnormalities. Am J Gastroenterol 2005; 100:1185–94.

Andrews NC. Disorders of iron metabolism. N Eng J Med 1999; 341:1986–95.

Lieu PT, Heiskala M, Peterson PA, et al. The roles of iron in health and disease. Mol Aspects Med 2001; 22:1–87.

Siah CW, Trinder D, Olynyk JK. Iron overload. Clin Chim Acta 2005; 358:24–36.

Tavill AS. Diagnosis and management of hemochromatosis. Hepatology 2001; 33:1321–8.

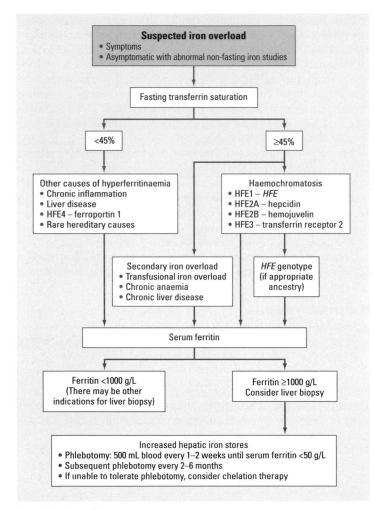

FIGURE 37.1: Clinical pathway for evaluation of suspected iron overload.

Chapter **38**

CHRONIC NON-VIRAL HEPATITIS

KEY POINTS

- Chronic non-viral hepatitis is a clinicopathologic liver syndrome most commonly due to autoimmune hepatitis.
- Other causes include cryptogenic hepatitis, and drug or toxin induced hepatitis.
- Autoimmune hepatitis is characterised by the presence of smooth muscle antibodies, antinuclear antibodies and hypergammaglobulinaemia, and histologically by the presence of interface hepatitis and lymphoplasmacytic infiltrate.
- Key management objectives are to establish the cause and degree of hepatic inflammation and fibrosis.
- Corticosteroids alone or in combination with azathioprine are the treatment of choice for autoimmune hepatitis and may play a role in cryptogenic hepatitis and select cases of drug-induced hepatitis.

INTRODUCTION

Chronic non-viral hepatitis is a clinicopathological liver syndrome due to causes other than chronic viral infection. The most common causes are autoimmune hepatitis, cryptogenic hepatitis and drug or toxin-induced hepatitis. Symptoms are typically non-specific and include fatigue, malaise and right upper quadrant discomfort. Signs of chronic liver disease, hepatosplenomegaly and portal hypertension may be present. The most important histologic feature is interface hepatitis with piecemeal necrosis in the periportal region. Autoimmune hepatitis is the most important differential diagnosis.

Definition

Chronic non-viral hepatitis is a disease of the liver characterised by chronic inflammation and liver cell necrosis, that is due to non-viral causes and which persists without improvement for at least 6 months. However, in autoimmune hepatitis, the 6-month requirement is no longer required to establish chronicity as the condition may present acutely. Also, drug or toxin-induced liver disease is sometimes considered a chronic disease when the duration of liver inflammation extends beyond 3 months.

CAUSES

The causes of non-viral chronic hepatitis are listed in Table 38.1. The principal cause is autoimmune hepatitis. Less common causes include drug-induced hepatitis and cryptogenic hepatitis. The hereditary metabolic liver diseases, Wilson's disease and alpha$_1$-antitrypsin deficiency, may also cause a chronic hepatitis-like picture. Diseases mimicking chronic hepatitis include non-alcoholic steatohepatitis, sclerosing cholangitis and primary biliary cirrhosis.

TABLE 38.1: Non-viral causes of chronic hepatitis

Cause	Specific histology
Autoimmune hepatitis	Interface and lobular hepatitis, plasma cell and lymphocytic infiltrate, rosette formation, bridging and confluent necrosis
Drugs and toxins	Similar to chronic viral hepatitis; may be autoimmune hepatitis-like; ± eosinophils; ± granulomas
Cryptogenic	Similar to autoimmune hepatitis
Wilson's disease	Copper deposits
Alpha$_1$-antitrypsin deficiency	Eosinophilic globules in periportal zones

Autoimmune hepatitis

Autoimmune hepatitis (AIH) accounts for about 20% of cases of chronic hepatitis. The disease has a female preponderance, affects all ages and has a worldwide distribution. There is a genetic association with the human leucocyte antigens B8, DR3 and DR4. The cause of AIH is unknown. Autoantibodies including antinuclear antibody (ANA) and anti-smooth muscle antibody (SMA) are very common but not specific for the disease or of pathogenetic significance. At least two types of AIH are recognised.

Type 1 AIH is the most common form representing 80% of cases. It is characterised by the presence of ANA and/or SMA and hypergammaglobulinaemia. The peak incidence occurs between the ages of 16 and 30 years, with 70% being females younger than 40 years. Around 30%–50% of patients have concurrent immune diseases including ulcerative colitis, autoimmune thyroiditis and synovitis. The clinical course is often indolent. Symptoms may start abruptly in 40% of patients, but an acute fulminant presentation occurs rarely. Cirrhosis may be present at diagnosis in 25% of cases.

Type 2 AIH is a rare disorder that predominantly affects children aged between 2 and 14 years. It is characterised by the presence of antibodies to liver-kidney microsome type 1 (anti-LKM-1). The target autoantigen is the drug metabolising enzyme, cytochrome mono-oxygenase P450 IID6 (CYP2D6). Extrahepatic immune diseases occur more commonly than in type 1 AIH. There is an association with autoimmune polyglandular syndrome type 1. The clinical course is more aggressive than type 1 AIH with a higher frequency of progression to cirrhosis.

Drug-induced hepatitis

Drugs associated with inducing hepatitis are listed in Table 38.2. For more information on drug-induced hepatotoxicity, see Chapter 41.

TABLE 38.2: Drugs reported to cause chronic hepatitis	
• Paracetamol	• Minocycline
• Dantrolene	• Nitrofurantoin
• Diclofenac	• Papaverine
• Isoniazid	• Perhexilene
• Lisinopril	• Propylthiouracil
• Methyldopa	• Sulfonamides

Cryptogenic hepatitis

Around 10%–20% of patients with chronic hepatitis have no definable cause and are classified as cryptogenic hepatitis. It is a diagnosis of exclusion. It may be due to an unknown virus, burnt-out non-alcoholic steatohepatitis or an autoimmune process.

The condition may clinically resemble type 1 AIH in age and sex distribution, necroinflammatory activity, HLA status and response to therapy.

Inherited metabolic liver diseases

Wilson's disease may cause chronic hepatitis in about 5%–30% of patients. Liver inflammation typically manifests in older children, and adults under the age of 35 years. Chronic hepatitis is an uncommon manifestation of alpha$_1$-antitrypsin deficiency. It occurs in both children and adults and is usually mild. Globular eosinophilic deposits in the cytoplasm of hepatocytes on haematoxylin and eosin (H&E) or periodic acid-Schiff (PAS) staining after diastase are characteristic of the disease.

CLINICAL FEATURES

General

Chronic non-viral hepatitis may present with asymptomatic liver function test abnormalities, non-specific symptoms or overt manifestations of liver failure.

Autoimmune hepatitis

The clinical features of severe AIH are shown in Table 38.3. An acute onset is observed in about 25% of patients. Fulminant hepatitis occurs rarely. Common extrahepatic associations are autoimmune thyroid disease, ulcerative colitis and synovitis.

TABLE 38.3: Clinical features of severe autoimmune hepatitis

Clinical features at presentation	Frequency (%)
Symptoms	
• Fatigue and loss of energy	85
• Dark urine and/or light stools	77
• Abdominal pain/discomfort	48
• Anorexia, nausea	30
• Pruritus	36
• Polymyalgias	30
• Diarrhoea	28
• Amenorrhoea (women)	89
• Cosmetic changes (facial rounding, hirsutism, acne)	19

TABLE 38.3: Clinical features of severe autoimmune hepatitis *(continued)*

Clinical features at presentation	Frequency (%)
Clinical signs	
• Hepatomegaly	78
• Spider naevi	58
• Palpable spleen	32–56
• Scleral icterus/jaundice	46
• Ascites	20
• Encephalopathy	16

Diagnostic approach

The key objectives in the assessment of chronic hepatitis are to establish:

- the cause
- degree of hepatic necroinflammation and fibrosis
- severity of chronic liver disease.

The diagnostic tests for chronic hepatitis are listed in Table 38.4.

TABLE 38.4: Diagnostic tests for viral and non-viral causes of chronic hepatitis

Cause	Diagnostic investigations
Viral	
• Chronic hepatitis B	HBsAg, HBeAg, HBV DNA
• Chronic hepatitis C	Anti HCV Ab, HCV RNA
• Chronic hepatitis D	Anti-HDV IgM, HDV RNA
Non-viral	
• Autoimmune hepatitis	ANA, SMA, LKM-1; IgG or gammaglobulin level; HLA B8, Drw3, Drw4
• Wilson's disease	Serum caeruloplasmin level, serum and urinary copper studies, hepatic copper concentration
• Alpha₁-antitrypsin deficiency	Serum alpha₁-antitrypsin level, protease inhibitor phenotype
• Drug-induced	Careful drug history
• Cryptogenic	Exclusion of above causes

Ab = anitbody; ANA = antinuclear antibodies; HBeAg = hepatitis B e antigen; HBsAg = hepatitis B surface antigen; HBV = hepatitis B virus; HCV = hepatitis C virus; HDV = hepatitis D virus; HLA = human leucocyte antigen; IgG = immunoglobulin G; LKM-1 = antibodies to liver-kidney microsome type 1; SMA = anti-smooth muscle antibody.

INVESTIGATIONS

Liver function tests: in AIH, serum levels of alanine aminotransferase (ALT) and aspartate aminotransferase (AST) are elevated: serum aminotransferase levels reflect the severity of inflammatory activity and prognosis (Table 38.5). Most patients with AIH have serum AST levels <500 U/L at presentation. Serum alkaline phosphatase (ALP) levels are usually normal to less than 2-fold elevated. Hyperbilirubinaemia is common in severe AIH. A reduced serum albumin concentration and/or prolonged international normalised ratio (INR) indicate an advanced stage of liver disease.

Serum globulins: hypergammaglobulinaemia is present in more than 80% of cases of AIH and is a marker of disease severity (Table 38.5). A polyclonal increase in serum immunoglobulins is also common, particularly the IgG fraction. Elevated serum globulin concentrations are also a feature of most cases of cryptogenic hepatitis.

Immunoserological tests: ANA titres of ≥1:40 are found in 75% of AIH cases. Both homogeneous and speckled patterns of immunofluorescence are seen. SMA is the principal marker of type 1 AIH. It coexists with ANA ≥85% of cases but may be the only marker of the disease. Antibodies to LKM-1 characterise type 2 AIH, but are also seen in hepatitis C infection.

Other investigations: serum caeruloplasmin, copper and alpha$_1$-antitrypsin levels particularly if patients are ≤40 years. Serum caeruloplasmin and copper concentrations are typically low in Wilson's disease. Low serum alpha$_1$-antitrypsin concentrations should prompt protease inhibitor (Pi) phenotyping. Other standard tests include full blood count, thyroid function tests (due to the association with thyroiditis) and INR, while serum alpha-fetoprotein levels should be done in patients with suspected cirrhosis.

Liver imaging: liver ultrasound with Doppler should be done in patients suspected of having cirrhosis. Triphasic abdominal computed tomography (CT) or magnetic resonance imaging (MRI) is reserved for patients with suspicious lesions on ultrasound.

Liver biopsy: percutaneous liver biopsy is generally recommended in the absence of contraindications. To confirm the clinical diagnosis, grade the severity of necroinflammation, stage the degree of fibrosis and, in the case of AIH, monitor treatment response. A simple scoring system for classifying necroinflammatory activity and fibrosis in chronic hepatitis is shown in Table 38.6. Histology plays an important role in establishing the diagnosis of AIH (see Table 38.7). Classic features are interface hepatitis with lymphocytic infiltrates, plasma cells and piecemeal necrosis. Bridging and confluent necrosis indicate severe AIH and a poor prognosis if untreated. Key histologic features of the other differential diagnoses are shown in Table 38.1.

TABLE 38.5: Markers of severity of inflammation in autoimmune hepatitis

Inflammatory activity	
Severe	*Mild–moderate*
• AST ≥10-fold • AST ≥5-fold plus gammaglobulin >2-fold • Bridging necrosis • Confluent necrosis	• AST <10-fold • Gammaglobulin <2-fold • Periportal hepatitis

TABLE 38.6: Simple scoring system for chronic hepatitis

Grade	Necroinflammatory activity	Fibrosis
0	None or minimal	None
1	Portal inflammation; lobular inflammation with no necrosis	Expanded fibrotic portal tracts
2	Mild piecemeal necrosis; focal lobular necrosis	Periportal or portal-portal septa but intact architecture
3	Moderate piecemeal necrosis; severe focal cell damage in lobules	Fibrosis with architectural distortion
4	Severe piecemeal necrosis, bridging necrosis in lobules	Cirrhosis

TABLE 38.7: Scoring system for diagnosis of autoimmune hepatitis parameter

Autoimmune hepatitis parameter	Score
Gender	
Female	+2
Male	0
Serum biochemistry	
Ratio of elevation of serum alkaline phosphatase vs aminotransferase	
>3.0	−2
1.5–3	0
<1.5	+2
Total serum globulin, gammaglobulin, or IgG times upper limit of normal	
>2.0	+3
1.5–2.0	+2
1.0–1.5	+1
<1.0	0
Autoantibodies (titres by immunofluorescence)	
ANA, SMA, LKM-1	
>1:80	+3
1:80	+2
1:40	+1
<1:40	0
Antimitochondrial antibody	
Positive	−4
Negative	0
Hepatitis viral markers	
Negative	+3
Positive	−3
Other aetiological factors	
History of drug usage	
Yes	−4
No	+1
Alcohol usage	
<25 g/day	+2
>60 g/day	−2
Genetic factors: HLA DR3 or DR4	+1
Other autoimmune diseases	+2

TABLE 38.7: Scoring system for diagnosis of autoimmune hepatitis parameter *(continued)*

Autoimmune hepatitis parameter	Score
Response to therapy	
Complete response	+2
Complete response with relapse	+3
Liver histology	
Interface hepatitis	+3
Predominant lymphoplasmacytic infiltrate	+1
Rosetting of liver cells	+1
None of the above	−5
Biliary changes	−3
Other changes	−3
Seropositivity for other defined autoantibodies	+2

ANA = antinuclear antibodies; HLA = human leucocyte antigen; LKM-1 = antibodies to liver-kidney microsome type 1; SMA = anti-smooth muscle antibody.

DIAGNOSIS

Autoimmune hepatitis

A diagnosis of AIH requires:

- exclusion of viral, alcohol, drug-related and hereditary liver diseases
- demonstrable hepatitis (predominantly raised AST and ALT)
- features of immune reactivity (autoantibodies, high globulin levels)
- compatible histology.

A scoring system that grades individual components of the syndrome may be applied to confirm the diagnosis (Table 38.7). Using this system, a definite diagnosis of AIH can be made with aggregate scores of >15 before treatment and >17 after treatment. Probable AIH corresponds to pre- and post-treatment scores of 10–15 and 12–17 respectively.

Other conditions

Cryptogenic hepatitis is a diagnosis of exclusion requiring negative viral and autoantibody markers in the absence of relevant drug or toxin exposure. Drug-induced chronic hepatitis requires a compatible drug-history and the exclusion of viral and other non-viral causes. Wilson's disease is diagnosed on the basis of low serum caeruloplasmin levels, elevated 24-hour urinary copper and hepatic copper overload as demonstrated by staining and/or measurement of hepatic copper concentration.

TREATMENT

Autoimmune hepatitis

Treatment of AIH significantly improves life expectancy. Indications for treatment are sustained severe inflammation or persistent symptoms (e.g. fatigue, arthralgia) associated with mild–moderate disease. Treatment is not indicated in those with inactive cirrhosis, asymptomatic portal or mild interface hepatitis and those with decompensated liver disease.

Standard treatment regimens are prednisolone alone or prednisolone combined with azathioprine (Table 38.8). Prednisolone monotherapy is preferred in pregnancy and those with cytopenias or active malignancy.

TABLE 38.8: Treatment of autoimmune hepatitis

	Monotherapy regimen	**Combination regimen**
Induction		
• Prednisolone	60 mg for 1 week, 40 mg for 1 week, 30 mg for 2 weeks; 15–20 mg for maintenance	30 mg for 1 week, 20 mg for 1 week, 15 mg for 2 weeks; 10 mg for maintenance
• Azathioprine	None	50–100 mg for maintenance
*Upon remission**		
• Prednisolone	Taper by 2.5 mg every week	Taper by 2.5 mg every week
• Azathioprine	NA	Reduce by 25 mg every 3 weeks
Relapse		
• Prednisolone	Same as induction schedule	Same as induction schedule
• Azathioprine	None	50–100 mg maintenance

* Treatment should be for 12–24 months and for at least 3–6 months after clinical and biochemical remission is achieved.

The goal of treatment is to induce remission as defined in Table 38.9. For both treatment schedules, remission rates are around 65% after 18 months' therapy. Treatment should be continued for between 12 and 24 months and at least 3–6 months after clinical and biochemical remission is achieved. Prednisolone is then slowly withdrawn over 6 weeks with regular monitoring of liver function tests and globulin levels during follow-up. Relapse occurs within 6 months in up to 50% of cases. This rate is reduced to 20% if histologic remission is documented prior to drug withdrawal. Treatment of relapse is with the original treatment schedule.

Other treatment end-points that may occur are an incomplete response, treatment failure and intolerance of drug therapy (Table 38.9). Patients with an incomplete response typically require long-term maintenance immunosuppressive therapy at the lowest possible dose to maintain AST levels <5-fold normal. Treatment

TABLE 38.9: End points of treatment and appropriate management response

End point	Definition	Response
Remission	Asymptomatic and AST levels ≤2-fold times normal and/or normal liver or portal hepatitis or inactive cirrhosis on biopsy	Taper off prednisolone over 6–12 weeks and monitor
Incomplete response	No remission within 2 years of treatment	Continue drug(s) on lowest possible dose to keep AST ≤5-fold normal or achieve histologic remission
Treatment failure	Clinical and/or biochemical deterioration despite treatment compliance	Prednisolone 60 mg/day or prednisolone 30 mg/day plus azathioprine 150 mg/day for at least 1 month
Drug intolerance	Severe side effects of treatment: marked weight gain, psychosis, symptomatic osteoporosis, unstable diabetes (prednisolone); and/or severe cytopenia, fever, neoplasm, rash, nausea/vomiting (azathioprine)	Dose reduction by 50%; complete withdrawal if no improvement or toxicity severe

failure occurs in 10%–15% of patients and requires a trial of high-dose corticosteroids or combination therapy in higher doses (Table 38.9). Liver transplantation should be considered in those who fail to respond and/or develop liver failure, or are fulminant cases. Therapeutic options for drug intolerance are dose reduction by 50% or withdrawal of the implicated drug and to use a higher dose of the tolerated agent. New therapies for difficult-to-treat patients include tacrolimus, cyclosporin A, mycophenolate mofetil, ursodeoxycholic acid and budesonide.

Drug-induced hepatitis

Prevention is the best form of therapy. Biochemical monitoring is appropriate to detect early injury during isoniazid and dantrolene therapy. Management of established chronic hepatitis is with immediate withdrawal of the offending drug. Corticosteroid therapy may be considered on an individual case basis.

Cryptogenic hepatitis

Patients with cryptogenic hepatitis and autoimmune features, such as raised serum IgG hypergammaglobulinaemia and concurrent immunologic disorders, often respond well to corticosteroid therapy. In such patients, an empirical trial of corticosteroids is worthwhile using one of the two treatment schedules outlined in Table 38.8.

SUMMARY

Chronic non-viral hepatitis is a clinicopathological liver syndrome due to causes other than chronic viral infection. The most common cause is autoimmune hepatitis. Other causes are cryptogenic hepatitis and drug or toxin-induced hepatitis. Symptoms are typically non-specific and include fatigue, malaise and right upper quadrant discomfort. Signs of chronic liver disease, hepatosplenomegaly and portal hypertension may be present. The most important histologic feature is interface hepatitis with piecemeal necrosis in the periportal region.

Key objectives in the assessment are to establish the cause, the degree of hepatic necroinflammation and fibrosis and the severity of the chronic liver disease (Figure 38.1). Treatment depends on the cause. Steroids are important in autoimmune hepatitis (together with azathioprine) and may play a role in drug- or toxin-induced hepatitis and cryptogenic hepatitis.

Causes	Diagnostic tests	Histology	Treatment
Autoimmune hepatitis (AIH)	ANA, SMA, LKM-1, IgG or gammaglobulins, HLA B8, Drw3, Drw4	Interface and lobular hepatitis, plasma cell and lymphocyte infiltrate, rosette formation, bridging and confluent necrosis	Prednisolone Azathioprine
Wilson's disease	Serum caeruloplasmin Serum and urine copper Hepatic copper concentration	Copper deposits	Diet Pharmacotherapy (see Chapter 42)
Alpha$_1$-antitrypsin deficiency	Serum alpha$_1$-antitrypsin level Protease inhibitor phenotype	Eosinophilic globules in periportal zones	Liver transplant Avoid cigarette smoking (lung disease) See Chapter 42
Cryptogenic	Exclusion of above causes	Similar to AIH	Empirical trial of steroids
Drugs/toxins	Detailed drug history	Similar to chronic viral hepatitis; may be like AIH $\pm$ eosinophils; $\pm$ granulomas	Exclude drug or toxin Consider steroids on individual case basis

FIGURE 38.1: Chronic non-viral hepatitis.

AIH = autoimmune hepatitis; ANA = antinuclear antibodies; HLA = human leucocyte antigen; IgG = immunoglobulin G; LKM-1 = antibodies to liver-kidney microsome type 1; SMA = anti-smooth muscle antibody.

FURTHER READING

Czaja AJ. Current concepts in autoimmune hepatitis. Am Hepatol 2005; 4:6–24.

Czaja AJ, Carpenter HA. Distinctive clinical phenotype and treatment outcome of type I autoimmune hepatitis in the elderly. Hepatology 2006; 43:532–8.

Hall PD. Chronic hepatitis: an update with guidelines for histopathological assessment of liver biopsies. Pathology 1998; 30:369–80.

Heneghan MA, McFarlane IG. Current and novel immunosuppressive therapy for autoimmune hepatitis. Hepatology 2002; 35:7–13.

Manns MP, Strassburg CP. Autoimmune hepatitis: clinical challenges. Gastroenterology 2001; 120:1502–17.

Chapter **39**

OBESITY AND ABNORMAL LIVER FUNCTION TESTS

KEY POINTS

- Non-alcoholic fatty liver disease (NAFLD) is the most common cause of abnormal liver function tests in the Western world.

- NAFLD encompasses the spectrum of liver disease from bland steatosis to steatosis with inflammation and variable degrees of fibrosis (non-alcoholic steatohepatitis).

- NAFLD is associated with a variety of clinical conditions including obesity, hyperlipidaemia and hyperglycaemia, which are all, in turn, associated with the presence of insulin resistance.

- A proportion of patients with non-alcoholic steatohepatitis (NASH) progress to cirrhosis, hepatic decompensation and hepatocellular carcinoma.

- The main therapeutic modality is lifestyle change, including slow, steady weight loss and exercise.

- Lipid-lowering agents and oral antidiabetic agents that make hepatocytes more insulin sensitive are the main therapeutic agents used to manage NASH.

- Patients with NAFLD are at increased risk of type 2 diabetes mellitus and cardiovascular mortality.

INTRODUCTION

Fatty liver or steatosis refers to the accumulation of fat within the liver. The fatty liver disorders are the most common cause of disturbances of liver function tests in the Western world. While there are several causes of fatty liver, including that of excessive consumption of alcohol (see Chapter 40), the commonest cause is that of insulin resistance usually (but not always) associated with one or a combination of obesity, hyperlipidaemia and/or hyperglycaemia. Non-alcoholic fatty liver disease (NAFLD) is the term used to describe steatosis unrelated to excessive alcohol consumption. NAFLD is a form of metabolic liver disease nearly always associated with insulin resistance and very often with the metabolic, or insulin resistance (IR), syndrome.

NAFLD encompasses the entire pathological spectrum from bland steatosis to decompensated cirrhosis. It therefore includes:

- Steatosis
- Non-alcoholic steatohepatitis (fatty liver is accompanied by hepatocyte inflammation and liver cell injury [hepatitis]), with or without fibrosis
- Cirrhosis.

The term non-alcoholic steatohepatitis (NASH) is defined by histological features resembling those of alcoholic hepatitis that are present in patients who have not consumed excessive quantities of alcohol. Most studies define the latter as alcohol consumption less than 20 g per day (i.e. less than 2 standard alcoholic drinks per day).

Prevalence

The commonest cause of unexplained liver function test abnormalities is associated with the fatty liver disorders. The prevalence of such unexplained liver function abnormalities (most commonly an elevated alanine aminotransferase [ALT] or aspartate aminotransferase [AST]) in patients with NAFLD is approximately 7%–20% of the adult population (based on American studies). It is thought that 2%–3% of adults have NASH, and that approximately 20% of these patients with NASH are at risk for developing cirrhosis and subsequently dying from end-stage liver disease. There are, to date, no Australian prevalence data, but prevalence is thought to be similar based on the knowledge of the prevalence of underlying insulin resistance and obesity. Given the significance of obesity and diabetes as risk factors, and the fact that these conditions are increasing in prevalence, it is estimated that the prevalence of NASH is likely to increase in the coming decades.

Risk factors

NAFLD is associated with central adiposity, obesity, hyperlipidaemia (particularly hypertriglyceridaemia, insulin resistance, the metabolic syndrome and type 2 diabetes—all conditions associated with insulin resistance (see Table 39.1). In addition, NAFLD is associated with rapid weight loss, particularly that observed after jejunoileal bypass surgery (Table 39.2).

TABLE 39.1: When to think about the insulin resistance syndrome

---

- Obesity (central)
- Hypertension
- Hyperlipidaemia
- Microalbuminuria
- Type 2 diabetes or a family history of type 2 diabetes
- Polycystic ovary syndrome
- Hyperuricaemia

TABLE 39.2: Non-alcoholic fatty liver disease (NAFLD) and its clinical associations

---

- Type 2 diabetes (including family history) or the insulin resistance syndrome
- Rapid and profound weight loss
- Some forms of obesity reduction surgery
- Dyslipidaemia, particularly hypertriglyceridaemia
- Gallstone disease
- Polycystic ovary syndrome
- Gout
- Family history of NAFLD

Natural history and prognosis

In the absence of steatohepatitis, NAFLD does not appear to cause fibrosis or progressive liver disease. In contrast, NASH may be associated with disease progression. The proportion of patients with NAFLD in the community who have cirrhosis is not known. Among those referred to liver clinics and selected for liver biopsy, the proportion with significant fibrosis is in the range of 20%–45%. NASH is a slowly progressing liver disorder. Factors associated with more severe disease include obesity, type 2 diabetes, age over 45 years and hypertriglyceridaemia. The role of gender is contentious. Some, studies have suggested that female gender is an independent risk factor for more severe liver disease.

Only those with advanced liver disease are likely to develop significant liver-related morbidity and mortality. Among those with cirrhosis, there is a risk of decompensation and liver failure.

Obesity and fatty liver disorders have been associated with the development of hepatocellular carcinoma, however the exact risk is not known. In a high proportion of patients with cryptogenic cirrhosis, the cirrhosis appears to be related to 'burnt out' NASH. That is, these patients fulfil the clinical profile of a patient with an underlying clinical profile of insulin resistance.

It is important to be aware that, as a consequence of insulin resistance, patients with NAFLD are at increased risk of type 2 diabetes mellitus and cardiovascular mortality.

CLINICAL PRESENTATION

The majority of patients are asymptomatic. They come to medical attention because of abnormal liver function tests or an incidental finding of diffusely increased echogenicity on hepatic ultrasound, which is suggestive of fatty liver. Patients may complain of fatigue and right upper quadrant discomfort. Some patients may have hepatomegaly. The consistency of the liver is usually firm, but not hard, and may be slightly tender. Peripheral stigmata associated with this form of liver disease are uncommon, and their presence may indicate the presence of cirrhosis.

A high proportion of patients have an elevated body mass index (BMI) and waist circumference. Patients of Asian background develop NAFLD at lower BMIs than their Caucasian counterparts.

PATHOGENESIS

Underlying insulin resistance favours lipolysis in adipose tissue with the release of free fatty acids. These are taken up by the liver and stored as lipid. In addition, there is increased lipid synthesis, reduced fat burning and reduced lipid export by the liver. The net effect is accumulation of fatty acids in hepatocytes. Fatty acids may directly injure liver cells or favour the development of oxidative stress and cytokine release. It is thought that genetic factors, at least in part, lead to individual susceptibility and disease severity.

DIAGNOSIS

NAFLD is a clinicopathological diagnosis that requires the exclusion of other liver disorders. In particular, significant alcohol consumption (>20 g ethanol per day) must be excluded. Other common conditions that need to be excluded are chronic viral hepatitis (B and C), drug-induced liver disease, haemochromatosis, Wilson's disease and autoimmune liver disease. Certain drugs cause steatohepatitis (Table 39.3).

TABLE 39.3: Drugs that cause steatohepatitis

- Tamoxifen
- Oestrogens
- Corticosteroids
- Amiodarone

INVESTIGATIONS

Liver biochemistry: ALT and gamma-glutamyltransferase (GGT) elevations are the commonest disturbances, although minor elevations of AST and alkaline phosphatase (ALP) may also occur. The value for ALT is usually greater than the AST level (the opposite is observed with alcoholic hepatitis). When the AST is greater than the ALT level this could indicate cirrhosis. Minor abnormalities of serum albumin and bilirubin may indicate cirrhosis.

Blood count: Low platelet count is common in cirrhosis, otherwise no abnormalities observed.

It is important to be aware that a disproportionate elevation of GGT with an elevated mean corpuscular volume (MCV) should raise concerns of excessive alcohol intake.

Tests of insulin resistance: These are increasingly regarded as important in the work-up of patients with NAFLD. Simple tests that may indicate insulin resistance include fasting blood glucose and fasting insulin levels. In the presence of an abnormal result, an oral glucose tolerance test to diagnose diabetes or impaired glucose tolerance is recommended.

Measurement of lipids: Hyperlipidaemia is frequently observed in patients with NAFLD. Elevated cholesterol and triglyceride levels are commonly detected, usually with a disproportionate elevation of the triglyceride levels.

Elevated serum ferritin: An isolated elevated serum ferritin is very common in patients with NAFLD; however significant iron overload is rare.

Hepatic imaging: An abnormal ultrasound with a pattern of increased echogenicity is commonly observed. However, while NAFLD is the most common cause of increased echogenicity, this phenomenon may also be observed in significant fibrosis from any aetiology. Computed tomography (CT) scanning is generally not required to evaluate NAFLD. Imaging cannot distinguish between steatosis and steatohepatitis (only liver histology can).

Liver biopsy: Liver histology allows the clinician to confirm the diagnosis of NAFLD, to exclude other pathology and to differentiate steatosis from NASH. Histology also facilitates staging of the disease, including providing an assessment on the severity of hepatic fibrosis (the main determinant of prognosis). The issue of when and who to biopsy is not conclusive.

The following is a useful guide:
- Unless there are features to suggest more severe liver disease, a period of lifestyle modification for 3–6 months is recommended for patients with suspected NAFLD prior to proceeding with a biopsy.

Who to biopsy?
Consideration should be given for the following criteria:
- Patients in whom liver tests fail to correct after lifestyle changes whereby biopsy is reasonable for the reasons indicated above
- Persons aged >45 years
- BMI >30 kg/m^2
- Type 2 diabetes
- Features suggestive of cirrhosis
- If having a laparoscopic cholecystectomy.

Note: specific ALT levels are not an indication for biopsy.

Pathology
Steatosis or fatty infiltration is required to be present for a diagnosis of NAFLD. NASH, in addition, requires the presence of inflammation, liver cell injury and/or fibrosis. The extent of fibrosis is the most important prognostic variable when looking at severity and does not necessarily parallel liver enzyme levels.

MANAGEMENT

Lifestyle modifications

Lifestyle change, including healthy eating and increasing physical activity, is core to the management of NAFLD.

The dietary treatment for NASH is based upon reversing insulin resistance. The added benefits of this healthy lifestyle approach include benefits to morbidity associated with diabetes and cardiovascular disease. Furthermore, early intervention may delay the onset of diabetes.

Weight loss is recommended (ideally aiming for a BMI within normal limits), however this should be achieved gradually (e.g. 0.25–0.5 kg/week), as a rapid weight loss (e.g. with 'fad' diets) may result in further deterioration of liver function. This weight loss should be sustained. Weight loss reduces steatosis, liver cell injury and inflammation. There is some evidence to suggest that sustained weight loss may also improve the severity of fibrosis. To optimally manage obesity, it may be necessary to refer the patient to a specialist accredited dietitian. Weight loss options have to emphasise appropriate dietary interventions associated with an increase in physical activity. When appropriate, this may be supplemented by the use of lipase inhibitors. Bariatric surgery (e.g. gastric banding) is a safe and effective method for achieving durable weight loss for patients with morbid obesity and has been shown to reverse steatohepatitis.

Physical activity in its own right is able to improve insulin sensitivity, even in the absence of weight loss. Furthermore, the addition of physical activity to an energy-restricted diet has been shown to be more effective in promoting weight loss than an energy-restricted diet alone.

Optimising diabetes and lipid control appears to improve liver biochemistry. Fatty liver disease does not appear to predispose patients to increased hepatotoxicity from most lipid-lowering, obesity and antidiabetic pharmacological agents, and they should be prescribed as medically indicated. Lipid modulating and insulin sensitising agents appear the most promising therapeutic agents. While insulin sensitising agents appear beneficial in managing the steatohepatitis, they may be associated with weight gain.

Minimising alcohol consumption (even abstaining) is very important. Alcohol consumption aggravates the formation of steatosis and induces pro-oxidant cofactors. This further enhances cellular injury. Interestingly, obesity and insulin resistance are now known to be important risk factors for fibrotic progression in alcoholic liver disease. The latter reflects the fact that many patients happen to have both heavy alcohol consumption and risk factors for NASH (obesity, insulin resistance, etc) and, consequently, the fatty liver disease has multiple aetiologies (both alcoholic liver disease and NAFLD).

Medications

Only a few large scale clinical trials have been published. The use of medication is also important because the diabetes, hyperlipidemia and obesity may all need therapeutic intervention. Nevertheless, all the following medications have been used to treat NAFLD and NASH in particular, despite the fact that none has an approved indication for this purpose.

- Biguanides: e.g. metformin, acts on liver as well as peripheral tissues to improve insulin sensitivity. There is no evidence of a long-term beneficial effect.
- Thiazolidinediones: PPARgamma agonists (e.g. rosiglitazone, pioglitazone) increase insulin receptor expression in adipocytes and hepatocytes. Recent studies suggest that they improve liver function tests and they may result in improvement in liver pathology, but unfortunately are associated with an increase in body weight.
- Hypolipidaemics:
  - HMG-CoA reductase inhibitors have been shown to improve liver function tests in NASH. These agents are used mainly when elevated cholesterol and triglycerides are an issue.
  - Fibrates (e.g. gemfibrozil) are used mainly in the context of hypertriglyceridaemia.
- Antioxidants: some animal studies support the role of vitamin E supplementation, however there are no good human data.
- Lipase inhibitors: these are an adjunct to dietary therapy to assist weight loss.

SUMMARY

NAFLD is already the most common cause of abnormal liver function tests in the Western world. This acronym includes bland steatosis, steatosis with inflammation and/or fibrosis. Obesity, hyperglycaemia and hyperlipidaemia are frequently associated with NAFLD. Therefore, it is not surprising that most patients

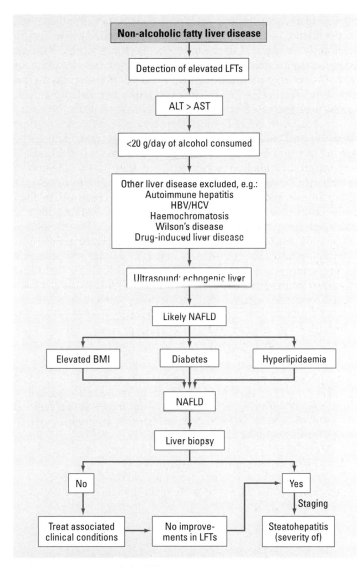

FIGURE 39.1: Diagnosis of non-alcoholic fatty liver disease.

ALT = alanine aminotransferase; AST = aspartate aminotransferase; BMI = body mass index; HBV = hepatitis B virus; HCV = hepatitis C virus; NAFLD = non-alcoholic fatty liver disease; LFTs = liver function tests.

with NAFLD have underlying insulin resistance. Furthermore, the prevalence of NAFLD is increasing, paralleling the rise in the obesity epidemic observed in the Western world. Patients usually come to medical attention because of the detection of elevated liver enzymes, particularly elevated transaminases with an ALT >AST (Figure 39.1). Liver ultrasound frequently reveals a pattern of increased echogenicity. It is important to be aware that patients with NAFLD have an increased prevalence of type 2 diabetes and cardiovascular disease. Investigations include the need to measure lipid and blood glucose levels. Liver biopsy is frequently performed to confirm the diagnosis of NAFLD, to differentiate steatosis from NASH and to stage the disease. A proportion of patients with NAFLD develop progressive liver disease, ultimately leading to the development of cirrhosis, hepatic decompensation and (less commonly) hepatocellular carcinoma. The basis of management is that of slow and steady weight loss with appropriate dietary measures and exercise. Hyperlipidaemia and hyperglycaemia may require pharmacotherapy including the use of HMG-CoA reductase inhibitors, fibrates, biguanides and thiazolidinediones.

FURTHER READING

Farrell GC, Larter CZ. Nonalcoholic fatty liver disease: from steatosis to cirrhosis. Hepatology 2006; 43(2 Suppl 1):S99–112.

Grant LM, Lisker-Melman M. Nonalcoholic fatty liver disease. Ann Hepatol 2004; 3:93–9.

McCullough AJ. The clinical features, diagnosis and natural history of nonalcoholic fatty liver disease. Clin Liver Dis 2004; 8:521–33, viii.

Neuschwander-Tetri B. Fatty liver and the metabolic syndrome. Curr Opin Gastroenterol 2007; 23:193–8.

Chapter 40

ALCOHOLIC LIVER DISEASE

KEY POINTS

- Alcohol is one of the most common causes of liver disease—alcoholic liver disease (ALD).
- The clinical and pathological spectrum of ALD includes fatty liver, hepatitis and cirrhosis, which may lead to complications including portal hypertension, liver failure and hepatocellular carcinoma.
- Recent and past alcohol consumption should be assessed in all cases of liver disease.
- The most useful laboratory marker for alcohol abuse is gamma-glutamyltransferase (GGT), but this is only moderately sensitive.
- Hepatitis C virus (HCV) infection in ALD is associated with more severe liver disease.
- Liver biopsy is a very useful diagnostic tool, but is infrequently required.
- Abstinence from alcohol is the major factor that influences survival.
- Severe alcoholic hepatitis is uncommon with a mortality of 1 in 3 in the first 30 days.
- Corticosteroids and pentoxifylline are effective for short-term treatment of severe alcoholic hepatitis.
- Liver transplantation may be considered in highly selected cases where liver disease progresses despite sustained abstinence.

Alcohol remains one of the most common causes of liver disease and contributes to 1000 deaths and 64,000 hospital admissions per year in Australia. National per capita alcohol consumption correlates with mortality from alcoholic liver disease (ALD), has fallen from a peak in 1985 but has been relatively static for the last decade.

PATHOLOGY AND CLINICAL PRESENTATION

Symptoms and signs are not reliable indicators of the presence or severity of ALD. There may be no symptoms even in the presence of cirrhosis. In other cases, clinical features do allow a confident diagnosis. The clinical and pathological spectrum of alcoholic liver disease includes fatty liver, hepatitis and cirrhosis, but these commonly coexist.

Alcoholic fatty liver

Alcoholic fatty liver results from accumulation of fat droplets within hepatocytes (steatosis) without inflammation or fibrosis. It may commence after a few days of heavy drinking and manifests as anorexia, nausea and right upper quadrant discomfort. The liver is enlarged, firm and may be tender. There are typically no other signs.

Alcoholic hepatitis

Alcoholic hepatitis is defined pathologically by polymorphonuclear infiltration with hepatocyte injury (ballooning necrosis and apoptosis), accumulation of Mallory's hyaline (derived from intermediate filaments) and variable hepatic fibrosis. It presents with anorexia, nausea and abdominal pain, with jaundice, bruising and encephalopathy in association with alcohol abuse. Hepatomegaly may be marked and associated with tenderness, splenomegaly, signs of liver failure and ascites. Systemic disturbances include fever and neutrophilic leucocytosis. The gamma-glutamyltransferase (GGT) is the predominant abnormality. The AST generally exceeds the ALT, but both are only moderately raised. Values for aspartate aminotransferase (AST) or alanine aminotransferase (ALT) above 500 U/L suggest another disorder that may coexist with ALD, most often viral hepatitis or paracetamol (acetaminophen) toxicity.

TABLE 40.1: Using the Maddrey score to assess the severity of alcoholic hepatitis

Maddrey score = 4.6 × (prolongation of prothrombin time above control in seconds) + bilirubin (μmol/L)/17
Interpretation: Short-term (30 day) mortality is related to the Maddrey score
Maddrey score >32 is associated with mortality of 30%–50%
Maddrey score <32 is associated with minimal mortality

Example: Patient prothrombin time 16 s, bilirubin 150 μmol/L, laboratory control prothrombin time 12 s
Maddrey score = 4.6 × (16 − 12) + 150/17 = 26. This indicates a low likelihood of mortality during the current admission

Mild cases are common and typically manifest with abnormal serum biochemistry, and hepatomegaly. Severe alcoholic hepatitis is relatively rare and carries a short-term mortality of approximately 50%. The severity of alcoholic hepatitis can be assessed using a number of simple quantitative indices (Maddrey score, MELD Score, Combined Clinical and Laboratory Index). Of these, the Maddrey Discriminant Function (MDF) is the simplest (Table 40.1).

Alcoholic cirrhosis

Alcoholic cirrhosis may present with fatigue, anorexia, nausea, malaise or weight loss but typically presents with complications such as portal hypertension leading to variceal bleeding and/or ascites, liver failure and hepatocellular carcinoma. Alcoholic cirrhosis is a recognised risk factor for hepatocellular carcinoma

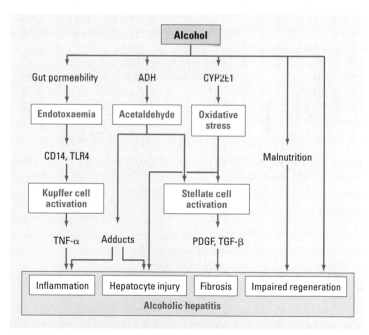

FIGURE 40.1: Overview of the pathogenesis of alcoholic hepatitis.

ADH = alcohol dehydrogenase; PDGF = platelet-derived growth factor; TGF-β = transforming growth factor beta; TLR4 = toll-like receptor 4; TNF-α = tumor necrosis factor alpha.

but it is not clear that there is an association between alcohol abuse and hepatocellular carcinoma in the absence of cirrhosis.

Physical examination may be normal in compensated cirrhosis. Peripheral signs include spider naevi, palmar erythema and Dupuytren's contracture (a sign of alcohol use but not cirrhosis). Among hospitalised patients, hepatomegaly is the most common finding. Jaundice, ascites and encephalopathy are found in about half and alcohol withdrawal is evident in 29% of patients.

Pathogenesis

The risk of cirrhosis correlates with daily average consumption above a threshold of 20 g per day for women and 40 g per day for men. ALD is a multi-step chronic disease process (Figure 40.1).

The risk of liver disease is related to the amount of alcohol consumed, but female gender, other undefined genetic factors, chronic viral hepatitis, hepatotoxins, obesity and other nutritional impairment all accelerate the disease process. Hepatitis C is more common in alcoholics than in the general community and when the two are combined, liver disease progresses more rapidly.

Excessive drinkers are at increased risk of some types of drug-induced liver injury. For example, paracetamol in apparently therapeutic doses has led to acute liver failure in alcoholics and methotrexate accelerates hepatic fibrosis in heavy drinkers.

DETECTION OF ALCOHOL ABUSE

A quantitative alcohol history should be recorded for all patients. Average daily consumption is expressed in grams of alcohol or standard drinks (each containing 10 g ethanol). Consumption is frequently underreported. In some cases, alcohol abuse may be recognised via other typical medical or psychosocial problems such as depression, neurological toxicity, abdominal pain, relationship difficulties, poor work performance, trauma and violence.

Several brief questionnaires have been validated for the detection of alcohol abuse (Table 40.2). If a screening test is positive, more detailed assessment is indicated.

Laboratory markers such as gamma-glutamyltransferase (GGT) and mean corpuscular volume (MCV) are only moderately sensitive and specific for drinking problems in general. In ALD, the GGT level is almost invariably elevated. However, elevated levels may also be seen in other liver diseases and with some drugs

---

TABLE 40.2: Screening questions for excessive alcohol consumption

---

A positive response on screening indicates the need for further assesssment

a. AUDIT (original version has 10 questions, but question 3 on its own is very useful)

How often do you have six or more drinks on one occasion? (positive response is monthly or more)

b. The CAGE screening questions: two or more positive responses suggest alcohol dependence

C – Have you ever felt the need to **c**ut down your drinking?

A – Have you ever felt **a**nnoyed by criticism of your drinking?

G – Have you ever felt **g**uilty about your drinking?

F – Have you ever taken a drink (**e**ye-opener) first thing in the morning?

(notably anticonvulsants). The MCV is generally less sensitive and less specific than GGT. Combined assessment of MCV and GGT detects 70% of the alcohol-dependent population. The carbohydrate-deficient transferrin (CDT) test may be more specific than GGT, but the test is not widely available at present and there are false positives in any form of advanced liver disease. Several other laboratory parameters may be elevated, including uric acid, triglycerides and high-density lipoprotein cholesterol. These are not adequately sensitive or specific for use as a screening test.

NATURAL HISTORY

In the short term, the mortality of alcoholic hepatitis is closely related to the severity of illness on presentation. For severe cases, the short-term mortality remains close to 50%. Overall, the mortality is approximately 15% in the first 30 days and 40% by 1 year. Hepatic encephalopathy, ascites, hepatorenal syndrome and bleeding oesophageal varices contribute to mortality. Extrahepatic mortality in alcoholics is related to trauma and the common comorbidities of depression and tobacco dependence.

Abstinence from alcohol consumption is the major factor influencing survival. In those who continue to drink, alcoholic hepatitis progresses rapidly to cirrhosis. The survival benefit with abstinence is less clear for advanced liver disease, as the outcome may be determined by irreversible liver damage and complications such as portal hypertension rather than by continuing alcohol consumption.

The prognosis for alcoholic hepatitis is worse for women than for men. In addition, women suffer from higher levels of psychological comorbidity, primarily depression.

Other liver diseases influence the outcome of patients with alcoholic hepatitis, most notably chronic hepatitis C. Hepatitis C virus (HCV) infection in patients with alcohol-induced liver disease is associated with more severe liver disease.

DIAGNOSIS

Assessment of alcohol use disorder

The alcohol use disorder is assessed according to International Classification of Diseases (ICD-10) criteria. Harmful consumption refers to continuing consumption despite harms recognised by the patient. Dependence refers to the presence of three or more of the following symptoms: drinking despite harm, a strong desire to drink, loss of control over drinking, withdrawal symptoms, tolerance and salience (giving a higher priority to drinking than to other activities).

Role of liver biopsy

Biopsy is the definitive diagnostic tool, but typically is not required, as the results infrequently alter diagnosis or therapy. Biopsy is desirable if the alcohol aetiology cannot be clarified clinically and to confirm diagnosis before starting specific therapy. In most severe cases, coagulopathy precludes percutaneous biopsy, but the transjugular route can be safely used where available.

Histological features of alcoholic hepatitis include steatosis, ballooning necrosis, acidophil bodies, Mallory's hyaline with cellular infiltration and fibrosis. Fibrosis commences in zone 3 of the hepatic lobule around the central vein as a result of relative hypoxia and is termed perivenular. 'Chicken-wire' fibrosis surrounds lobular hepatocytes.

MANAGEMENT

Fatty liver and mild alcoholic hepatitis almost invariably recover with abstinence from alcohol. Severe disease is associated with poor outcomes and warrants specific treatment, but the available options are limited (Table 40.3).

TABLE 40.3: Management options for alcoholic liver disease

Interventions to reduce alcohol consumption
- Brief intervention
- Counselling, e.g.:
  - Motivational interviewing
  - 12-step programme, including Alcoholics Anonymous
- Pharmacotherapy
  - Acamprosate
  - Naltrexone
  - Disulfiram
- Residential rehabilitation

Treatment of liver injury
- Nutritional supplementation
- Corticosteroids
- Propylthiouracil
- Pentoxifylline

Transplantation

Management of alcohol use disorder

Goal setting

In all cases, a period of 1–3 months abstinence is advisable to allow liver injury to resolve and to break the habit of daily drinking. For those with severe liver disease, lifelong abstinence is the appropriate goal. Those with minimal liver abnormalities and without alcohol dependence in whom liver tests normalise may eventually return to moderate consumption within National Health and Medical Research Council of Australia (NHMRC) guidelines.

How can abstinence be achieved?

Treatment for alcohol abuse is moderately effective. For non-dependent drinkers, brief intervention may be effective. It does not require specialised staff and can be done in 5–10 min. The FLAGS acronym summarises one approach (Table 40.4). Follow-up is recommended with repeated intervention if necessary.

For alcohol dependence, the initial step is to manage the risk of withdrawal. The risk is higher if there have been previous

TABLE 40.4: Brief intervention for alcohol abuse—FLAGS	
Feedback	The nature and extent of alcohol-related problems
Listen	To patient concerns
Advise	Patient clearly to reduce consumption
Goals	Negotiate clinically appropriate goals acceptable to the patient
Strategies	Specific suggestions to modify drinking

withdrawal episodes, and with more severe and longstanding alcohol dependence. Diazepam is usually the drug of choice, but in the presence of liver failure, active metabolites of diazepam can precipitate hepatic encephalopathy. In this setting, oxazepam is the preferred drug as it does not have active metabolites. Symptom-triggered treatment involves regular monitoring (every 1–6 hours depending on severity) with an alcohol withdrawal scale if hospitalised (AWS or the CIWA) and administration of a benzodiazepine according to the score (Table 40.5). This provides more intensive treatment when symptoms are severe and lessens the duration of treatment once symptoms settle. Benzodiazepines should not be used for more than 1 week due to the risk of dependence. All patients should receive thiamine initially parenterally, then orally until sustained abstinence is achieved.

Once withdrawal has settled, continuing management to prevent relapse to heavy drinking may be implemented by an interested general practitioner, if available, or via a specialist alcohol treatment service. Treatment options include counselling of various types, naltrexone, acamprosate, peer support and residential rehabilitation. There is no clear evidence to favour one treatment modality over the others. Naltrexone is an orally

TABLE 40.5: Typical regimen for alcohol withdrawal		
Score	**Diazepam dose**	**Oxazepam dose**
Low (AWS 0–3)	0	0
Moderate (AWS 3–5)	10 mg	30 mg
High (AWS >5)	20 mg	60 mg
Repeat assessment 2–6-hourly depending on severity. All patients should receive adequate doses of thiamine.		

active opioid antagonist that reduces the psychological reward provided by alcohol, leading to reduced desire to drink. Naltrexone has hepatotoxic potential, typically at higher doses than are used routinely. Hepatic naltrexone clearance is reduced in cirrhosis, but no increased risk of hepatotoxicity has been reported. Acamprosate inhibits central nervous system N-methyl-D-aspartate receptors and GABA transmission. Side effects are uncommon and mild and include diarrhoea, dizziness and pruritus. Acamprosate is not metabolised by the liver and its pharmacokinetics are not altered in liver failure. Disulfiram inhibits aldehyde dehydrogenase (ALDH), leading to accumulation of acetaldehyde after alcohol consumption, which causes an aversive reaction with nausea and vomiting. Directly supervised treatment (by family member or health professional) may be very effective but unsupervised treatment is ineffective. It is occasionally hepatotoxic and is not recommended in severe liver disease. Pharmacotherapy is typically commenced once the patient is well enough to contemplate resumption of alcohol consumption and ideally before discharge from hospital. Counselling models include motivational interviewing and cognitive behaviour therapy, which can be offered for individuals, families or groups. Alcoholics Anonymous (AA) is a peer fellowship that conceptualises 'alcoholism' as a medical disease that can be controlled by adopting a 12-step approach. The duration of abstinence correlates with the number of AA meetings attended. Residential rehabilitation services should be considered for severe cases with medical and social disintegration.

Psychological comorbidities such as depression and anxiety are very common. Recognition and specific treatment for these comorbidities increases the chance of controlling alcohol consumption.

Monitoring alcohol intake

Monitoring alcohol intake by self-report provides adequate information in most cases. Alcohol may be measured in blood, breath or urine and positive results indicate consumption within the last few hours. Trace levels in blood (up to 0.01%) have been reported from endogenous ethanol production. In abstinent patients, levels of GGT fall with an apparent half-life of 2 weeks and are usually normal within 6 weeks. The MCV falls over several months and is insensitive to drinking relapse. Rising CDT levels have been reported to precede self-report of relapse.

Management of liver disease

Hospital admission is required for severe disease, complications and failed out patient management.

Corticosteroids

Corticosteroids are the most studied treatment for severe alcoholic hepatitis and have been shown to reduce short-term mortality, but their role remains controversial. In alcoholic hepatitis, corticosteroid therapy generally produces few complications, but gastrointestinal (GI) bleeding and serious infections have been reported. Prednisolone is preferred to prednisone, because of reduced activation of prednisone in active liver disease. Indications for prednisolone are an MDF >32 or spontaneous encephalopathy, failure to improve during the first few days of hospitalisation and no contraindications such as active gastrointestinal bleeding, hepatorenal syndrome, sepsis or viral hepatitis. These individuals are seen infrequently. The usual dose is 40 mg for one month.

Nutritional supplementation

Alcohol provides 30 kJ (7 calories) of energy per gram, but is nutritionally 'empty', lacking in protein, vitamins and minerals. In patients with ALD, alcohol may provide up to 50% of calories, so that some evidence of malnutrition may be found in almost all patients. Nutritional supplementation attempts to correct this deficiency and provides the substrates needed for hepatic regeneration and systemic nutrition. Maintaining a positive nitrogen balance correlates with an improved outcome of severe ALD, but is difficult to achieve. In practice, it is essential that all patients with alcoholic hepatitis are adequately nourished and should receive the standard daily requirements of at least 30 kcal/kg/day and 1 g protein/kg/day. Supplements should be given first via oral or enteral routes, but if difficulties arise, the parenteral route may be used.

Pentoxifylline

Pentoxifylline is a dimethylxanthine derivative used for peripheral vascular disease because it decreases blood viscosity (via increasing erythrocyte deformity) and improves blood flow. It also attenuates tumour necrosis factor-alpha (TNF-α) release and action and exerts an antifibrinogenic action. Pentoxifylline (400 mg t.d.s.) has recently been shown to improve short-term (4 week) survival in a prospective randomised controlled trial of 96 patients with severe alcoholic hepatitis. This survival benefit was related to a significant decrease in the rate of development of hepatorenal syndrome. Replication of this result by other clinical units is required before its use can be confidently recommended. The only significant side effects were nausea, epigastric pain and vomiting, and these resolved soon after discontinuation of treatment. The drug is inexpensive and widely available. Use of this drug in patients with sepsis and active gastrointestinal bleeding has not been evaluated.

New approaches to therapy

These agents show promise but are not readily available. S-adenosylmethionine (SAMe) is a source of cysteine for the production of glutathione (GSH). In cirrhosis, SAMe synthase activity is reduced. Treatment with SAMe has been shown to lead to increased survival of patients with alcoholic cirrhosis in one study. The drug is available from health food stores but long-term treatment is costly. Studies in experimental animals have shown that polyenylphosphatidylcholine (PPC) reverses a number of the adverse effects of ethanol on the liver. Polyenylphosphatidylcholine acts as an antioxidant, downregulates CYP2E1 activity, restores SAMe synthase activity and reduces stellate cell activation and collagen synthesis. A large cooperative Veterans Affairs study of PPC in ambulatory patients with ALD has shown a trend towards protection against cirrhosis, but PPC is not readily available. Glutathione depletion is common to the toxicity of both paracetamol and alcohol but a controlled study of N-acetylcysteine found no benefit in patients with alcoholic hepatitis. In view of the central role of TNF-α in alcoholic hepatitis, inhibition of TNF-α with a monoclonal antibody (infliximab) might be useful clinically. A recent case series noted increased survival compared with historical controls but a controlled trial was abandoned due to an excess of deaths due to sepsis. Preliminary data have been reported from a controlled trial of interleukin-10 documenting a beneficial effect in alcoholic hepatitis.

Liver transplantation

Alcoholic liver disease is now an accepted indication for orthotopic liver transplantation (OLT). When carefully selected cases are offered transplantation, clinical outcomes are comparable to those of patients transplanted for other liver diseases.

The ideal candidate is neither too sick nor too well, has evidence of psychosocial stability, accepts the role of alcohol in causing their liver disease and expresses a commitment to lifelong abstinence from alcohol. Most transplantation units require a minimum of 6 months of abstinence before consideration for transplantation. One advantage of this approach is that a number of patients with advanced liver disease who achieve stable abstinence will recover sufficiently so as to not require transplantation. Patients with alcoholic hepatitis are unlikely to meet the above criteria for transplantation. They have been drinking to the time of admission and are typically difficult to assess from a psychosocial perspective as they are severely ill and often encephalopathic.

Once good health is restored after transplantation, there is a risk of recurrent alcohol abuse that may lead to recurrent ALD in the graft, non-compliance with immunosuppression and other alcohol-related problems. About one-third of survivors return to alcohol consumption, but often consumption remains at very moderate levels. Periodic re-assessment of alcohol use is indicated during follow-up.

SUMMARY

In the management of alcoholic liver disease, remember the following:
- Alcohol abstinence (consider specific measures, e.g. disulfiram)
- Nutritious diet (consider supplementation where indicated)
- Corticosteroids or pentoxifylline for severe alcoholic hepatitis
- Liver transplantation for highly selected cases.

FURTHER READING

Haber PS, Warner R, Seth D, et al. Pathogenesis and management of alcoholic hepatitis. J Gastroenterol Hepatol 2003; 18:1332–44.

Hulse G, White J, Cape G, eds. Management of alcohol and drug problems. Melbourne: Oxford University Press; 2002.

Chapter 41

DRUGS AND LIVER DISEASE

KEY POINTS

- Drugs have become the leading cause of acute liver failure in Western countries.
- The liver plays a central role in elimination of many drugs through a sophisticated series of metabolic enzymes.
- Clinical presentation varies from asymptomatic elevations of liver function tests to coma secondary to fulminant hepatic failure.
- Drug-related hepatotoxicity can mimic clinically and histologically almost any type of liver disease.
- Diagnosis is based on:
  - Detailed drug history
  - Thorough clinical examination
  - Temporal relationship of exposure and symptoms and signs of liver disease
  - Exclusion of other causes.
- Treatment: potential causative drugs must be stopped immediately.

INTRODUCTION

The liver plays a central role in the elimination of a large number of medications. It has an elaborate mechanism of transporters that can transfer drugs from the circulation into the hepatocyte and then their metabolic products into bile or back into the circulation for renal clearance.

The liver also has a sophisticated series of metabolic enzymes, which, in general, convert drugs from lipophilic substances to hydrophilic substances that can be more easily eliminated. The cytochrome P450 enzymes, which play the major role in drug metabolism, may produce reactive metabolites during this process and these are thought to be the mechanism by which many adverse hepatic reactions occur.

Epidemiology

Drug-induced hepatotoxicity is the leading cause of acute liver failure and liver transplantation in Western countries.

RISK FACTORS FOR DRUG HEPATOTOXICITY

Several environmental and genetic mechanisms may influence individual susceptibility to drug hepatotoxicity.

Age: older persons appear to be more susceptible to drug-induced hepatotoxicity.

Gender: women are more affected by the toxic adverse effects on the liver than men.

Alcohol: can modulate the hepatotoxic potential of drugs through CYP induction, inhibition or substrate competition.

Underlying preexisting liver disease: hepatotoxicity caused by isoniazid is more common in patients with viral hepatitis and/or HIV infection. Also HIV patients undergoing antiretroviral treatment have a higher risk of severe hepatotoxicity when co-infected with hepatitis B or C viruses, and an increased risk of hepatotoxicity from sulfamethoxazole/trimethoprim.

Genetic factors: genetic variations in human leucocyte antigen (HLA) molecules can predispose individuals to immunoallergic drug hepatotoxicity. Certain HLA class II alleles are important in explaining why a given drug may cause different patterns of liver damage in certain individuals. Susceptibility to isoniazid hepatotoxicity in predisposed individuals may be due to a relationship between N-acetyltransferase 2 deficiency and the propensity to develop hepatotoxicity.

PRESENTATION

In general, adverse hepatic drug reactions are 'idiosyncratic'—that is, they are unpredictable. The clinical spectrum of drug-induced liver disease varies greatly.

Drug-related hepatotoxicity can mimic clinically and histologically almost any type of liver disease (Table 41.1). Presenting symptoms are similarly diverse, from asymptomatic elevations of liver function tests to coma secondary to fulminant hepatic failure. Anorexia and tiredness can be the presentations of hepatitic reactions while itch, dark urine and jaundice occur in more severe cholestatic syndromes.

TABLE 41.1: Drug-induced liver disease	
Condition	**Drug**
Acute hepatocellular necrosis	Isoniazid, cloxacillin, halothane, methyldopa, paracetamol
Fatty liver	Tetracycline, valproic acid, corticosteroids, non-steroidal antiinflammatory drugs, perhexiline, amiodarone
Granulomatous reactions	Hydralazine, allopurinol, carbamazepine
Acute cholestasis	Oral contraceptive steroids, anabolic androgens, chlorpromazine, flucloxacillin
Chronic cholestasis	Chlorpromazine, flucloxacillin, amitriptyline
Chronic hepatitis/necrosis	Methyldopa, nitrofurantoin, dantrolene
Fibrosis and cirrhosis	Methotrexate
Vascular disorders	Oral contraceptive steroids, anabolic androgens, azathioprine

History
A thorough drug history has to be taken in all patients presenting with symptoms or investigations suggesting liver disease. This needs to include all medications taken over the previous 3 months, including over-the-counter preparations and complementary medicines. If the suspicion of hepatic drug reaction is high, the patient may need to be questioned again and the local medical officer and the local pharmacist called to ascertain all medications taken.

In general, patients with preexisting liver disease are not more susceptible to adverse hepatic drug reactions, but once one occurs it may lead to more severe liver dysfunction.

Physical findings
Patients with suspected hepatic adverse reactions need to be closely examined for jaundice and signs of chronic liver disease such as spider naevi and palmar erythema. The size and consistency of the liver is important as it may suggest other causes for the liver dysfunction such as cirrhosis or secondary tumours.

INVESTIGATIONS

Liver function tests are the initial investigations to confirm a liver abnormality. It should be remembered that a number of drugs, including phenytoin and rifampicin, induce cytochrome P450 enzymes and may lead to significant elevations of gamma-glutamyltransferase (GGT) without reflecting liver cell damage. As drug-induced liver disease can cause a wide spectrum of liver abnormalities, liver function tests may show a hepatitic, cholestatic or a mixed picture.

It is always important to exclude other causes of liver abnormality with abdominal ultrasound and serology for viral hepatitis and autoimmune liver disease should be performed in most cases.

Liver biopsy

A liver biopsy is not usually required to establish a diagnosis of hepatic drug reaction. However, it should be performed if there is sufficient doubt about the diagnosis, a severe liver reaction or if the patient is not improving with cessation of the offending medication.

There are features on histology, which may suggest a drug reaction including the presence of eosinophils or a mixed hepatitic, cholestatic pattern. A second opinion from an experienced liver histopathologist may be helpful in difficult cases.

DIAGNOSIS

The diagnosis of hepatic drug reactions should be considered in all patients presenting with abnormal liver function tests. The diagnosis is usually made when other causes of liver dysfunction are excluded, such as viral hepatitis, autoimmune hepatitis and bile duct obstruction. All drugs, including alternative medicines, should be considered as potential causes of liver abnormalities. Although some drugs more commonly produce adverse hepatic reactions, Table 41.2 lists the drugs with hepatotoxicity most commonly reported in Australia to ADRAC (Adverse Drug Reactions Advisory Committee). Table 41.3 lists the complementary medicines most commonly reported with hepatotoxicity. Clinicians cannot be expected to remember all drugs that produce adverse hepatic reactions, but there are a number of reference texts that can be consulted to see if the reaction has been reported before.

In most cases the diagnosis is confirmed when the liver abnormality resolves on the cessation of the offending agent. This usually occurs over 1–2 weeks, but occasionally prolonged abnormalities can occur (i.e. flucloxacillin-induced cholestasis). As mentioned, a liver biopsy has a definite but limited role in the management of these patients.

Finally, hepatic failure can occur secondary to drug use, and referral to a liver transplant unit should be made in these situations.

TABLE 41.2: Most commonly reported drugs with hepatotoxicity

Drug	No. of reports	No. of reports with sole suspected drug	No. of reports with fatal outcome
Flucloxacillin	601	281	22
Amoxycillin/clavulanate	471	281	15
Erythromycin	300	191	5
Carbamazepine	281	183	7
Simvastatin	202	125	7
Ranitidine	198	73	12
Methyldopa	186	133	9
Paracetamol/codeine	173	15	10
Sulfamethoxazole/ trimethoprim	165	90	1
Diclofenac	156	91	9
Phenytoin	153	80	8
Allopurinol	115	46	15
Rifampicin	115	27	9
Roxithromycin	113	55	5
Sulindac	106	79	1
Sulfasalazine	97	56	6
Amoxycillin	97	10	2
Ketoconazole	96	72	–
Nitrofurantoin	91	62	5

TABLE 41.3: Most commonly reported complementary medicines with hepatotoxicity

Medicine	No. of reports	No. of reports with sole suspected drug
Kombucha tea	8	7
Echinacea	7	4
Evening primrose oil	5	3
Valerian	3	–

SUMMARY

Drug-induced hepatotoxicity is the leading cause of acute liver failure and liver transplantation in Western countries. This is in accord with the central role of the liver in drug metabolism and elimination.

It can be difficult to diagnose drug-induced hepatotoxicity as it can mimic almost any type of liver disease. It is vital to take a detailed drug history and to have a high index of suspicion (Figure 41.1). A temporal relationship between the taking of the drug and clinical signs and symptoms may be an important clue. Exclusion of other causes is mandatory.

Treatment is the immediate stoppage of the suspected causative drug.

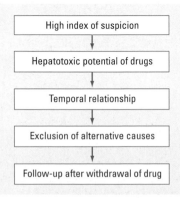

FIGURE 41.1: Approach to diagnosis of suspected drug-induced hepatotoxicity.

Chapter **42**

A FAMILY HISTORY OF LIVER DISEASE

SUMMARY

- The current status in the understanding of genetic and environmental factors in selected hepatobiliary diseases is discussed.
- These include Wilson's disease, alpha₁-antitrypsin deficiency, hereditary haemochromatosis, the hepatic porphyrias, cystic fibrosis, Gaucher's disease, polycystic liver disease and Gilbert's syndrome.
- Discussion embraces the genetics, clinical characteristics, diagnosis and treatment of the above disorders.

INTRODUCTION

Human genomics, the study of structure, function and interactions of all genes in the human genome, promises to improve the diagnosis, treatment and prevention of disease. It is predicted that genomics will influence the practice of medicine in the future. The overall aim is to be able to better predict an individual's risk of developing common complex disease, so that prevention and treatment can be optimised.

WILSON'S DISEASE

KEY POINTS

- An autosomal recessive genetic disorder characterised by accumulation of copper in liver, brain and cornea, secondary to impaired intrahepatic trafficking and biliary excretion of copper.
- Clinically, Wilson's disease (WD) involves:
  - Liver—cirrhosis, chronic hepatitis or fulminant hepatic failure
  - Neurologic—Kayser-Fleischer rings, parkinsonian characteristics and intellectual disturbances
  - Miscellaneous: Fanconi's syndrome, osteoporosis, haemolytic anaemia.

- Diagnosis: caeruloplasmin ↓; free copper ↑;
  urinary copper excretion ↑; hepatic copper concentration ↑.
- Treatment: D-penicillamine is first-line therapy. Other
  drugs include trientine and zinc tetrathiomolybdate. Liver
  transplantation may be appropriate.

Genetics and pathophysiology

Wilson's disease (WD) is an autosomal recessive disorder characterised by accumulation of copper (Cu) in liver, brain and cornea, secondary to impaired intrahepatic trafficking and biliary excretion of Cu. The WD gene (on chromosome 13) codes for a Cu transporting P-type ATPase (*ATP-7B*), which can be altered by multiple mutations. An impaired or deficient WD gene product is responsible for the lack of Cu incorporation into caeruloplasmin and the defective biliary excretion of Cu in WD resulting in increased hepatic stores of Cu. Free Cu is released into the serum and deposited into end organs.

Epidemiology

WD is a rare disorder, affecting approximately 3 people per 100,000.

Clinical features

Clinical symptoms are rarely observed before the age of 5 years and most untreated patients become symptomatic by the age of 40 years. The main organ systems involved are the liver, brain, eyes, kidneys and joints.

Hepatic

- Cirrhosis which may be either micronodular or a mixed macro-micronodular histologic pattern.
- Chronic hepatitis characterised by raised serum aminotransferases in the presence of severe hepatocellular necrosis and inflammation.
- Fulminant hepatic failure. Elevated serum aminotransferases with marked elevation of serum bilirubin, low alkaline phosphatase level and Coombs'-negative haemolytic anaemia. Serum caeruloplasmin may be normal but 24-h urinary Cu and free serum Cu are usually raised.

Neurologic

Kayser-Fleischer rings (KF) (on ophthalmic slit-lamp examination) are present in most patients with neurological symptoms and over half of those without. Neurologic symptoms are varied and include parkinsonian characteristics. Intellectual disturbances include mild memory impairment and overt psychosis.

Miscellaneous

Fanconi's syndrome with proximal tubular acidosis, osteoporosis with spontaneous fractures and Cu-induced haemolytic anaemia.

Diagnosis

- Requires a combination of clinical and biochemistry tests.
- Serum caeruloplasmin. Low serum levels of caeruloplasmin.
- Non-caeruloplasmin serum copper is elevated. Normal free Cu level is under 10 µg/dL. In WD it is greater than 25 µg/dL.
- Urinary Cu excretion (normal 40 µg/24 h). Most WD patients have a urinary Cu excretion greater than 100 µg/24 h.

Liver biopsy: hepatic Cu concentration >250 µg/g dry tissue (normal less than 50 µg/g).

Genetic studies: molecular genetic analysis is of limited value as there are more than 200 mutations. Mutation or haplotype analyses are the only reliable tools for screening the families of an index case.

Treatment

D-penicillamine: first-line drug in Wilson's disease. In 20% of patients, hypersensitivity reactions (neutropenia, thrombocytopenia, rash and arthritis) can occur.

Trientine: second-line therapy. Less potent Cu chelator. Sideroblastic anaemia a major side effect.

Zinc: used mainly in presymptomatic patients as maintenance therapy and in combination therapy.

Tetrathiomolybdate: mainly used to avoid neurologic deterioration that accompanies chelation treatment in some patients.

Liver transplantation: transplant recipients have an excellent long-term prognosis because the underlying biochemical defect is corrected.

ALPHA₁-ANTITRYPSIN DEFICIENCY (A₁-ATD)

KEY POINTS

- Autosomal recessive genetic disorder that predisposes to liver disease and chronic obstructive pulmonary disease (COPD).
- Main function of alpha₁-antitrypsin is to protect tissues against proteases such as neutrophil elastase.
- Clinically involves liver: chronic hepatitis, cirrhosis and hepatocellular carcinoma.
- Investigations: serum concentration of alpha₁-antitrypsin: detection of defective α_1-ATZ alleles.
- Treatment: no specific therapy. 4-phenyl butyric acid is promising. Other strategies include liver transplantation and reconstitution of the normal genotype through gene therapy.

Alpha₁-antitrypsin deficiency (α_1-ATD) is a genetic disorder (autosomal/recessive) that predisposes to chronic liver disease and chronic obstructive pulmonary disease (COPD). It affects 1 in 2,000–5,000 individuals.

α_1-ATD is a glycoprotein mainly produced by hepatocytes in the liver. Its main function is to protect tissues against proteases, such as neutrophil elastase.

Pathogenesis and genetics

A mutation in codon 342 of the α_1-ATD gene, changing a single amino-acid from lysine to glutamate is the primary cause of α_1-ATD. This results in a defective α_1-antitrypsin molecule (α_1-ATZ) that aggregates in the endoplasmic reticulum of the hepatocyte, leading to a cascade of events causing injury to the liver. There is variation in the severity of the disease because of gene modifiers and environmental factors, which modulate the hepatocyte deposition of α_1-ATZ.

Clinical manifestations

Liver disease

Liver disease encompasses chronic hepatitis, cirrhosis and hepatocellular carcinoma. α_1-ATD should be considered in any adult who presents with the above diseases of unknown aetiology. α_1-ATD is usually diagnosed early in life (4–8 weeks of life) presenting as persistent jaundice with raised liver transaminases and bilirubin.

Investigations: serum concentrations of α_1-AT and detection of defective α_1-ATZ alleles.

Treatment: no specific therapy is available, though 4-phenyl butyric acid is a promising drug. Other treatment strategies include orthoptic liver transplantation, somatic gene therapy and replacement therapy.

Other diseases

An increased prevalence of pulmonary disease (emphysema, panniculitis, vasculitis) is noted, which require specific treatment.

HEREDITARY HAEMOCHROMATOSIS

KEY POINTS

- Autosomal recessive. Most patients homozygous for C282Y mutation of the *HFE* gene. A small percentage have the mutation C282Y:H63D.
- Arises from an imbalance between Fe absorption and excretion (inappropriate increased absorption of dietary iron).
- The most important clinical characteristics are:
  - Asymptomatic—incidentally discovered
  - Arthralgias/arthritis
  - Chronic liver disease
  - Alcohol is a key factor in determining clinical expression.
- Biochemical abnormalities include elevated transferrin saturation and ferritin.
- Liver biopsy indicated in the presence of hepatomegaly, raised liver enzymes, very high ferritin levels.
- Imaging studies. MRI is the preferred modality for quantification of hepatic iron.
- Ultrasonography important in staging of liver disease.
- Treatment: phlebotomy—monitor haemoglobin and haematocrit.
- Avoid alcohol and high doses of ascorbic and citric acids.

Hereditary haemochromatosis (HH) is inherited as an autosomal recessive disorder. Most adult patients are homozygous for the C282Y mutation of the *HFE* gene (C282Y: C282Y). A small but significant percentage of HH patients have the mutation C282Y:H63D termed the compound heterozygote state (see Chapter 37).

Prevalence
HH is the most common genetic disease in white persons of Northern European descent—approximately 1:250.

Molecular pathogenesis
Haemochromatosis arises from an imbalance between iron (Fe) absorption and excretion. It is generally accepted that pathologic Fe in HH arises from inappropriately increased absorption of dietary Fe.

The molecular pathophysiology of HH is unknown. There is increasing evidence that hepcidin (an 'iron hormone') might serve as a signalling molecule because it is produced by the liver and released into the blood in response to iron loading or acute infections. Hepcidin is thus emerging as an important regulator of Fe metabolism. Low hepcidin expression and secretion is a unifying feature of all primary overload syndromes.

Clinical presentation
The most common presenting symptoms are:
- Asymptomatic – incidental diagnosis because of discovery of elevated serum Fe markers (↑ serum transferrin Fe saturation, ↑ ferritin) and/or raised aminotransferase levels
- Joint pains (arthritis or arthralgias)
- Chronic liver disease (often associated with diabetes mellitus). The liver disease may progress from fibrosis to cirrhosis and hepatocellular carcinoma.
- Heavy alcohol intake can accelerate liver damage in homozygous HH.

Investigations
- Biochemical abnormalities: elevated transferrin saturation and ferritin. *Note*: ferritin is an acute phase reactant and, when used alone, is often raised in other disease states such as hepatitis, fatty liver, inflammatory conditions and malignancy. Other parameters that should be assessed include: serum Fe, transferrin, full blood count, liver function tests, coagulation studies.
- Genetic testing: predisposition to HH is indicated if there is homozygosity for C282Y or compound heterozygosity for C282Y and H63D. Several less common mutations in the *HFE* gene may occur (Table 42.1).

TABLE 42.1: Causes of iron overload	
Inherited	**Acquired**

Hereditary haemochromatosis
• Type I *HFE*-related:
  – C282Y homozygotes
  – C282Y:H63D compound
    heterozygotes
• Rare alternative *HFE* mutations
• Types 2, 3, 4, non-*HFE* mutations
	Chronic liver diseases
	• End-stage cirrhosis
	• Hepatitis B and C
	• Alcoholic liver disease
	• Non-alcoholic steatohepatitis
	• Porphyria cutanea tarda
	Dietary iron overload
	Haematological disorders
	• Iron-loading anaemias:
	  – Thalassaemia major
	  – Sideroblastic anaemia
	  – Chronic haemolytic anaemia
	  – Parenteral iron overload
	Inherited/acquired?
	• African iron overload
	• Neonatal haemochromatosis

- Imaging studies: Magnetic resonance imaging (MRI) is the preferred modality. Quantification of Fe storage can be assessed. Computed tomography (CT) scan sensitivity for quantification of hepatic Fe is lower than MRI. Ultrasonography has a poor sensitivity for iron but is important in the staging of liver disease and portal hypertension, and for surveillance of malignant tumours.
- Liver biopsy: indicated for patients with hepatomegaly and raised liver enzymes. Extreme elevation of ferritin (>1000 mg/L) has been associated with cirrhosis. Fe stains, Fe quantification and histopathology should be assessed.
- Other causes of Fe overload due to increased Fe absorption: chronic liver diseases (hepatitis B and C; alcoholic liver disease, non-alcoholic fatty liver disease, porphyria cutanea tarda), dietary Fe overload, miscellaneous causes (African iron overload, neonatal Fe overload, atransferrinaemia) (Table 42.1).

Treatment

Phlebotomy at weekly intervals with regular monitoring of haemoglobin and haematocrit values. The target ferritin level should be 25–50 mg/L. Once Fe stores have been mobilised, phlebotomy 3 or 4 times per year may be adequate.

High doses of ascorbic and citric acid and dietary supplements containing Fe should be avoided.

Alcohol should be avoided.

All first-degree relatives of homozygous HH patients should be screened as the expressivity of *HFE* gene mutation is higher in family members of patients with HH.

HEPATIC PORPHYRIAS

KEY POINTS

- Inherited metabolic disorders due to deficiencies of specific enzymes in haem biosynthesis.
- The hepatic porphyrias are: acute intermittent porphyria, variegate porphyria, hereditary coproporphyria; porphyria cutanea tarda; ALA dehydratase porphyria.
- The hepatic porphyrias are autosomal dominant except for ALA dehydratase deficiency which is autosomal recessive.
- Clinical features include abdominal pain, neurological symptoms and cutaneous lesions.
- Precipitating factors: environmental agents (alcohol, smoking, dietary restriction and infection), pharmacological agents (anticonvulsants, antimicrobials, diuretics, cardiovascular drugs and substance abuse).
- Management: identify and avoid precipitating factors, treat pain with opiates (not oxycodone), correct fluids and electrolytes, glucose, intravenous haem for severe attacks. Protoporphyria requires liver transplantation.

Hepatic porphyrias are inherited metabolic disorders due to deficiencies of specific enzymes in haem biosynthesis.

The hepatic porphyrias are: acute intermittent porphyria, variegate porphyria, hereditary coproporphyria, porphyria cutanea tarda, ALA dehydratase porphyria (Table 42.2).

Hepatoerythropoietic porphyria and erythropoietic protoporphyria involve the liver and bone marrow.

TABLE 42.2: Hepatic porphyrias

Disorder	Enzymatic defect	Inheritance	Abdominal pain	Skin lesions	Biochemical markers
Acute intermittent porphyria	PBG deaminase	Autosomal dominant	Yes	No	Urine: ALA < PBG
Variegate porphyria	Protoporphyrinogen oxidase	Autosomal dominant	Yes	Yes	Urine: ALA > PBG coproporphyrin
Hereditary coproporphyria	Coproporphyrinogen	Autosomal dominant	Yes	Yes	Urine: ALA > PBG, coproporphyrin Stool: coproporphyrin
Porphyria cutanea tarda	Uroporphyrinogen III decarboxylase	Autosomal dominant	No	Yes	Urine: uroporphyrin, 7-carboxylate porphyrin Stool: isocoproporphyrin
ALA dehydratase deficiency	ALA dehydratase	Autosomal dominant or acquired	Yes	No	Urine: ALA

* ALA = 5 aminolevulinic acid; PBG = porphobilinogen.

Clinical features

Acute porphyrias

- Characterised by potentially life-threatening neurologic symptoms.
- Females more frequently affected, often in the fourth decade of life. Symptoms rarely occur before puberty.
- Attacks usually last for several days, often require hospitalisation and are followed by complete recovery. Abdominal pain is the most common symptom, often accompanied by nausea, constipation and symptoms of sympathetic overactivity and neuropsychiatric disturbances.
- Attacks are often precipitated by environmental agents (alcohol, smoking, infection, stress, low-energy diets) or pharmacologic compounds (anticonvulsants, barbiturates, various antimicrobial agents, cardiovascular drugs, diuretics, substance abuse).

Photocutaneous porphyrias

- Characterised by variety of severe skin lesions.
- Porphyrin accumulation leads to photosensitisation and skin damage following exposure to sunlight.
- Presents with subepidermal bullae, pigmentation and hypertrichosis.
- Sporadic porphyria cutanea tarda (PCT): associated with chronic alcoholic liver disease, hepatitis C infection and Fe overload.
- High rates of hepatocellular carcinoma occur in PCT patients with chronic liver disease.

Treatment

Acute attacks

- Avoid drugs and other precipitating factors. Treat pain with opiates (not oxycodone).
- Aggressive management of fluid and electrolyte disturbances (glucose inhibits ALA synthetase activity).
- Intravenous haematin in severe attacks (haematin is a stable form of haem that inhibits ALA synthetase and subsequent ALA and porphobilinogen accumulation).
- Haematin can have a dramatic effect on neurologic symptoms.
- Liver transplantation is indicated for patients with protoporphyria.

Photocutaneous porphyrias

- Avoid ultraviolet exposure.
- Sunscreens and protective clothing.
- In PCT phlebotomy and chloroquine may be useful.

CYSTIC FIBROSIS (CF)

KEY POINTS

- Autosomal recessive disease of epithelial cell ion transport.
- The gene encodes for the cystic fibrosis transmembrane regulator (*CFTR*).
- Focal biliary cirrhosis is the pathognomonic lesion. Biliary tree abnormalities include gallstones, micro-gallbladder and mucocele. Sclerosing cholangitis and cholangiocarcinoma occur in higher frequency in cystic fibrosis patients.
- Liver biochemical tests may not correlate with severity of the disease.
- Treatment: ursodeoxycholic acid may hep to improve clinical status.

Cystic fibrosis (CF) is an autosomal recessive disease of epithelial cell ion transport. The gene involved is on the long arm of chromosome 7 and encodes for the cystic fibrosis transmembrane regulator (*CFTR*). In this discussion, the hepatic complications of CF will be reviewed.

Hepatobiliary characteristics

Focal biliary cirrhosis, a patchy distribution of cirrhotic transformation with inspissation of the small bile ducts, which occurs predominately in the portal tracts, is the pathognomonic lesion in CF-associated liver disease. Biliary tree abnormalities include gallstones, micro-gallbladder and mucocele.

Sclerosing cholangitis, and cholangiocarcinoma occur with higher frequency in patients with CF.

- Biochemistry: liver biochemical tests may remain relatively normal and do not correlate with the severity of the liver disease.
- Liver biopsy: sampling error may occur because of the focal distribution of the lesions.
- Imaging: ultrasonography may detect the presence of abnormalities.

- Gene testing: useful, although cirrhosis and portal hypertension affect only a very small proportion of the total CF population.

Treatment

Ursodeoxycholic acid has been shown to improve the biochemical indices of liver injury and may help to improve overall clinical status. Portal hypertension can be treated with portosystemic shunts.

GAUCHER'S DISEASE

KEY POINTS

- Gaucher's disease is an autosomal recessive condition resulting in a deficiency of glucocerebrosidase.
- This leads to an accumulation of sphingolipids in the reticuloendothelial system including the liver and spleen.
- There are 3 forms:
  - Type 1—hepatosplenomegaly
  - Type 2—hepatosplenomegaly plus neuropathic features and is often fatal by age 2 years
  - Type 3—hepatosplenomegaly and a later onset of neuropathic features.

POLYCYSTIC LIVER DISEASE

KEY POINTS

- Dominant inheritance.
- Characterised by presence of four or more liver cysts of biliary epithelial origin in individuals over 40 years of age.
- Often associated with autosomal dominant polycystic kidney disease.
- Diagnosis: imaging studies of the abdomen; ultrasonography, CT scan and MRI.
- Clinical: often asymptomatic. Symptoms may develop due to mass effect of the cyst or complications (intracystic haemorrhage, infection or cyst rupture).
- Treatment: fenestration of the cyst.

Polycystic liver disease (PCLD) is a dominantly inherited condition characterised by the presence of four or more liver cysts of biliary epithelial origin in individuals older than 40 years. PCLD can exist as a specific clinical entity separate from autosomal dominant polycystic kidney disease (ADPKD) and is termed autosomal dominant polycystic liver disease (ADPLD). However, it is common for PCLD to be associated with polycystic kidney disease with patients presenting initially with kidney cysts first followed by hepatic cysts. The prevalence of hepatic cysts in ADPKD is age-related, ranging from 0% at 20 years to 80% at 60 years. The mutant gene (*PRKCSH*) is usually located on chromosome 19 and encodes for a protein called hepatocystin.

Diagnosis

Diagnosis is made by imaging studies of the abdomen: ultrasonography, CT and MRI.

Clinical

Often asymptomatic. Symptoms develop during fourth or fifth decade due to mass effect of the cyst or complications such as intracystic haemorrhage, or infection and cyst rupture.

Treatment

Therapy of cysts is surgical with fenestration of the cysts the usual procedure.

GILBERT'S SYNDROME

Gilbert's syndrome is a common cause of unconjugated hyperbilirubinaemia that affects 3% to 8% of the population and is inherited in an autosomal recessive pattern. Average age at presentation is 18 years and it is rarely recognised before puberty. Splenomegaly and a mild haemolytic anaemia may be present.

Pathogenesis

There is a defect in the hepatic uptake of bilirubin by the hepatocyte and a partial defect in conjugation of bilirubin. There is a reduction in the enzyme bilirubin UDP-glucuronosyltransferase 1 (B-UGT), the enzyme responsible for formation of conjugated bilirubin in the hepatocyte. This is from a mutation in the gene encoding B-UGT (in the promoter region upstream to exon-1) that reduces production. Gilbert's syndrome arises in those homozygous for the variant promoter.

Wilson's disease	α_1-ATD	Hereditary haemochromatosis
Autosomal recessive ↓ ↑ Cu in liver, brain, cornea ↓ **Clinical** **Liver:** Cirrhosis, chronic hepatitis: hepatic failure **CNS:** K-F rings: parkinsonian features, intellectual disturbances **Miscellaneous:** Fanconi's syndrome Osteoporosis, anaemia ↓ **Diagnosis** ↓ Caeruloplasmin ↑ Free Cu ↑ Urinary Cu excretion ↑ Hepatic Cu concentration ↓ **Treatment** D-penicillamine, trientine, zinc tetrathiomolybdate Liver transplant	Autosomal recessive ↓ α_1-antitrypsin protects tissues against proteases ↓ **Clinical** **Liver:** Chronic hepatitis, cirrhosis and HCC ↓ **Diagnosis** ↓ Serum α_1-antitrypsin Defective α_1-ATZ alleles ↓ **Treatment** No specific therapy	Autosomal recessive ↓ Homozygous C282Y mutation of *HFE* gene Imbalance between Fe absorption and excretion Hepcidin important regulator ↓ **Clinical** • Symptomatic arthralgias • Arthralgias/arthritis • Chronic liver disease ↓ **Diagnosis** ↑ Transferrin saturation and ferritin imaging, MRI, ultrasonography ↓ **Treatment** Phlebotomy Avoid alcohol, high doses of ascorbic and citric acid

FIGURE 42.1: A background of liver disease in a family.

α_1-ATD = alpha$_1$-antitrypsin deficiency; α_1-ATZ = the defective α_1-antitrypsin molecule; AIP = acute intermittent porphyria; ALA = 5 aminolevulinic acid; B-UGT = bilirubin UDP-glucuronosyltransferase 1; CNS = central nervous system; Cu = copper; Fe = iron; HCC = hepatocellular carcinoma; HP = hepatic porphyrias; IV = intravenous; K-F = Kayser-Fleischer; MRI = magnetic resonance imaging; PCT = porphyria cutanea tarda; RES = reticuloendothelial system.

Hepatic prophyrias	Gilbert's syndrome	Polycystic liver disease
Autosomal dominant except for ALA dehydratase deficiency ↓ HP includes PCT, hereditary coproporphyria, AIP, variegate porphyria, ALA dehydratase deficiency ↓ **Clinical** Abdominal pain CNS symptoms Cutaneous lesions ↓ Precipitating factors Environmental and pharmacological agents ↓ **Treatment** Avoid precipitants Pain—opiates Correct fluid and electrolytes Glucose IV haem Liver transplant for protoporphyria	Autosomal recessive ↓ Common cause of unconjugated hyperbilirubinaemia ↓ Deficiency of enzyme D-UGT ↓ **Clinical** Mostly asymptomatic Jaundice evoked by stress, fatigue, illness ↓ **Treatment** Benign. No treatment necessary	Autosomal dominant ↓ **Clinical** Often associated with polycystic kidneys Often asymptomatic ↓ **Treatment** Fenestration of cyst
	Cystic fibrosis	**Gaucher's disease**
	Autosomal recessive ↓ **Clinical** Focal biliary cirrhosis pathognomonic lesion ↓ **Treatment** Ursodeoxycholic acid may improve condition	Autosomal recessive ↓ **Clinical** Accumulation of sphingolipids in RES Three types: • Hepatosplenomegaly • Hepatosplenomegaly plus CNS signs • Hepatosplenomegaly and later onset of CNS signs

Clinical characteristics

Most patients are asymptomatic and jaundice develops with intercurrent illness, fasting, stress, fatigue, ethanol, nicotinic acid intake and premenstrually.

Diagnosis

Rise in bilirubin with fasting is a good diagnostic test. Total bilirubin levels are usually less than 3 mg/mL and may rise to 5–6 mg/mL during illness or stress.

Gilbert's syndrome is a benign condition and no therapy is required.

FURTHER READING

Ferenci P. Wilson's disease. Clin Gastroenterol Hepatol 2005; 3:726–33.

Lazaridis KN, Petersen GM. Genomics, genetic epidemiology and genomic medicine. Clin Gastroentrol Hepatol 2005; 3:320–8.

Stoller JK, Aboussouan LS. α1-antitrypsin deficiency. Lancet 2005; 365:2225–36.

Zoller H, Cox T. Haemochromatosis: genetic testing and clinical practice. Clin Gastroenterol Hepatol 2005; 3:945–58.

Chapter 43

GRANULOMATOUS LIVER DISEASE

KEY POINTS

- The hallmark of granulomatous liver inflammation is the epithelioid granuloma.
- The aetiology is multifactorial. infections (e.g. tuberculosis), sarcoidosis, primary biliary cirrhosis, drugs, Crohn's disease and neoplasms.
- The cause is unknown in approximately 50% of cases.
- Work-up for hepatic granulomas includes a detailed history (including drugs), biochemical and serologic testing (alkaline phosphatase, angiotensin converting enzyme and antimitochondrial antibodies are particularly important) and microbiological evaluation.

INTRODUCTION

Often granulomas are found on liver biopsy and the clinical case needs to be reviewed to try and find the cause. The causes of granulomas are multifactorial and include tuberculosis, sarcoidosis, primary biliary cirrhosis, various drugs, neoplasms (e.g. Hodgkin's lymphoma) and Crohn's disease. The cause is unknown in approximately 50% of cases.

PRESENTATION AND CLINICAL EXAMINATION

Typical presentations include pyrexia of unknown origin or incidental abnormal liver function tests. Often the clinical examination is normal, though there may be symptoms and signs of an associated systemic disease (Figure 43.1). Infrequently, hepatomegaly, splenomegaly or lymphadenopathy may be detected.

Biochemical liver tests

Generally, liver function testing is non-specific, but a predominant alkaline phosphatase (ALP) elevation may be present.

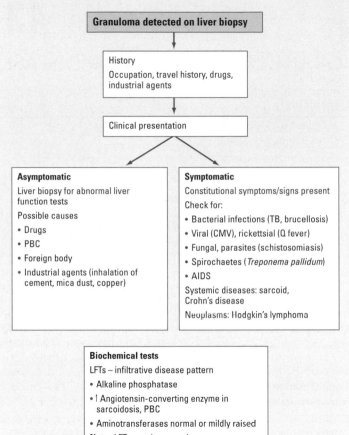

FIGURE 43.1: Diagnosis of granulomas.

AIDS = aquired immunodeficiency syndrome; CMV = cytomegalovirus; LFTs = liver function tests; TB = tuberculosis; PBC = primary biliary cirrhosis.

Histopathology

Hepatic granulomas are found in 0.8%–15% of liver biopsies. The epithelioid granuloma may be associated with distinguishing morphological pathological features. These can include duct involvement (primary biliary cirrhosis), periductal location with acute inflammatory changes (large duct obstruction with cholangitis), parenchymal and perivenular location (tuberculosis), caseation (tuberculosis), fibrin-ring pattern with central fat vacuole (Q fever), schistosome ova (schistosomiasis) or a positive fungal stain.

Lipogranulomas should be differentiated from epithelioid granulomas. Lipogranulomas are found in non-steatotic livers as a response to ubiquitous exogenous mineral oils used in food preparation.

CAUSES OF GRANULOMAS

The most common causes of hepatic granulomas where primary biliary cirrhosis has been excluded are sarcoidosis, chronic liver disease, biliary tract disease, tuberculosis, Q fever, other infections, drug hepatotoxicity, neoplasms and idiopathic (Table 43.1).

Sarcoidosis

Between 50%–90% of patients with sarcoidosis have hepatic involvement with granulomas. The frequency of granulomas is greatest in lymph nodes followed by lung and liver. There is no evidence of liver dysfunction in the majority of cases. Portal hypertension is rare but may occur without cirrhosis. The granulomas may recur following liver transplantation.

Primary biliary cirrhosis

Primary biliary cirrhosis (PBC) is a slowly progressive form of autoimmune liver disease that predominantly affects middle-aged women.

Epidemiological, clinical and biochemical features
- Female to male ratio is 9:1
- Peak incidence in fifth decade of life
- High serum alkaline phosphatase levels should raise suspicion
- Patients may be asymptomatic in the early phase of the disease
- Fatigue and pruritus may become troublesome
- Once symptoms develop, patients have a limited life expectancy with a median survival time around 10 years
- High serum bilirubin, low serum albumin and prolonged prothrombin time are all associated with a poor prognosis

TABLE 43.1: Causes of granulomas

Associated with pyrexia of unknown origin	Sarcoidosis, tuberculosis (miliary and pulmonary, caseation important), atypical mycobacterium, Q fever, brucellosis, cat-scratch disease, mycoses, drugs, idiopathic granulomatous hepatitis
Human immunodeficiency virus (HIV)	*Mycobacterium avium* complex, idiopathic, other mycobacteria, *Mycobacterium tuberculosis*, *Cryptococcus*, *Histoplasma*, medications (trimethoprim-sulfamethoxazole)
Infectious diseases	Bacteria: actinomycosis, brucellosis, cat-scratch disease, listeriosis, syphilis, tularaemia, Whipple's disease Mycobacteria: tuberculosis, leprosy (lepromatous and tuberculoid) Rickettsia: Q fever Chlamydia: lymphopathia venereum, psittacosis Fungi: aspergillosis, blastomycosis, candidiasis, cryptococcosis, histoplasmosis Viruses: cytomegalovirus, Epstein-Barr virus, infectious mononucleosis Parasites: amoebiasis, capillariasis, fascioliasis, schistosomiasis, toxoplasmosis, visceral leishmaniasis (kala-azar)
Hypersensitivity and immunological diseases	Metals: beryllium, copper, gold Hypogammaglobulinaemia, primary biliary cirrhosis, primary sclerosing cholangitis, systemic lupus erythematosus Vascular diseases: disseminated visceral giant cell arteritis, polyarteritis nodosa, temporal arthritis, Wegener's granulomatosis
Foreign materials	Anthracotic pigments, barium, cement and mica dust; mineral oil—radiocontrast media, food additives; silica, suture material, talc
Neoplasms	Hodgkin's disease, non-Hodgkin's lymphoma
Miscellaneous diseases	Biliary tract obstruction, bile granulomas, chronic inflammatory bowel disease, eosinophilic gastroenteritis, jejunoileal bypass, porphyria cutanea tarda, sarcoidosis, idiopathic
Drugs	Allopurinol, amiodarone, amoxicillin/clavulanic acid, chlorpromazine, chlorpropamide, diltiazem, gold salts, halothane, hydralazine, methyldopa, benzylpenicillin, phenoxymethylpenicillin, phenylbutazone, phenytoin, procainamide, quinidine, quinine, sulfonamides

- There is a strong association with other autoimmune diseases including Sjögren's syndrome, scleroderma, CREST syndrome, autoimmune thyroiditis
- Patients may have associated histological feature of autoimmune hepatitis and, in these situations, the term 'overlap syndrome' is used

Investigations
- The presence of anti-mitochondrial antibodies in the serum is characteristic
- A liver biopsy is vital for both diagnostic and prognostic purposes
- Histologically is characterised by inflammatory destruction of the interlobular and septal bile ducts, which leads to chronic cholestasis and biliary cirrhosis Ultimately non-caseating granulomas will develop

Management issues
- Ursodeoxycholic acid (UDCA) is the only proven medical therapy
- May require medical attention for the associated complications of pruritus, osteoporosis, fat-soluble vitamin deficiency, hypercholesterolaemia and steatorrhoea
- There is a substantial increased risk of hepatocellular carcinoma
- Patients may require liver transplantation for end-stage liver disease
- Overlap syndrome patients will require a combination of UDCA and corticosteroid therapy

Idiopathic granulomatous hepatitis
This group accounts for 5%–10% of hepatic granulomas.

Presentation
- Prolonged or recurrent fever
- Weight loss
- Myalgia and arthralgia
- Vague abdominal pain
There is seldom hepatocellular damage. It is usually a diagnosis of exclusion.

TREATMENT

Identified or suspected drugs or toxins should be withdrawn and the patient monitored. Specific infective diseases should be treated with appropriate antibiotics, antifungals or other specific drugs.

Patients diagnosed with idiopathic granulomatous hepatitis can be treated with corticosteroids starting with prednisolone 40 mg daily and steroids should be weaned over 2–4 weeks depending on the observed response. Most patients can be treated with a defined course of steroids and retreated as necessary if symptomatic relapse occurs. Treatment should be dictated by symptoms rather than biochemical response or relapse.

Patients refractory to steroid therapy can be treated with other immunosuppressive therapy, such as methotrexate at a dose of 0.20 mg/kg/week, and steroids gradually withdrawn. Methotrexate should be discontinued over a 12–18-month period.

SUMMARY

Hepatic granulomas are found in 0.8%–15% of liver biopsies. The causes of granulomas are multifactorial and include tuberculosis, sarcoidosis, primary biliary cirrhosis, various drugs, neoplasms (e.g. lymphoma) and Crohn's disease. The cause is unknown in approximately 50% of cases. A detailed history is essential in establishing the cause. The hallmark of granulomatous inflammation is the epithelioid granuloma. The clinical manifestations, treatment and prognosis are those of the underlying disease.

FURTHER READING

Kaplan MM, Gershwin ME. Primary biliary cirrhosis. N Engl J Med 2005; 353:1261–73.

Knox TA, Kaplan MM, Golfand JA, et al. Methotrexate treatment of idiopathic granulomatous hepatitis. Ann Int Med 1995; 122:592–5.

Lefkowitch JH. Hepatic granulomas. J Hepatol 1999; 30:40–5.

Matheus T, Muñoz S. Granulomatous liver disease and cholestasis. Clin Liver Dis 2004; 8:229–46.

Sandor M, Weinstock JV, Wynn TA. Granulomas in schistosome and mycobacterial infections: a model of local immune responses. Trends Immunol 2003; 24:44–52.

Chapter **44**

MASS IN THE LIVER

KEY POINTS

- Widespread use of modern imaging modalities has resulted in frequent identification of incidental focal liver masses/nodules.
- Advances in imaging techniques now allow most masses to be diagnosed without the need for surgical resection.
- Imaging techniques useful for differential diagnosis include ultrasound (with or without colour Doppler), triphasic contrast-enhanced computed tomography (CT), CT angiography (with or without iodised oil), gadolinium-enhanced magnetic resonance imaging (MRI), and imaging-guided biopsy.
- Incidentally found liver masses usually represent benign pathology and many, particularly simple cysts and typical haemangiomas, can be successfully diagnosed with ultrasound alone.
- Liver masses in the cirrhotic patient have a high risk of being hepatocellular carcinoma and require thorough investigation.
- A multidisciplinary approach is recommended for difficult cases and for malignant masses.

APPROACHES TO THE LIVER MASS

The diagnostic approach to a mass in the liver differs according to the medical history of the patient. Patients can be separated into three groups:
- Previously well with a mass found incidentally on abdominal imaging
- A background of chronic liver disease or known cirrhosis
- A history of extrahepatic malignancy or symptoms suggestive of malignancy.

Incidental liver mass in the well patient

With the widespread use of ultrasound for the investigation of a wide range of abdominal symptoms, focal liver masses are frequently identified. Most of these represent benign pathology, and further imaging is only required if there is doubt as to the nature of the mass on the initial study. Patients with a simple cyst can be reassured and no further investigation is needed. A recent study has shown that if a focal mass has the typical appearance of a haemangioma on ultrasound the risk of missing a malignant lesion is less than 0.5%, so further imaging is not required. Other focal lesions usually require further investigation, depending on the initial form of imaging employed.

The patient with chronic liver disease or known cirrhosis

The risk of hepatocellular carcinoma (HCC) is greatly increased in the cirrhotic patient with lesions >3 cm diameter, having a >95% risk of being a HCC. All focal liver lesions in patients with significant chronic liver disease should be considered a HCC until proven otherwise and further investigation is always warranted.

The patient with extrahepatic malignancy or symptoms suggestive of malignancy

The liver is a common site for metastatic disease; the most common primary sites are within the gastrointestinal tract, lung, urogenital tract, breast followed by non-Hodgkin's lymphoma. The finding of multiple lesions of differing sizes that involve both lobes of the liver is a typical presentation of hepatic metastases. Solitary liver lesions, unless clearly benign, require further imaging or image-guided biopsy.

BENIGN LIVER MASSES

Cavernous haemangioma

Cavernous haemangiomas are the most common benign hepatic tumour, occur in 5% of the population and are female predominant. On ultrasound they are well circumscribed, uniform, hyperechoic lesions without a peripheral halo. When found incidentally in the otherwise well patient, classical ultrasound features are usually sufficient to establish the diagnosis and further investigation or treatment is unnecessary. Atypical haemangiomas can present a diagnostic challenge but triphasic computed tomography (CT) or, preferably, gadolinium-enhanced magnetic resonance imaging (MRI) will confirm the diagnosis in the majority of cases and have largely replaced ^{99m}Tc-labelled red blood cell studies (Table 44.1).

Focal nodular hyperplasia

Focal nodular hyperplasia (FNH) is a well circumscribed mass that typically displays a central stellate scar, a feature that is best seen with triphasic CT or gadolinium-enhanced MRI (Table 44.1). FNH is female predominant, usually asymptomatic and does not progress to malignancy. Ultrasound displays an isoechoic or hypoechoic lesion and colour Doppler may display vessels radiating outward from the artery within the central scar. Most lesions are less than 5 cm diameter and solitary. Occasionally differentiation from fibrolamellar HCC may be difficult.

Adenoma

Hepatic adenoma is an uncommon female-predominant benign liver mass with the potential for haemorrhage, rupture or malignant transformation. It is more common in women exposed to oral contraceptive steroids and men who have used anabolic steroids. Ultrasound appearance is variable, but adenomas are mostly isoechoic or hypoechoic with variable echodensity within the lesion. At triphasic CT adenomas are typically low density on pre-contrast images with rapid enhancement during the arterial phase, though differentiation from FNH and occasionally HCC is difficult (Table 44.1). Fat or blood products may be seen within the lesion on MRI. Surgical resection is recommended due to the significant complication rate associated with adenomas and the risk of misdiagnosis of HCC.

Simple cysts

Simple cysts occur in 2.5% of the population, are often multiple and appear on ultrasound as round or oval anechoic lesions with smooth, thin or imperceptible walls, showing posterior enhancement and no internal structure (Table 44.1). Usually no further investigation is required and the patient can be reassured as to the benign nature of the lesion.

Complex cysts

In contrast to simple cysts, complex cysts display internal echoes, irregular thick walls, thick septations more than 3 mm or mural nodularity on ultrasound. Differential diagnosis includes pyogenic abscess, hydatid disease and, rarely, neoplasms such as biliary cystadenoma and hepatic metastases. Further investigation is warranted, with the direction guided by associated clinical features.

TABLE 44.1: Relative utility of imaging modalities in providing a diagnosis of a hepatic mass

	Ultrasound ± colour Doppler	Triphasic CT	Gadolinium-enhanced MRI	CT angio ± iodised oil	99mTc-RBC SPECT	FDG PET
Simple cyst	++++	+++	+++	−	−	−
Haemangioma	+++	+++	++++	+++	+++	−
Focal nodular hyperplasia	+	+++	+++	++	−	−
Adenoma	++	+++	+++	+++	−	−
Hepatocellular carcinoma	++[1]	++++	++++	++++	−	+
Metastasis	+++[1]	++++	++++	+++	−	++++

[1]Frequently employed as a screening investigation in high-risk populations.

Angio = angiography; CT = computed tomography; FDG PET = fluorodeoxyglucose positron emission tomography; MRI = magnetic resonance imaging; RBC = red blood cell; SPECT = single photon emission computed tomography.

MALIGNANT LIVER MASSES

Hepatocellular carcinoma

Hepatocellular carcinoma (HCC) is the most common primary malignant tumour of the liver, exhibits male-predominance and usually occurs on a background of chronic liver disease. Either triphasic CT or gadolinium enhanced MRI are the investigations of choice (Table 44.1), depending on availability and institutional preference; with the typical lesion demonstrating arterial enhancement followed by rapid contrast washout in the portal venous and later phases. MRI has the advantage of better differentiating between regenerative nodules, dysplastic nodules and HCC. Other imaging modalities, such as CT angiography with iodised oil, are reserved for equivocal lesions, and may assist in differentiation from regenerative or dysplastic nodules. A raised serum alpha-fetoprotein is present in 50% of patients and aids diagnosis if present. Fine needle aspiration of suspected HCC is to be avoided due to the risk of tumour seeding if there is potential for curative surgical resection or hepatic transplantation.

Fibrolamellar hepatocellular carcinoma

Fibrolamellar HCC is a rare tumour that arises in non-cirrhotic liver in young patients and is slower growing than typical HCC. As the name suggests, there is often extensive fibrous tissue within the tumour and a central scar, giving a heterogenous appearance on imaging. Triphasic CT usually demonstrates a well circumscribed, lobular heterogenous mass that is hypervascular in the arterial phase. Differentiation from FNH or adenoma may be difficult, though FNH lesions are rarely >5 cm diameter, while fibrolamellar HCC are often larger at the time of first detection and have a more heterogeneous appearance. Surgical resection or liver transplantation is usually undertaken, though local recurrence rates with the former are high.

Cholangiocarcinoma

Cholangiocarcinoma is an uncommon tumour arising from the biliary tract often on a background of biliary disease, particularly sclerosing cholangitis. Masses may be peripheral or hilar and the diagnosis is suggested by the combination of a mass or biliary stricture with distal biliary obstruction. Diagnosis is often difficult and a combination of solid organ imaging, cholangiography and cytology is usually required. The tumour marker CA19.9 may be elevated but false positives are common, particularly if cholangitis is present.

Metastases to the liver

After the lymphatic system, the liver is the most common site for metastatic cancer. Hepatic metastases are often first detected on ultrasound as multiple nodules of differing sizes with a hypoechoic halo usually involving both lobes of the liver. Solitary lesions are observed in 10% of cases. Large tumours may outgrow their blood supply leading to central necrosis. As hepatic metastases may be derived from a wide range of primary cancers, their appearance on imaging is quite variable. Most lesions are hypovascular and are most obvious as areas of reduced attenuation during the portal venous phase of a triphasic CT (Table 44.1), sometimes exhibiting peripheral ring-like enhancement. Hypervascular metastases are less common and include renal cell carcinoma, carcinoid, islet cell carcinoma, thyroid carcinoma, melanoma, neuroendocrine tumours and some breast carcinomas. Additional evaluation by way of MRI (Table 44.1) or (^{18}F) fluorodeoxyglucose positron emission tomography (FDG PET) may be undertaken if surgical resection or percutaneous ablation is being considered. Management is influenced by the nature of the primary cancer, if known, with colorectal metastasis being resected if feasible. For unresectable lesions, imaging-guided fine needle aspiration cytology confirms the diagnosis and may help guide cytotoxic therapy.

THE DIAGNOSTIC DILEMMA

Some liver masses prove difficult to diagnose, even when multiple imaging modalities are employed and the results interpreted by a specialist experienced in hepatic investigation. This is particularly true of small (<1 cm) lesions. In these situations, the following may be helpful.

- Has the patient had abdominal imaging in the past? If studies from several years back show a similar mass then the lesion is benign.
- Repeat imaging in 4–6 months. If there has been no change in appearance, benign pathology is likely, though further follow-up imaging may be required.
- Undertake fine needle aspiration cytology, unless the lesion is highly vascular or a potentially resectable HCC or metastasis is likely.
- Undertake surgical resection.

Some liver masses may represent non-neoplastic processes, such as focal fatty infiltration in the liver, focal fat sparing in a fatty liver or haematoma. MRI can characterise blood products and focal areas of fat or fatty sparing within and out of phase imaging.

The differential diagnosis and management of a subset of liver masses can be difficult and is best addressed by a multidisciplinary approach. A team typically consists of:

- Gastroenterologist or hepatologist
- Upper gastrointestinal surgeon
- Oncologist
- Radiologist and/or interventional radiologist.

Decision making not only includes reaching a diagnosis, but selecting patients with malignant disease who are candidates for liver transplantation or surgical resection as well as for less invasive procedures, including percutaneous radiofrequency ablation (RFA), ethanol injection, cryogenic ablation, transarterial chemoembolisation (TACE) or ^{90}Y microsphere embolisation.

FURTHER READING

American College of Radiology. ACR appropriateness criteria: liver lesion characterisation, and suspected liver metastases. Online. Available: http://www.acr.org/SecondaryMainMenuCategories/quality_safety/ app_criteria/pdf/ExpertPanelonGastrointestinalImaging/LiverLesion CharacterizationDoc9.aspx

Choi BY, Nguyen MH. The diagnosis and management of benign hepatic tumors. J Clin Gastroenterol 2005; 39:401–12.

Kinkel K, Lu Y, Both M, et al. Detection of hepatic metastases from cancers of the gastrointestinal tract by using noninvasive imaging methods (US, CT, MR imaging, PET): a meta-analysis. Radiology 2002; 224:748–56.

Leifer DM, Middleton WD, Teefey SA, et al. Follow-up of patients at low risk for hepatic malignancy with a characteristic hemangioma at US. Radiology 2000; 214:167–72.

Li D, Hann LE. A practical approach to analyzing focal lesions in the liver. Ultrasound Q 2005; 21:187–200.

Mortele KJ, Praet M, Van Vlierberghe H, et al. CT and MR imaging findings in focal nodular hyperplasia of the liver: radiologic-pathologic correlation. Am J Roentgenol 2000; 175:687–92.

Szklaruk J, Silverman PM, Charnsangavej C. Imaging in the diagnosis, staging, treatment, and surveillance of hepatocellular carcinoma. Am J Roentgenol 2003; 180:441–54.

Taylor M, Forster J, Langer B, et al. A study of prognostic factors for hepatic resection for colorectal metastases. Am J Surg 1997; 173:467–71.

Chapter 45

NUTRITION IN PATIENTS WITH LIVER DISEASE

KEY POINTS

- Malnutrition is prevalent among patients with liver disease.
- Malnutrition is associated with higher risk of developing complications of cirrhosis.
- Malnutrition prior to transplant increases the risk of post-transplant complications such as infections and intensive care stay.
- The aetiologies of malnutrition in cirrhosis include low intake, malabsorption, medication effects, protein and salt dietary restriction, inattention to dietary intake in the hospital and possible increased requirements.
- Encourage increased oral intake, preferably in small frequent meals.
- Encephalopathy should be managed with medication while reserving protein restriction for difficult to control cases.
- Enteral feeding is feasible and as effective as parenteral nutrition (PN) in the immediate post-transplant period.
- Central obesity and insulin resistance are risk factors for the development of non-alcoholic steatohepatitis (NASH).
- Weight loss and increased physical activity improve insulin resistance and may be helpful in NASH.
- Antioxidants such as vitamin E may be helpful in NASH.
- NASH and progression to hepatic fibrosis are major complications of prolonged parenteral nutrition (PN) dependence in patients with short bowel syndrome.
- Recommendations to decrease parenteral nutrition-associated liver disease (PNALD) include avoiding overfeeding, cycling PN (12–16 hours rather than continuous) and limiting intravenous lipids to less than 1 g/kg/day.
- PNALD remains a serious complication of prolonged PN and is one of the indications for small bowel transplant in intestinal failure.

NUTRITIONAL ASSESSMENT IN CIRRHOSIS

Many of the commonly used parameters to assess nutrition are not as useful in advanced liver disease. Weight is complicated by ascites and oedema, which will mask the extent of lean and adipose tissue loss. Albumin and prealbumin levels may reflect decreased hepatic synthesis rather than malnutrition. Several techniques may be more useful in cirrhosis. Subjective global assessment (SGA) involves the assessment of several factors including weight loss during the previous 6 months, dietary intake, the presence of gastrointestinal symptoms and physical ailments that may limit intake and physical signs of malnutrition such as muscle wasting and peripheral oedema. This technique has been validated as a reliable technique for the assessment of nutritional status in cirrhosis and a useful predictor of outcome after liver transplant. Bioelectrical impedance (BIE) is a predictor of body cell mass and its validity has been confirmed in cirrhosis with and without ascites. Handgrip strength is a sensitive measurement of malnutrition and, compared with other measures (SGA and the prognostic nutritional index), is associated with the development of complications such as ascites, hepatic encephalopathy, hepatorenal syndrome and spontaneous bacterial peritonitis whereas SGA and prognostic nutritional index are not. Decreased handgrip strength prior to transplant is also associated with longer stay in the intensive care unit and more infection post transplant.

Protein–energy malnutrition

Protein–energy malnutrition (PEM) is a common problem in liver disease patients with significant loss of body cell mass and total body fat reported in all stages of liver diseases. Its prevalence increases with progression of liver disease with reported rates of 20% in patients with Child-Pugh A and 50%–60% in Child-Pugh C. The reported rate among patients awaiting liver transplant ranges between 18% and 100%. Although active alcoholism is a major risk factor for malnutrition, the prevalence may not be different among alcoholic and non-alcoholic aetiologies of liver cirrhosis.

Multiple factors may be involved in the development of PEM in advanced liver disease (Figure 45.1). Inadequate dietary intake has been described in up to 87% of patients. This may be caused by anorexia and dysgeusia, which may be related to zinc and vitamin A deficiencies. Commonly prescribed salt and protein dietary restrictions may also affect appetite. In addition, patients with large ascites may experience early satiety and abdominal pain, limiting food intake, and generalised weakness and encephalopathy may limit physical access to adequate intake. In the hospital, deficient intake is commonly iatrogenic. Malabsorption may be another factor contributing to PEM. Steatorrhoea has been reported in both cholestatic and non-cholestatic liver disease and may be caused by decreased intestinal bile salt pool, pancreatic insufficiency and bacterial overgrowth associated with impaired intestinal motility. The use of lactulose and neomycin in encephalopathy may exacerbate malabsorption. It has been suggested that increased nutritional requirement may exacerbate malnutrition in cirrhosis. However, studies comparing measured energy expenditure using indirect calorimetry and that calculated by Harris Benedict equations (Table 45.1) suggest the presence of large variability among patients with cirrhosis, with both hypermetabolism and hypometabolism equally observed in about one-third of patients (more than 20% discrepancy). Of significance, patients with increased energy expenditure experienced increased rates of morbidity and mortality. The mechanism of hypermetabolism in some cirrhotic patients may be related to infection, ascites and portal hypertension. Both the removal of ascites and the reduction of portal hypertension by transjugular intrahepatic portosystemic shunt (TIPS) have been associated with reduction of energy expenditure.

Malnutrition in cirrhotic patients is associated with increased risk of complications including variceal bleeding, ascites, encephalopathy and infections. Malnutrition was also found to be an independent predictor of mortality in cirrhosis. In addition, some studies indicate that malnutrition prior to transplant is associated with increased risk of post-transplant infections, variceal bleeding, prolonged hospital stay and longer ventilatory support time.

TABLE 45.1: Harris Benedict equations

Basal energy expenditure for women = $665 + (9.6 \times W) + (1.8 \times H) + (4.7 \times A)$
Basal energy expenditure for men = $66 + (13.7 \times W) + (5 \times H) + (6.8 \times A)$

W = weight in kg; H = height in cm; A = age in years.

Energy and protein requirements

Harris Benedict equations (Table 45.1) can be utilised to estimate basal energy expenditure (BEE) and most cirrhotic patients require 120% of the BEE. It is recommended that the ideal rather than the actual body weight be used in the calculations to avoid overfeeding. In general, most patients require 25–35 kcal/kg/day. Indirect calorimetry may be helpful in determining energy requirements of patients with possible hypermetabolism failing to respond to regular nutritional recommendations. This involves measurement of oxygen consumption and CO_2 output at the mouth using metabolic cart. Another simpler estimate of energy expenditure is based on O_2 consumption as follows:

Energy expenditure = O_2 consumption (mL/min) × 7.

Most cirrhotic patients tolerate 1–1.2 g/kg protein intake. In the presence of portosystemic encephalopathy, pharmacological therapy should be aggressively attempted prior to resorting to dietary protein restriction.

Fuel consumption

Cirrhotic patients develop hyperinsulinaemia and glucose intolerance and up to one-third develop diabetes mellitus. Fuel consumption in cirrhosis reflects a pattern that is similar to that observed in starvation. Measurements of respiratory quotient (rate of CO_2 production/O_2 consumption) during fasting in cirrhotic patients demonstrate accelerated shift to fat oxidation, possibly reflecting a decrease in glycogen reserves, compared with normal subjects. Essential fatty acid deficiencies and low serum concentration of fatty acids are common. Therefore, feeding should not be withheld for extended periods of time. It is generally recommended that cirrhotic patients consume 4–5 meals a day including a late evening snack. The latter was shown to improve nitrogen balance in cirrhotic patients.

TREATMENT

Can nutrition intervention improve nutritional status in patients with advanced liver disease and improve clinical outcome? In patients with alcoholic cirrhosis, oral nutrition supplement providing 1000 calories and 34 grams of protein improved nutritional parameters including mid-arm circumference,

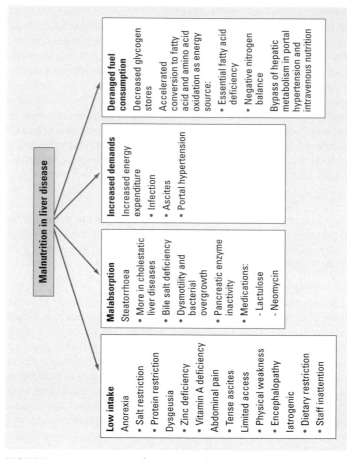

FIGURE 45.1: Factors contributing to malnutrition in liver disease.

albumin level and handgrip strength along with fewer episodes of hospitalisations. Both late-evening meals and nocturnal feeding have been shown to improve nitrogen balance. However, oral nutritional supplement may not increase total energy and protein intake, probably reflecting compensatory decrease in voluntary food intake. Aggressive nutritional support with enteral tube feeding was associated with faster clinical improvement, decreased bilirubin and hepatic encephalopathy and decreased in-hospital mortality in patients with alcoholic liver disease. Early enteral feeding has been successfully attempted post transplant and was associated with improved nitrogen balance and decreased viral infections and is as effective as total parenteral nutrition in maintaining nutritional status post transplant with lower cost and complications.

Branched-chain amino acids

Decreased branched-chain amino acid (BCAA) levels and increased ratio of aromatic amino acid (AAA) to BCAA may be involved in the development of encephalopathy probably via increased passage of AAA across the blood–brain barrier promoting the development of false neurotransmitters. A recent review of 11 randomised trials concluded that BCAA supplements are associated with improved encephalopathy, particularly when provided enterally compared with the intravenous route. However, most of these studies were small and of short-term duration. Specialised BCAA-rich tube feeding formulas are generally not recommended for management of encephalopathy, except in cases where encephalopathy is not easily controlled and patients cannot tolerate the recommended protein intake without developing encephalopathy.

There is growing evidence of beneficial effects of BCAA supplementation on malnutrition in cirrhosis. In two multicentre randomised studies, 12 g oral BCAAs for 1 and 2 years was associated with improved nutritional parameters and decreased rate of mortality, advance to liver failure and hospital admissions compared with lactalbumin or maltodextrin control. However, there was a low compliance rate, probably related to the poor palatability of oral BCAAs. Four grams of BCAA at breakfast and 8 g at bedtime resulted in improved albumin compared with 4 g BCAA three times during daytime.

Non-alcoholic fatty liver disease

Non-alcoholic fatty liver disease (NAFLD) represents a spectrum of liver diseases, characterised mainly by macrovesicular steatosis in the absence of significant alcohol ingestion. It is now known to lead to progressive fibrosis and cirrhosis. Major risk factors include overweight (specifically central obesity), sedentary lifestyles and insulin resistance. Lipid peroxidation and high levels of reactive oxygen substrates are thought to be key mediators in the progression from simple steatosis to NASH providing the rationale for using antioxidants such as vitamin E in non-alcoholic steatohepatitis (NASH). Diets low in processed carbohydrates and saturated fats with a goal to achieve a 500–1000 cal/day deficit improve insulin sensitivity, reduce serum aminotransferases and decrease hepatic steatosis. As an antioxidant and inhibitor of fibrosing cytokine and transforming growth factor, vitamin E has been tested in several clinical trials. Some trials showed improvement in transaminases with vitamin E supplement of 400–1200 IU/day, particularly among children. Current recommendations limit vitamin E supplement to no more that 400 IU/day, as recent studies suggest a possible increase in the rate of all-cause mortality and cardiac complications with vitamin E supplements >400 IU/day.

Parenteral nutrition-associated liver disease

The risk of developing parenteral nutrition-associated liver disease (PNALD) increases with longer parenteral nutrition (PN) dependence. Steatosis and progression to steatohepatitis with fibrosis is the predominant histological picture observed in adults and older children, while cholestasis is more predominant in infants. Abnormal liver tests are observed in 55%, 64% and 72% of patients and cirrhosis with complications is observed in 26%, 39% and 50% after 2, 4 and 6 years of PN dependence, respectively. PNALD is more predominant in infants with reported prevalence up to 85% after 6 weeks of PN dependence. In addition, the risk of PNALD is higher among patients with shorter remnant intestine, those with diseased remnant intestine and those totally dependent on PN with no enteral intake. Several mechanisms have been postulated for the pathogenesis of PNALD, including essential fatty acid and carnitine deficiency, although the former is unlikely unless lipids are totally omitted from PN. In addition, carnitine supplementation has not been associated with improvement in PNALD. Intravenous nutrition bypasses the liver where most of transsulfuration of amino acids occurs. In support of this, taurine and choline deficiencies have been observed in PN dependence, and taurine supplementation in infants reduced the rate of PNALD, although their roles in adults are not clear. Overfeeding results in higher insulin:glucagon ratio, promotes free fatty acid mobilisation and the development of steatosis. Increased oxidative stress and lipid peroxidation may be involved. Lack of enteral nutrition has been associated with intestinal mucosal atrophy, which may be associated with bacterial translocation and the induction of systemic inflammation. In addition, higher risk of PNALD has been reported in association with higher rate of lipid perfusion above 1 g/kg/day. Therefore, recommendations to decrease the risk of PNALD include encouraging enteral nutrition as much as clinically possible, avoiding overfeeding, limiting lipid infusion to less than 1 g/kg/day and cycling of PN (over 12–16 hours versus continuous). However, PNALD remains one of the more serious complications of PN in patients with short bowel syndrome and is a major indication for small bowel transplant in these patients.

Liver transplant

As previously described, malnutrition prior to transplant is a risk factor for increased post-transplant complications. However, randomised studies of the effects of nutritional support on transplant outcome are lacking. In a prospective study enteral nutrition supplement providing 750 cal and 20 g protein to transplant candidates with less than the 25th percentile of mid-arm circumference had no impact on outcome although there was a tendency towards decreased mortality. In a pilot study, 15 liver transplant candidates given an immunomodulatory enteral formula orally had a lower rate of infection (33% versus 71%, respectively) and improved total body protein, compared with standard nutrition. In post-transplant patients, energy requirements are about 20% above resting energy expenditure. Protein catabolism with nitrogen loss is observed in the immediate post-transplant period when protein intake should be 1.5–2 g/day. Water and electrolyte imbalances are also common in the post-transplant patients and may be exacerbated by gastric and biliary drainage. In addition, cyclosporin and tacrolimus increase magnesium loss. In the first few days after transplant, oral intake may be limited by ileus. Therefore, PN is utilised in many centres. PN was shown to improve nitrogen balance and shorten intensive care unit stay. BCAA-enriched solution was not superior to the standard solution. Significantly, enteral nutrition using intraoperative jejunostomy tube or nasojejunal tube has been used successfully post transplant. In a prospective study of 50 liver transplantation patients, enteral nutrition resulted in greater calorie and protein intakes, better nitrogen balance, quicker recovery in grip strength and fewer infections compared with control patients.

SUMMARY

Malnutrition plays a significant role in liver disease. Protein–calorie malnutrition is prevalent in cirrhosis, is commonly iatrogenic and is associated with increased complications. On the other hand, central obesity and insulin resistance are risk factors for NASH, increasingly the aetiology for cirrhosis and liver transplant. In addition, parenteral-nutrition dependence is associated with progressive liver disease and is one of the indications for small intestine transplant in short bowel syndrome. Attention to nutrition management may help improve outcomes in liver disease.

FURTHER READING

Buchman AL, Lyer K, Fryer J. Parenteral nutrition-associated liver disease and the role for isolated intestine and intestine/liver transplantation. Hepatology 2006; 43:9–19.

Cabre E, Gassull MA. Nutrition in liver disease. Curr Opin Clin Nutr Metab Care 2005; 8:545–51.

Campos AC, Matias JE, Coelho JC. Nutritional aspects of liver transplantation. Curr Opin Clin Nutr Metab Care 2002; 5:297–307.

Chang CY, Argo CK, Al-Osaimi AM, et al. Therapy of NAFLD: antioxidants and cytoprotective agents. J Clin Gastroenterol 2006; 40: S51–60.

DiCecco SR, Francisco-Ziller N. Nutrition in alcoholic liver disease. Nutr Clin Pract 2006; 21:245–54.

Marchesini G, Marzocchi R, Noia M, et al. Branched-chain amino acid supplementation in patients with liver diseases. J Nutr 2005; 135:1596S–601S.

Chapter 46

END-STAGE LIVER DISEASE

KEY POINTS

- End-stage liver disease is a complication of cirrhosis that is due to a variety of aetiologies, including chronic viral hepatitis, alcoholic liver disease, non-alcoholic fatty liver disease, autoimmune disease and metabolic disease.
- The manifestations of end-stage liver disease are a consequence of hepatic synthetic failure and portal hypertension.
- Common manifestations of end-stage liver disease include portal hypertensive bleeding, fluid retention and ascites, spontaneous bacterial peritonitis, hepatorenal syndrome and hepatic encephalopathy.
- Patients with cirrhosis should be monitored for manifestations of end-stage liver disease so that appropriate measures can be implemented to prevent and treat complications. This includes screening for oesophageal varices and hepatocellular carcinoma, introduction of prophylactic antibiotics in select circumstances and regular monitoring of renal and liver function. Concomitant therapies should be monitored carefully.

INTRODUCTION

End-stage liver disease is also known as decompensated liver disease. It develops in patients with underlying cirrhosis due to a wide variety of causes, including chronic hepatitis C, chronic hepatitis B, alcoholic liver disease, non-alcoholic fatty disease, autoimmune liver diseases (autoimmune hepatitis, primary biliary cirrhosis, primary sclerosing cholangitis) and genetic or metabolic liver diseases (alpha$_1$-antitrypsin deficiency, genetic haemochromatosis, Wilson's disease). Despite the wide aetiological processes involved in the development of cirrhosis, the manifestations of end-stage liver disease are common to all, and are consequent to the combination of portal hypertension and hepatic synthetic failure (Table 46.1). Extrahepatic manifestations of end-stage liver disease include hepatopulmonary syndrome and portopulmonary hypertension. In addition, the presence of cirrhosis predisposes to hepatocellular carcinoma (HCC), bone disease and malnutrition.

TABLE 46.1: Manifestations of end-stage liver disease
Complications of portal hypertension and portosystemic shunting
• Ascites
• Spontaneous bacterial peritonitis
• Hepatorenal syndrome
• Oesophageal and gastric varices
• Hepatic encephalopathy
• Hepatopulmonary syndrome and portopulmonary hypertension
Consequences of hepatic synthetic failure
• Hypoalbuminaemia
• Hypoprothrombinaemia and coagulopathy
• Hyperbilirubinaemia

ASSESSMENT

History

The essential elements of history taking for patients with end-stage liver disease (Figure 46.1) include:
- Likely aetiology and duration of liver disease:
  - History of alcohol intake (age of onset, daily intake, last use)
  - History of injection drug use (age of onset, last use)
  - Ethnicity and country of birth
  - Family history of liver disease
  - History of obesity, features of metabolic syndrome.
- Precipitants of recent deterioration:
  - Recent alcohol abuse
  - Recent illness, including infections, diarrhoea, vomiting, constipation
  - Recent medication history, including diuretics, sedatives, analgesics, non-steroidal antiinflammatories
  - History of gastrointestinal bleeding
  - Nutritional intake, including salt intake, protein intake.

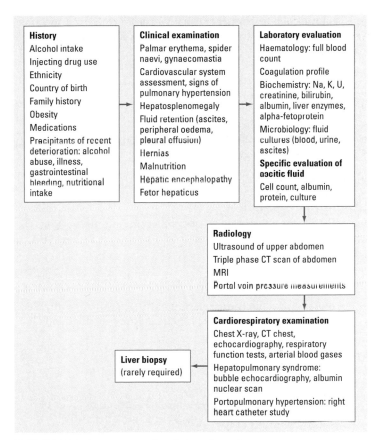

FIGURE 46.1: Assessment of end-stage liver disease.

CT = computed tomography; K = potassium, MRI = magnetic resonance imaging; U = urea.

Physical examination

Assessment of patient with end-stage liver disease (Figure 46.1) should include examination for:

- Palmar erythema
- Finger clubbing (presence indicative of hepatopulmonary syndrome)
- Spider naevi
- Gynaecomastia, loss of body hair, testicular atrophy (in males)

- Cardiovascular assessment (usually reveals hyperdynamic circulation, with warm peripheries and mild tachycardia and hypotension)
- Signs of pulmonary hypertension (may be present in 2%–10% of patients with portal hypertension)
- Hepatosplenomegaly
- Fluid retention (ascites, peripheral oedema, pleural effusion)
- Hernias (periumbilical, inguinal)
- Malnutrition (loss of subcutaneous fat deposits, muscle wasting)
- Signs of hepatic encephalopathy (flapping tremor, cognitive changes)
- Fetor hepaticus.

Laboratory evaluation

In addition to the investigations listed, other specific investigations will be required to determine the cause of liver disease (Figure 46.1).

Haematology

- Full blood count (leucopenia and thrombocytopenia reflect portal hypertension).
- Coagulation profile (prolongation of international normalised ratio [INR] reflects hepatic synthetic failure or inadequate vitamin K absorption).

Serum biochemistry

- Sodium, potassium, urea, creatinine.
- Bilirubin, albumin, liver enzymes.
- Serum alpha-fetoprotein (elevation may reflect HCC, or be related to liver inflammation in chronic viral hepatitis).

Microbiology

- Fluid cultures (blood, urine, ascites, etc, if sepsis suspected, or change in clinical condition).

Evaluation of ascitic fluid

- A diagnostic paracentesis involves the removal of 20–40 mL of ascitic fluid.
- Fluid should be sent for a cell count, albumin, protein and culture (by inoculation into blood culture bottles).
- An ascitic white cell count (WCC) >500 cells/mm^3 or neutrophil count >250 cells/mm^3 indicates the presence of infection (usually spontaneous bacterial peritonitis).

- A serum to ascites albumin gradient (SAAG) of >11 g/L is consistent with ascites due to portal hypertension, rather than malignancy or infection.
- An ascites protein concentration of <10 g/L is associated with a high risk for spontaneous bacterial peritonitis.

Radiologic investigations

- Ultrasound of upper abdomen: a screening test to identify space occupying lesions in the liver, portal vein patency, the presence of ascites, splenomegaly.
- Triple-phase computed tomography (CT) scan of the abdomen: a more sensitive test for identification of hepatocellular carcinoma (classically displays enhancement on arterial phase, and a defect on portal phase), lymphadenopathy, ascites, vascular shunts.
- Magnetic resonance imaging (MRI): can be used safely in patients with renal impairment. More sensitive than ultrasound for detection of hepatocellular carcinoma.
- Portal vein pressure measurements, used in some specialist centres for quantitation of portal hypertension. Involves hepatic vein cannulation, usually via the right external jugular vein. Clinically significant portal hypertension is a hepatic vein–portal vein pressure gradient (HVPG) >10 mmHg (normal 3–6 mmHg). Varices rarely bleed until HVPG >12 mmHg.

Cardiorespiratory evaluation

Shortness of breath is a common symptom in patients with end-stage liver disease. Specific investigations of the cardiorespiratory systems may include:

- Chest X-ray
- CT chest
- Echocardiography
- Full respiratory function tests
- Arterial blood gases on room air
- If hepatopulmonary syndrome is suspected then:
  - Contrast-enhanced 'bubble' echocardiography
  - Technetium-99-labelled macroaggregated albumin nuclear scan
- If portopulmonary hypertension is suspected then:
  - Right heart catheter study.

Liver biopsy

Liver biopsy is rarely required in patients with end-stage liver disease as a diagnosis of cirrhosis can usually be established with a combination of history, physical examination, laboratory testing and imaging. Where an aetiology is not apparent, liver biopsy may occasionally provide additional information, although this would rarely influence further management. In most cases, percutaneous biopsy is precluded because of ascites, coagulopathy or thrombocytopenia, and a transjugular route should be considered.

In patients with end-stage liver disease and a space occupying lesion, ultrasound- or CT-guided biopsy is usually not required to establish a diagnosis of hepatocellular carcinoma if this diagnosis can be made on characteristic imaging and an elevated alpha-fetoprotein level. Patients with small hepatocellular carcinoma lesions will remain amenable to liver transplantation regardless of confirmation of hepatocellular carcinoma.

Severity scores in end-stage liver disease

A number of scoring systems are used to assess severity of liver failure, and are used to determine prognosis, priority for liver transplantation and risks of procedures such as general anaesthesia or portosystemic shunt procedures. The two most commonly used systems are the Child-Pugh (Child-Turcotte-Pugh) classification (Table 46.2) and the Model for End-stage Liver Disease (MELD).

$$\text{MELD score} = 0.957 \times \text{Creatinine (mg/dL)}^* + 0.378$$
$$\times \text{Bilirubin (mg/dL)}^* + 1.12 \times \text{INR} + 0.643$$

* To convert μmol/L to mg/dL, multiply by 0.01652. INR = international normalised ratio.

TABLE 46.2: Child-Pugh score for severity of liver disease.
Child-Pugh A: 5–6; Child-Pugh B: 7–9; Child-Pugh C: 10–15

	1 point	**2 points**	**3 points**
Ascites	None	Slight	Mod/severe
Encephalopathy	None	Grade 1–2	Grade 3–4
Bilirubin (μmol/L) • non-cholestatic • cholestatic	<35 <70	35–50 70–170	>50 >170
Serum albumin (g/L)	>35	35–28	<28
International normalised ratio (INR)	<1.7	1.7–2.3	>2.3

MANAGEMENT

Oedema, ascites and pleural effusions

Cirrhosis is associated with abnormal extracellular fluid volume regulation, which results in accumulation of fluid as oedema, ascites, or pleural effusion. This abnormality in volume regulation is associated with significant changes in the splanchnic circulation and renal circulation that induce sodium and water retention.

The management of fluid retention in decompensated liver disease usually involves a step-wise approach.

- Salt restriction, aiming for 50–100 mmol sodium/day. It is often useful for the patient to consult a dietitian for advice regarding salt content of specific foods.
- Avoid medications associated with salt and fluid retention, including non-steroidal antiinflammatory drugs, antacids, effervescent preparations.
- Fluid restriction is usually only recommended in the presence of hyponatremia with normal serum creatinine.
- Introduction of diuretics, initially with spironolactone, and later with addition of frusemide. Doses should be increased gradually, and patients should be carefully monitored for the development of renal impairment or electrolyte disturbance (hyponatraemia, hyper/hypokalaemia). Maximum doses of diuretics are spironolactone 400 mg, frusemide 120 mg, although few patients can achieve these doses without development of complications. Diuretics should be reduced or even stopped in the presence of hyponatraemia (sodium <125 mmol/L) or a rising creatinine.
- Patients are considered to have refractory ascites when the ascites cannot be mobilised with reasonable doses of diuretics (diuretic-resistant) or if diuretics cannot be tolerated (diuretic-intolerant) because of cramps, hyponatraemia or renal impairment.
- Management options in refractory ascites include:
  - Repeated large volume paracentesis (with intravenous volume expansion, e.g. concentrated albumin 10 g/L ascites removed)
  - Transjugular intrahepatic portosystemic shunt (TIPS)
  - Refractory ascites may be an indication for liver transplantation.

- Nutritional intake and status should be assessed in patients with ascites, and protein and calorie intake increased in malnourished patients (the majority). This may require use of nutritional supplements. Protein intake of 1–1.5 g protein/kg/day is recommended.
- Pleural effusions in cirrhotic patients (hepatic hydrothorax) are thought to occur when ascitic fluid traverses the diaphragm via small congenital or acquired defects in the diaphragm. They occur more commonly in the right pleural cavity. Management options include:
  - Salt and fluid restriction
  - Diuretic therapy
  - Repeated thoracocentesis
  - Insertion of pleural drains and thoracoscopic or operative procedures should be avoided as they are associated with high mortality
  - TIPS
  - Liver transplantation.

Hyponatraemia

Dilutional hyponatraemia is a common manifestation of end-stage liver disease and may occur in the absence of diuretic therapy. Diuretic therapy is the most common precipitant of a falling serum sodium level. It is not uncommon for patients to develop progressive hyponatraemia following admission to hospital without any obvious change to their diuretic dosages. A variety of factors are probably responsible including: adherence to prescribed doses of diuretics, adherence to a salt-restricted diet and intravenous infusions of 5% dextrose while the patient is nil by mouth. Other causes of hyponatraemia should also be considered, such as therapy with other drugs known to cause hyponatraemia (such as SSRI [selective serotonin reuptake inhibitor] antidepressants) or other disease processes, including diarrhoea.

The management of hyponatraemia in patients with marked fluid retention can be extremely difficult. It should be remembered that despite often markedly low serum sodium levels, patients with oedema and ascites have increased levels of total body sodium. Thus attempts at correcting hyponatraemia by infusion of normal saline will result in further exacerbation of the oedema state, but usually with little change in serum sodium level. Appropriate management should include:

- Cessation of diuretics (although further fluid retention is likely to result)
- Fluid restriction (800–1200 mL daily)
- Avoidance of normal saline infusion (use only 5% dextrose if IV fluids are necessary, noting fluid restrictions)
- Dietary salt restriction
- Avoidance of high sodium-containing antibiotics
- Hypertonic saline infusion should not be used, as central pontine myelinolysis may occur on rapid correction of serum sodium.

Patients with renal impairment and hyponatraemia are particularly difficult to manage and should be managed as for hepatorenal syndrome (see below).

Muscle cramps

Painful muscle cramps are a common problem in patients with end-stage liver disease and are often worse during diuretic therapy. Treatment is empirical and no therapies are of proven value. Stretching and massaging the affected muscles may provide relief. Some patients respond to cessation or dose reduction of diuretics or correction of hypomagnesaemia or hypozincaemia. Clinical efficacy of drugs such as quinine has not been established.

Spontaneous bacterial peritonitis

Spontaneous bacterial peritonitis (SBP) is a common life-threatening complication of end-stage liver disease. Patients may be asymptomatic, develop a fever or have worsening encephalopathy. Rarely are there obvious features of peritonitis with fever, chills, abdominal pain and tenderness.

A diagnosis of SBP is made when the ascitic white cell count or neutrophil count is elevated (as discussed previously). Identification of an organism on culture or Gram stain is not required to establish a diagnosis.

Prophylaxis

Prophylaxis with regular daily antibiotics (e.g. norfloxacin, sulfamethoxazole/trimethoprim) should be given in the following situations:

- A previous episode of SBP
- Patients with ascites and very low ascitic protein concentration (less than 10 g/L)

- Patients with ascites who are admitted to hospital with upper gastrointestinal bleeding.

Treatment

Most infections are due to Gram-negative organisms and treatment should be with broad-spectrum intravenous antibiotics, such as a third-generation cephalosporin. In patients receiving prophylactic antibiotics, Gram-positive infection is more common, which will affect choice of antibiotics. The specific choice of antibiotic used will vary according to hospital policy and availability.

The concomitant administration of intravenous concentrated albumin has been shown to significantly reduce the rate of acute renal failure and improve survival in patients with SBP.

Hepatorenal syndrome

Hepatorenal syndrome is a functional renal failure that occurs in patients with end-stage liver disease, almost always in the setting of severe ascites and hyponatraemia. It develops because of marked renal vasoconstriction and concomitant extrarenal vasodilatation that occurs in end-stage liver disease.

Diagnosis

Diagnostic criteria include:
- Low glomerular filtration rate (rising serum creatinine, creatinine clearance <40 mL/min)
- Oliguria, <500 mL/day
- Low urinary sodium concentration, <10 mmol/L.

Hepatorenal syndrome is classified as type 1 (rapid onset of progressive oliguria and rising serum creatinine, associated with extremely high mortality) and type 2 (insidious onset, better prognosis).

Other causes of renal failure should be excluded. These include acute tubular necrosis, hepatitis C- or B-related renal disease (e.g. glomerulonephritis), IgA nephropathy (in alcoholic liver disease), urinary obstruction, drug-induced interstitial nephritis (e.g. proton pump inhibitors, antibiotics).

Potential precipitants of renal failure should be avoided in patients with end-stage liver disease. They should be sought in patients who develop renal failure. These include:
- Infection, including SBP, pneumonia, urinary tract infection, bacteraemia

- Hypotension related to gastrointestinal bleeding
- Nephrotoxic medications, including non-steroidal antiinflammatory drugs and COX 2 inhibitors, aminoglycoside antibiotics, ACE inhibitors and angiotensin receptor antagonists
- Nephrotoxic contrast agents
- Hypovolaemia due to diuretics, limited oral intake, vomiting, diarrhoea, overuse of lactulose, large-volume paracentesis.

Management

- Careful assessment of volume status, including central venous pressure monitoring. Hypovolaemia should be corrected with isotonic saline, however, once euvolaemia has been obtained, sodium intake should be restricted.
- Intravenous antibiotics until infection can be excluded.
- Cessation of nephrotoxic medications.
- Use of splanchnic vasoconstrictors. Choice of agent will depend on availability, but include terlipressin with albumin infusion (the most widely studied), noradrenaline plus albumin or midodrine and albumin. For example:
  - Terlipressin 1 mg IV, 4- to 6-hourly with concentrated (20%) albumin 100 mL IV, twice daily for 7–14 days.
- TIPS has been shown to improve renal function in some patients with hepatorenal syndrome, but in very advanced liver disease may be associated with worsening of liver function and development of severe encephalopathy.
- Consideration of renal-replacement therapy (haemofiltration or haemodialysis) in patients with potentially reversible cause of deterioration, or in those being considered for liver transplantation.
- Liver transplantation is the only therapy associated with long-term survival.
- Primary prevention: all patients with cirrhosis and features of portal hypertension, such as platelet count below 100, splenomegaly, varices on abdominal imaging, should undergo endoscopy to assess for oesophageal varices and be considered for primary prevention. Strategies include:
  - Non-selective beta-blockers, aiming for reduction in heart rate of 25% or <60 beats/min, or
  - Endoscopic band ligation, aiming for eradication of varices.

- Initial management of bleeding:
  - Urgent evaluation of haemodynamic state
  - Fluid resuscitation, via large bore cannulas
  - Blood tests for full blood count, electrolytes and creatinine, liver function tests and cross-match
  - Central venous pressure, arterial monitoring
  - Consideration of endotracheal intubation depending on level of consciousness, and degree of bleeding
  - To reduce portal pressure, commence intravenous administration of:
    - Octreotide 50 μg IV, immediately, then 25–50 μg/h IV for 5 days, *or*
    - Terlipressin 2 mg IV, 6-hourly for 2–3 days
  - Urgent endoscopy to confirm source of bleeding and management with endoscopic band ligation.
- Continued or recurrent bleeding:
  - Repeat endoscopy and band ligation
  - Balloon tamponade
  - Emergency TIPS or surgical portosystemic shunt (depending on local expertise).
- Secondary prevention:
  - Repeated endoscopic band ligation to eradication of varices
  - Non-selective beta-blocker
  - Consider TIPS.

Hepatic encephalopathy

Hepatic encephalopathy is a common manifestation of end-stage liver disease. It has a spectrum of presentations from grade 1 (sleep inversion, poor concentration, personality change) through to grade 4 (deep coma). Sudden development or worsening of encephalopathy should prompt a search for a precipitant such as:

- Gastrointestinal bleeding
- Dehydration or electrolyte disturbance
- Renal impairment
- Use of sedatives or narcotics
- Sepsis, including SBP, urinary tract infection, respiratory infection, cellulitis
- Constipation
- Recent TIPS insertion
- Worsening of liver failure.

In the absence of a readily identifiable precipitant, infection should be assumed and the patient should be started on broad-spectrum intravenous antibiotics, such as a third-generation cephalosporin, according to hospital guidelines.

Management should be directed at correction of the precipitant, airway support if required and the use of lactulose at a dose required to promote two to three loose stools per day. In a deteriorating patient, lactulose 30 mL orally, rectally or via nasogastric tube, may be required every 1–2 hours to induce a rapid laxative effect. Care should be taken not to induce severe diarrhoea, and the patient should be monitored for development of bowel distension.

Protein restriction is not recommended in the management of hepatic encephalopathy. In acute, severe encephalopathy, protein should only be withheld for a maximum of 24–48 hours, then progressively increased to normal intake as recovery occurs. Protein intake should not be restricted in patients with chronic encephalopathy, as these patients are usually markedly malnourished. A protein intake of 1–1.5 g protein/kg/day is recommended.

Hepatocellular carcinoma
See Chapter 44.

Nutritional management
See Chapter 45.

SUMMARY

The manifestations of end-stage liver disease are common to all aetiologies and result from a combination of portal hypertension and hepatic synthetic failure. Clinicians should be aware of clinical signs and laboratory findings in end-stage liver disease, and actively seek precipitants when sudden deterioration occurs. A patient's status can change rapidly from being relatively stable, to being critically unwell. Management of bleeding gastro-oesophageal varices, hepatic encephalopathy, spontaneous bacterial assessment and acute renal failure for example, require rapid assessment and introduction of life-saving interventions. Less acute, long-term management requires careful attention to diet to ensure appropriate salt and fluid restrictions, and adequate protein and caloric intakes, as well as monitoring for complications such as hepatocellular carcinoma.

FURTHER READING

Cordoba J, Lopez-Hellin J, Planas M, et al. Normal protein diet for episodic hepatic encephalopathy: results of a randomized study. J Hepatol 2004; 41:38–43.

Garcia-Tsao G. Current management of the complications of cirrhosis and portal hypertension: variceal hemorrhage, ascites, and spontaneous bacterial peritonitis. Gastroenterology 2001; 120:726–48.

Gines P, Cardenas A, Arroyo V, et al. Management of cirrhosis and ascites. N Eng J Med 2004; 350:1646–54.

Gines P, Torre A, Terra C, et al. Review article: pharmacological treatment of hepatorenal syndrome. Aliment Pharmacol Ther 2004; 20 Suppl 3:57–62; discussion: 63–4.

Moore KP, Wong F, Gines P, et al. The management of ascites in cirrhosis: report on the consensus conference of the International Ascites Club. Hepatology 2003; 38:258–66.

Sharara AI, Rockey DC. Gastroesophageal variceal hemorrhage. N Engl J Med 2001; 345:669–81.

Wong F, Bernardi M, Balk R, et al. Sepsis in cirrhosis: report on the 7th meeting of the international ascites club. Gut 2005; 54:718–25.

Chapter 47

ACUTE LIVER FAILURE

KEY POINTS

- Acute liver failure (ALF) is defined as the rapid development of coagulopathy and mental status changes in a patient with deteriorating liver function tests with no known preexisting liver disease.
- The most common causes of ALF in the Western world include paracetamol hepatotoxicity, idiosyncratic drug toxicity and viral hepatitis.
- The clinical features of ALF result from reduced hepatocellular function and complications involving other organs, including hepatic encephalopathy, cerebral oedema and intracranial hypertension, coagulopathy and bleeding, sepsis, multiorgan failure syndrome and metabolic derangements.
- Initial evaluation is aimed at determining the underlying aetiology, assessing the severity of the illness and prognosis and identifying complications.
- Principles of management include intensive medical management with general supportive measures, aetiology-specific management when appropriate and consideration of early referral and transfer to a specialist transplant unit.
- Liver transplantation has dramatically improved outcomes for patients with ALF, with overall survival rates now greater than 60%.

DEFINITION

Acute liver failure (ALF), or fulminant hepatic failure, is defined as the rapid development of coagulopathy (INR ≥1.5) and mental status changes (encephalopathy) in a patient with rapidly deteriorating liver function tests without known preexisting liver disease. The presence of encephalopathy distinguishes ALF from severe acute hepatitis.

ALF is a broad term encompassing both fulminant hepatic failure (FHF) and subfulminant hepatic failure (or late-onset hepatic failure). FHF is generally used to describe the development of encephalopathy within 8 weeks of the onset of symptoms in a patient with a previously healthy liver. Subfulminant hepatic failure refers to patients with liver disease for up to 26 weeks prior to the development of hepatic encephalopathy. Some patients with previously unrecognised chronic liver disease decompensate and present with liver failure; although this is not technically FHF, discriminating this at the time of presentation may not be possible.

CAUSES OF ACUTE LIVER FAILURE

Acute liver failure represents a syndrome that is the final common pathway for a variety of liver insults. A cause for ALF can be established in approximately 60%–80% of cases. There is a marked worldwide variation in the relative incidence of the various underlying causes. For example, in Australia, the UK and the USA, medications (e.g. paracetamol) and idiosyncratic drug reactions are the most commonly identified aetiologies. In other parts of the world, including Asia, acute viral hepatitis is a leading cause of ALF.

Paracetamol (acetaminophen) hepatotoxicity

Paracetamol toxicity accounts for approximately 40% of cases of ALF in the UK and the US. Hepatotoxicity is dose-related; most ingestions leading to ALF exceed 10 g/day and mortality is higher with doses over 48 g. While most episodes result from deliberate acts of self-harm, a significant proportion of cases result from therapeutic use. Factors increasing susceptibility to hepatotoxicity include regular alcohol consumption, antiepileptic therapy, preexisting hepatic dysfunction and malnutrition.

Idiosyncratic drug toxicity

A variety of prescription drugs, including various antiepileptics (e.g. phenytoin, sodium valproate), non-steroidal antiinflammatory drugs (e.g. diclofenac) and antibiotics (e.g. isoniazid) have been implicated in acute liver failure (Table 47.1). Most cases occur within the first 4–6 weeks of initiating treatment, but can occur years after the drug is commenced. Certain herbal preparations and other nutritional supplements have been found to cause liver injury. In addition, a variety of illicit substances, including synthetic amphetamines, have been linked to ALF.

Viral hepatitis

Hepatitis A virus and hepatitis B virus are the chief causes of ALF in India and other parts of the developing world. However, ALF is an uncommon complication of viral hepatitis, occurring in 0.2%–4% of cases depending on the underlying aetiology. The risk of developing ALF from hepatitis E approaches 20% in pregnant women. Other viral aetiologies of ALF include hepatitis D virus coinfection or superinfection (Table 47.1), Epstein-Barr virus, cytomegalovirus, herpes simplex virus and varicella zoster.

Miscellaneous

There are a number of other less common causes of ALF. Pregnancy-related liver disease may result in ALF, usually in the third trimester. A variety of presentations may be seen with thrombocytopenia and features of pre-eclampsia often present. Wilson's disease may present as ALF, typically in young patients accompanied by the abrupt onset of haemolytic anaemia. The fulminant presentation carries a poor prognosis without transplantation. Autoimmune hepatitis, Budd-Chiari syndrome, toxins (mushroom poisoning, aflatoxins), ischaemic hepatitis and malignant infiltration of the liver are other infrequent causes of ALF (Table 47.1). A definite cause is unable to be identified in approximately 15%–40% of cases of ALF worldwide.

TABLE 47.1: Aetiologies of acute liver failure

Drug toxicity	*Other causes*
• Paracaetamol (acetaminophen)	• Autoimmune hepatitis
• Idiosyncratic drug reactions	• Viral hepatitis
– Halothane	– Hepatitis D virus
– Ampicillin-clavulanate	– Hepatitis B virus
– Doxycycline	– Hepatitis E virus
– Salicylates	– Hepatitis A virus
– Non-steroidal antiinflammatory drugs	• Wilson's disease
– Phenytoin	• Pregnancy
Herbal agents	• HELLP syndrome
• Ginseng	• Acute fatty liver of pregnancy
• Germander	• Ischaemic hepatitis
• Kava kava	• Heat stroke
	• Budd-Chiari syndrome
	• *Amanita phalloides* mushroom toxin

HELLP syndrome = haemolysis elevated liver enzymes low platelet syndrome.

CLINICAL FEATURES AND MAJOR COMPLICATIONS

The clinical features of ALF result from reduced hepatocellular function and from complications involving other organs. Non-specific symptoms such as nausea, vomiting and malaise are common initially, closely followed by the onset of jaundice.

Hepatic encephalopathy and cerebral oedema

Hepatic encephalopathy is a defining characteristic of ALF. Severity is graded on a scale of 1 to 4. In stage 1, patients have subtle impairments in concentration and altered sleep patterns. Stage 2 is marked by drowsiness and confusion often accompanied by asterixis or tremor. Stage 3 is marked by increasing somnolence and incoherence, which progresses to frank coma in stage 4. Hyperreflexia, clonus and muscular rigidity may be present in the latter stages.

Progressive cerebral oedema with the development of elevated intracranial pressure (ICP) plays a major role in the pathogenesis of this condition and has long been recognised as the most serious complication of ALF. The classic signs of raised ICP include systemic hypertension, bradycardia and irregular respirations (Cushing's triad). Intracranial hypertension can result in cerebral hypoperfusion and hypoxia leading to irreversible neurologic damage, uncal herniation and brain death. Direct intracranial pressure monitoring is commonly used in patients with ALF and severe encephalopathy.

Other complications of ALF, including hypoglycaemia, sepsis, fever, hypoxaemia and hypotension, may also contribute to neurologic abnormalities in these patients.

Coagulopathy and bleeding

Patients with ALF have a prolonged prothrombin time primarily because of decreased synthesis of clotting factors. Increased consumption of clotting factors and platelets may also occur, and platelet levels are often $<100,000/mm^3$. Clinically significant bleeding has been reported to occur in up to 20% of patients with ALF. The most common sources include the upper gastrointestinal tract, nasopharynx and skin puncture sites.

Infection

Patients with ALF are functionally immunosuppressed. Established bacterial and fungal infections occur in about 80% and 32% of patients, respectively. The major sites of infection are the respiratory and urinary tracts, and intravascular catheters. Localising signs of infection are frequently absent and a deterioration in mental status may be the only clue. Such patients are at increased risk of worsening encephalopathy and death.

Multiorgan failure syndrome

A hyperdynamic circulation with peripheral vasodilation and central volume depletion leading to hypotension are characteristic of ALF. Respiratory failure is common in these patients and may be due to pulmonary oedema, acute respiratory distress syndrome (ARDS) or pulmonary sepsis. Renal failure complicates up to 50% of cases of ALF and may be due to dehydration, hepatorenal syndrome or acute tubular necrosis.

Metabolic abnormalities

Metabolic derangements, including alkalosis and acidosis, hypoglycaemia and electrolyte depletion (phosphate, magnesium and potassium) are common in ALF. Enteral or parenteral feeding may be necessary to maintain adequate nutritional status.

INITIAL EVALUATION AND PROGNOSIS

The initial evaluation of patients with suspected ALF should be aimed at determining the underlying aetiology, assessing the severity of the disease and the underlying prognosis and identifying complications. The outcome of ALF is related to the aetiology, the degree of encephalopathy and related complications.

History taking should address possible exposure to viral infection and drugs (including herbal medications and other nutritional supplements) or other toxins; collateral history from family members is often necessary. It is also important to ask about the date of onset of jaundice and encephalopathy. Physical examination must include careful assessment and documentation of mental status and a search for stigmata of chronic liver disease (which should be absent). Jaundice is often, but not always, present. Right upper quadrant tenderness is variably present. Liver size may be small, indicating a loss of volume due to hepatic necrosis. Hepatomegaly should raise suspicion of viral hepatitis, malignant infiltration, congestive heart failure or acute Budd-Chiari syndrome. Patients frequently present with hypotension and tachycardia, which results from the reduced systemic vascular resistance accompanying FHF.

In addition to coagulation parameters, initial laboratory examination usually includes routine chemistry (liver function, renal function, electrolytes, blood glucose), arterial blood gas measurements (acid–base status, hypoxia, lactate), full blood count, paracetamol level, viral hepatitis serology, tests for Wilson's disease and autoimmune hepatitis and a pregnancy test in females. The serum ammonia level may be significantly elevated in patients with FHF. Liver ultrasound and Doppler may assist in determining hepatic vein flow and the presence of ascites. Any suspicion of an underlying infection should prompt a thorough search for an infective focus, including cultures of blood, sputum and urine and a chest radiograph. Cerebral computed tomography (CT) may be necessary to establish the presence of cerebral oedema. Liver biopsy is not always necessary, particularly in the context of a coagulopathy.

Determination of prognosis is important as it guides key management decisions, including the need for referral to a specialist transplant centre. However, assessment of prognosis in the individual patient is difficult and cannot be predicted by any single factor alone. The most important variables include the underlying aetiology (paracetamol toxicity, hepatitis A, ischaemic hepatitis and pregnancy-associated liver disease are associated with a more favourable outcome), the patient's age (<10 and >40 associated with poor prognosis) and the degree of encephalopathy (spontaneous recovery less likely with stages 3 or 4 encephalopathy). In general, the best prognoses occur in the absence of complications. Cerebral oedema, renal failure, ARDS, bleeding, and sepsis reduce the probability of survival.

In patients with FHF due to hepatitis A virus, survival rates are greater than 50%. The outcome for patients with FHF as the result of other causes of viral hepatitis is much less favourable.

In patients with Wilson disease, FHF is almost uniformly fatal without liver transplantation.

Rate of development and degree of encephalopathy is a useful predictor of outcome; a short time from jaundice (usually the first unequivocal sign of liver disease recognised by the patient or family) to encephalopathy is paradoxically associated with improved survival. When this interval is less than 2 weeks, the patient has hyperacute liver failure.

MANAGEMENT

The principles of management in patients with ALF include intensive medical management with general supportive measures, preferably in an intensive care setting, aetiology-specific management (when appropriate) and early referral and transfer to a specialist liver transplant unit. Unfortunately, despite aggressive treatment, many patients die from FHF. Prior to orthotopic liver transplantation (OLT) for FHF, the mortality rate was generally greater than 80%. Approximately 6% of OLTs performed in the USA are for FHF. However, with improved intensive care, the prognosis is much better now than in the past, with some series reporting a survival rate of approximately 60%.

Aetiology-specific treatment

Identification of the underlying aetiology not only provides useful prognostic information, but may also dictate specific management options. N-acetylcysteine should be used promptly in any case of known or suspected paracetamol overdose. Other specific therapies include corticosteroids for ALF due to autoimmune hepatitis, aciclovir for herpes simplex virus- or varicella zoster-hepatitis and rapid delivery for ALF due to pregnancy-related liver disease.

General measures

For those patients with ALF in whom no aetiology-specific therapy exists, treatment is limited to general supportive measures that anticipate and manage complications, allowing the liver time to regenerate. Patients with altered mentation should generally be admitted to an intensive care unit. These patients can deteriorate rapidly and require constant monitoring; early consideration of transfer to a transplant centre is important, as worsening encephalopathy increases the risk involved with transfer and may even preclude transfer. Specific criteria have been developed to guide decisions regarding transfer to a specialist liver transplant unit. Management issues relating to the most common complications seen in patients with ALF are outlined below.

Hepatic encephalopathy

The treatment of hepatic encephalopathy (HE) associated with ALF is directed at limiting the production of ammonia and avoiding precipitating factors, such as benzodiazepines. Lactulose may be useful in patients with grade 1 or 2 encephalopathy.

Cerebral oedema/intracranial hypertension

The risk of cerebral oedema in patients with ALF increases with the severity of encephalopathy. As patients progress to grades 3 or 4 encephalopathy, tracheal intubation is usually advised for airway protection and the head should be elevated to 30 degrees. Management issues include prompt recognition and treatment of associated seizures, invasive ICP monitoring and the use of mannitol and hyperventilation to reduce elevated ICP.

Coagulopathy and bleeding

Replacement therapy for thrombocytopenia and/or prolonged prothrombin time is recommended only in the setting of haemorrhage or prior to invasive procedures.

Infection

Routine antibiotic prophylaxis in patients with ALF has not been shown to improve survival. Periodic surveillance cultures should be performed to detect bacterial and fungal infections as early as possible and a low threshold for starting appropriate antimicrobial therapy is required.

Multiorgan failure syndrome

Hypotension resulting from volume depletion should be treated with blood or colloids. Care must be taken to avoid exacerbation of cerebral oedema with aggressive fluid replacement; a central venous catheter may be useful for monitoring intravascular volume status. Vasopressor agents may be required for reduced systemic vascular resistance. Endotracheal intubation and mechanical ventilation are often required for respiratory depression due to coma or impaired gas exchange resulting from pulmonary sepsis or ARDS. Renal function should be optimised by maintaining adequate haemodynamics while avoiding nephrotoxic medications and contrast agents. Dialysis support is sometimes required, with continuous venovenous haemofiltration preferred over intermittent modalities.

Nutrition

Maintaining adequate nutrition is critical in the management of ALF. Oral or enteral feeding is preferable in patients with mild–moderate encephalopathy. Parenteral nutrition should be considered early in patients with grade 3 and 4 encephalopathy.

Liver transplantation

The advent of orthotopic liver transplantation has dramatically improved overall survival rates for patients with ALF from less than 30% in the pre-transplant era to more than 60% presently. Post-transplant survival rates for ALF have been reported to be as high as 80%–90%. In the patient with ALF being considered for transplantation (Table 47.2), the likelihood of spontaneous recovery must be balanced against the risks of surgery and long-term immunosuppression. Approximately 40%–50% of patients with ALF will undergo transplantation. Despite the urgent listing assigned to these patients, a significant proportion will die on the waiting list or develop complications precluding transplantation due to a critical ongoing shortage of donor organs. Some centres utilise artificial liver support systems, although this is still considered experimental.

TABLE 47.2: King's College criteria for liver transplantation in acute liver failure

Paracetamol (acetaminophen) cases	Non-paracetamol (non-acetaminophen) cases
Arterial pH <7.3 or	INR >6.5 or
INR >6.5 and	Any three of the following;
Serum creatinine >301 μmol/L and	• Age <10 or >40 years
Stage 3 or 4 encephalopathy	• Duration of jaundice >7 days
	• Aetiology—idiosyncratic drug reaction, non-A, non-B hepatitis, halothane hepatitis, indeterminate
	• Serum bilirubin >308 μmol/L
	• INR >3.5
INR = international normalised ratio.	

A general approach to the management of patients with ALF is represented in Figure 47.1.

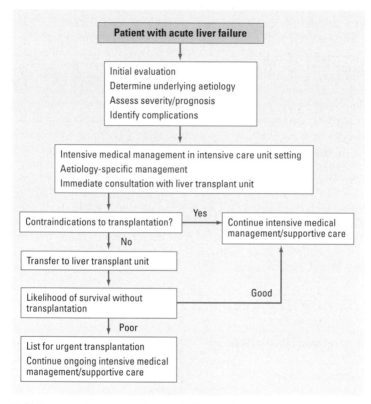

FIGURE 47.1: Management of acute liver failure.

SUMMARY

ALF is a term that encompasses both fulminant hepatic failure and subfulminant hepatic failure. It is defined as the rapid development of coagulopathy and encephalopathy in a patient with deteriorating liver function tests with no underlying liver disease. The most common causes include drug toxicity, acute viral hepatitis and pregnancy-related liver conditions. Patients may present with hepatic encephalopathy, coagulopathy, multiorgan failure and a variety of significant metabolic disturbances. Superimposed systemic infections often complicate the clinical scenario. Patients always require urgent evaluation and management, with the initial evaluation aimed at determining the underlying cause, assessing the severity of the illness and identifying complications. Such presentations necessitate intensive medical management. A high awareness of the need for early liver transplantation is warranted. Acute liver failure is associated with a high mortality rate, but with the advent of liver transplantation the overall survival rates are now greater than 60%.

FURTHER READING

Fontana RJ. Acute liver failure. In: Feldman M, ed. Sleisenger and Fordtran's gastrointestinal and liver disease. Philadelphia: Saunders; 2006:1993–2006.

Gill RQ, Sterling RK. Acute liver failure. J Clin Gastroenterol 2001; 33:191–8.

O'Grady JG. Acute liver failure. Postgrad Med J 2005; 81:148–54.

Polsen J, Lee WM. AASLD position paper: The management of acute liver failure. Hepatology 2005; 41:1179–97.

Sass DA, Shakil AO. Fulminant hepatic failure. Liver Transpl 2005; 11:594–605.

Chapter 48

PREGNANCY AND LIVER DISEASE

KEY POINTS

- During pregnancy expect a 10%–60% drop in serum albumin and a 2–4-fold increase in alkaline phosphatase.
- The transaminases and clotting times remain unchanged.
- Think of cholestasis of pregnancy in a woman who develops an itch mid to late pregnancy.
- Cholestasis of pregnancy is characterised by a rise in the bile acids, without evidence of biliary obstruction on imaging.
- Minor liver function test (LFT) changes can occur in severe hyperemesis gravidarum during the first trimester.
- Development of nausea, LFT abnormalities or right upper quadrant pain in late pregnancy could indicate serious liver problems, such as fatty liver of pregnancy.
- The timing of LFT abnormalities during pregnancy is the best guide to diagnosis, with most pregnancy-related disorders occurring in the third trimester.
- The risk of cholelithiasis increases during pregnancy and postpartum.

ABNORMAL LIVER FUNCTION TESTS IN PREGNANCY

Screening tests for women presenting with abnormal liver function tests (LFTs) in pregnancy should include serology for hepatitis A, B, C, Epstein-Barr virus (EBV), cytomegalovirus (CMV) and herpes simplex virus (HSV) as well as an upper abdominal ultrasound to exclude biliary disorders.

Determine the stage of pregnancy, and whether there is anything in the history to indicate a liver disorder. A pregnancy-related liver disorder should be considered in the event of any relevant past history, or history of medications or in the presence of features of pre-eclampsia.

NORMAL PHYSIOLOGICAL CHANGES IN PREGNANCY

Normal physiological changes in pregnancy are shown in Table 48.1. The mother's blood volume increases by 40%, and her total body water increases by 20%. This is reflected in a 10%–60% fall in serum albumin and also a fall in haemoglobin. Up to 50% of women develop spider naevi and palmar erythema during pregnancy, which is thought to be due to the increasing levels of oestrogen. This reverses quickly post delivery. Serum alkaline phosphatase increases 2–4-fold in the third trimester (placental) and gamma-glutamyltranspeptidase decreases slightly. No change is observed in the aminotransferases (alanine aminotransferase and aspartate aminotransferase) or the prothrombin time. A rise in the transaminases should lead to further investigation.

Up to 3% of pregnancies are complicated by abnormal LFTs at term. The best guide in determining the cause of abnormal LFTs is the timing of the problem during pregnancy (Figure 48.1). The differential diagnoses include:

• Liver diseases unique to pregnancy—generally occur in the third trimester (Table 48.2)

TABLE 48.1: Normal changes in liver function tests during pregnancy

Blood test	Change during pregnancy
Alkaline phosphatase	Increases 2–4-fold (placenta)
Gamma-glutamyl transpeptidase	No change or slightly decreases
Aspartate aminotransferase	No change
Alanine aminotransferase	No change
Bilirubin	No change or slightly increases
Bile salts	No change
Albumin	Decreases by 10%–60%
Globulin	Increases
Caeruloplasmin	Increases
Prothrombin time	No change
Cholesterol	2-fold increase
Triglycerides	2–3-fold increase

- Liver diseases occurring concomitantly—can occur anytime during pregnancy (Table 48.3)
- Preexisting chronic liver problems (Table 48.4).

Pregnancy is associated with an increased rate of gallstone formation. Hence cholecystitis and cholelithiasis need to be excluded in any pregnant woman presenting with right upper quadrant pain, nausea and abnormal LFTs. The differential diagnosis of right upper quadrant pain (Table 48.5) in late pregnancy includes pregnancy-related liver problems, such as liver involvement in pre-eclampsia, even hepatic infarction or rupture. It should be remembered that the gravid uterus pushes up the appendix, and appendicitis in late pregnancy can present with right upper quadrant pain.

Abnormal liver function tests in pregnancy

1st 2nd 3rd Trimester	Differential diagnosis:	Investigation:
	• Hyperemesis gravidarum	• UEC
	• Acute viral hepatitis	• HAV, HBV, HCV, EBV, CMV, HSV, (HEV) etc
	• Preexisting liver disorders	• Autoimmune serology • Chronic HCV, HBV • Past history/antenatal LFTs • US–structural changes • History of alcohol/insulin resistance
	• Cholelithiasis • Cholestasis of pregnancy • Liver involvement in pre-eclampsia • HELLP	• Upper abdominal US • Bile acids/no RUQ pain • Pre-eclampsia features– transaminase rise to fivefold • Microangiopathic haemolytic anaemia/thrombocytopaenia/ pre-eclampsia features
	• AFLP • Liver haematoma	• Encephalopathy/DIC/low BSL • US or CT liver. Large rise in transaminases
	• Budd-Chiari syndrome	• Doppler ultrasound/ascites

FIGURE 48.1: Abnormal liver function tests in pregnancy.

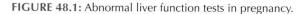

TABLE 48.2: Liver diseases unique to pregnancy

Liver disease	Incidence in pregnancy	Pathology	Maternal mortality	Fetal mortality	Postpartum recovery	Recurrence in subsequent pregnancies
Cholestasis of pregnancy	0.2% in Australia 14% in Chile	Centrilobular cholestasis, canalicular bile plugs	Unaffected	5-fold increase	Complete	Common
Pre-eclampsia	1%	Sinusoidal fibrin deposition, periportal haemorrhage and necrosis	Variable	Variable	Complete	Yes, rare
HELLP	0.2%–0.6%	Sinusoidal fibrin deposition, periportal haemorrhage and necrosis	1%–5%	35%	Complete	3%–19%
AFLP	1/6,000–1/13,000	Microvesicular fatty infiltration in zones 2 and 3	18%	36%	Complete	Very rare

AFLP = Acute fatty liver of pregnancy; HELLP = haemolysis elevated liver enzymes and low platelet syndrome.

TABLE 48.3: Liver disease occurring concomitantly during pregnancy

Disease	Change during pregnancy	Conception	Management	Effects on fetus
Acute hepatitis A, B and C	Acute hepatitis B may be severe in third trimester	Unchanged	Supportive	Depends on mother's health
Acute hepatitis E	Increase in fulminant cases in third trimester	No change	As for fulminant liver failure	Depends on maternal status
Herpes simplex virus	50% maternal mortality	No change	Viral swabs, intravenous aciclovir	Vertical transmission may occur
Focal nodular hyperplasia/hepatic adenomas	Increase in size, may rupture	Normal	Consider surgical removal before pregnancy	Relates to maternal health
Alcoholic liver disease	Probably none	Decreased fertility	Stop drinking	Fetal alcohol syndrome, liver dysfunction in some

TABLE 48.4: Liver disease existing before pregnancy

Disease	Change during pregnancy	Conception	Management	Effects on fetus
Cirrhosis and portal hypertension	10%–20% maternal mortality from liver failure, variceal haemorrhage	Decreased fertility	Close monitoring required	Increased prematurity and miscarriage
Extrahepatic portal hypertension	Probably increased risk of variceal haemorrhage in third trimester and labour	No change	May need oesophageal banding or beta-blockers	Fetal risk related to maternal risk of haemorrhage
Chronic hepatitis B	None	Normal fertility	Hyperimmune gamma globulin plus hepatitis B vaccine at birth	Very low chance of hepatitis B virus transmission in utero
Chronic hepatitis C	Decrease in aminotransferases	Contraindicated when taking interferon and ribavirin; normal fertility	No change	5% vertical transmission, 16% in babies of HIV-positive mothers
Autoimmune chronic active hepatitis	None, unless cirrhotic	Decreased fertility	Continue corticosteroids and/or azathioprine Close monitoring required	Azathioprine: slightly increased miscarriage and perinatal death
Wilson's disease	None, unless cirrhotic	Decreased fertility	Continue chelating agent (penicillamine) Close monitoring required	Some congenital defects on penicillamine
Non-alcoholic fatty liver	None	Unchanged	No change	Nil

HIV = human immunodeficiency virus.

TABLE 48.5: Differential diagnosis for right upper quadrant pain in the third trimester of pregnancy

Diagnosis	Incidence during pregnancy
Pyelonephritis	1%–2%
Cholelithiasis/cholecystitis	3%–5% have biliary sludge
Acute appendicitis	1/1500
Pancreatitis	1/1439
AFLP	1/10,000–1/15,000
Pre-eclampsia + liver involvement	<1%
HELLP syndrome	0.1%
Hepatic haematoma/rupture	1/45,000
Acute viral hepatitis	Same as in the general population
Acute Budd-Chiari syndrome	Rare

AFLP = Acute fatty liver of pregnancy; HELLP = haemolysis elevated liver enzymes and low platelet syndrome.

LIVER DISEASES UNIQUE TO PREGNANCY

Hyperemesis gravidarum

Hyperemesis gravidarum or extreme morning sickness is not a liver disease. However, one-quarter of women hospitalised for this condition have elevated aminotransferase levels. The condition classically occurs in the first trimester and resolves by about week 20, and is usually worse in twin pregnancies and during a first pregnancy. The LFT abnormalities improve on fluid and electrolyte management.

Cholestasis of pregnancy

Cholestasis of pregnancy is the most common liver disease unique to pregnancy. The incidence is about 1/500 pregnancies (0.2%) in Australia. A higher prevalence is seen in Scandinavia and South America (14% risk in Chile). The condition is characterised by pruritus, and an increase in the serum bile acid, and is usually seen in the third trimester. Women present with an itch, without any skin lesions (apart from scratch marks). There may be a history of mothers or sisters with the same problem, and it may have occurred in previous pregnancies. The itch normally goes within days after delivery.

Investigations

An itch is the only symptom; there should be no pain. Check for skin lesions as well as fasting bile acids, LFTs and an upper abdominal ultrasound (to exclude cholelithiasis). Make sure the expectant mother is not taking any drugs or herbs that could cause hepatotoxicity. Take a careful history, because any preexisting liver problem or hepatotoxic drug reaction will become more cholestatic during pregnancy. In addition, any form of cholestasis will cause an increase in serum bile acids. Rarely, thyrotoxicosis or primary biliary cirrhosis can present with an itch during pregnancy. These can be excluded by thyroid function tests and anti-mitochondrial antibody screening, respectively (especially if the problem doesn't resolve postpartum). The hallmark of the condition is normalisation of symptoms and LFT abnormalities within a few weeks post delivery. A liver biopsy is not necessary for the diagnosis, but histology would show intracanalicular cholestasis without inflammation, or liver damage.

The pathogenesis is not understood. Membrane layers of the hepatocytes and the bile canaliculi become slightly leaky during a normal pregnancy (an effect of oestrogen), and this is more pronounced in women with a family history. Genetic deficiencies of canalicular transport proteins are associated with this condition.

Risks to the mother

Apart from a severe itch, cholestasis of pregnancy does not affect the mother (excluding the increased risk of a postpartum haemorrhage). Some women develop LFT abnormalities—the bilirubin may rise to 100 µmol/L and serum aminotransferases increase to 2–10 times the upper limit of normal—but there is no associated increased risk of liver failure. There is a 70% chance of recurrence during a subsequent pregnancy.

Risks to the baby

There is a five-fold increase in the risk of preterm labour and stillbirth. Fetal monitoring does not predict the babies at risk, as there is no problem with placental blood flow. The fetal risk is not understood; high bile acids appear toxic to the baby, and cause myometrial irritability. When the total bile acids are 40 µmol/L or greater, fetal complications can occur. Women with this condition will usually have an induced delivery at 38 weeks, to decrease the fetal risk.

Treatment

Women in whom cholestasis of pregnancy occurs earlier than week 36 of pregnancy or who have high levels of bile acids should be offered treatment. The number of reported pregnant women on drug treatment for cholestasis of pregnancy is small. However studies have shown that ursodeoxycholic acid used at a dosage of 15–25 µg/kg/day in divided doses can improve both the mother's itch and the fetal outcome. Oral dexamethasone at 12 mg daily for 10 days has been used as salvage treatment. Other treatments, such as antihistamines, are not effective. Vitamin K supplements are necessary.

Pre-eclampsia and the HELLP syndrome

Pre-eclampsia occurs in 5%–10% of pregnancies. It occurs particularly with first pregnancies during the third trimester. About 10% of women with pre-eclampsia have minor LFT abnormalities. Pre-eclampsia is characterised by hypertension, oedema and proteinuria. Women with LFT abnormalities have a more severe form of pre-eclampsia.

The aetiology of pre-eclampsia is unknown. It is thought to relate to placental ischaemia, causing abnormal endothelial reactivity, and activation of the coagulation cascade, predisposing to fibrin deposition in small blood vessels. The clinical manifestations of the disease relate to which organs are involved (brain, kidney, liver or all of these).

Women with liver involvement may present with right upper quadrant pain or nausea in late pregnancy, along with other pre-eclamptic features. The transaminases are increased up to five-fold. Massive transaminase rises indicate hepatic infarction or rupture. Close monitoring and expedient delivery is required.

The haemolysis elevated liver enzymes and low platelet (HELLP) syndrome occurs in 0.2%–0.6% of all pregnancies, and in about 20% of women with severe pre-eclampsia. One-fifth of cases occur postpartum. Usually women present after week 32 with anorexia, nausea, right upper quadrant pain and/or bleeding from gums and intravenous access sites. The platelet count is $100,000 \times 10^9$/L or less. The blood film is consistent with microangiopathic haemolytic anaemia. Aminotransferases are elevated (>70U/L), lactate dehydrogenase >600 U/L and bilirubin slightly raised. The prothrombin time may be normal unless complicated by disseminated intravascular coagulation (DIC). The symptoms can be non-specific, and the condition may not be diagnosed until blood tests are done for pre-eclampsia. Characteristically, these women have rapid weight gain. If the diagnosis is suspected and the LFTs are unremarkable, they should be repeated in 4–6 hours, as things can change quickly.

The liver problem in the HELLP syndrome is the same as with pre-eclampsia, with microvascular blood vessel changes in the liver, leading to vasospasm and endothelial damage. This can cause hepatic infarcts. Microvascular ischaemia is exacerbated by thrombosis from DIC, worsening the problem. The histology demonstrates small vessel thrombosis and areas of haemorrhage and ischaemia. Some consider the HELLP syndrome a variant of pre-eclampsia, but it occurs in older multiparous women typically, and occasionally postpartum.

As with pre-eclampsia, the management is expedient delivery. If the condition occurs before 34 weeks' gestation, the mother needs to be monitored in an intensive care setting with intravenous dexamethasone for fetal lung maturity, and delivery as soon as practicable. The mother should be receiving magnesium sulfate, antihypertensives and blood products as required. As there is a risk of developing a hepatic haematoma, the liver needs to be imaged.

The differential diagnoses of liver involvement with pre-eclampsia and the HELLP syndrome include acute viral hepatitis, autoimmune thrombocytopenia and systemic lupus erythematosis, as well as acute fatty liver of pregnancy. Other possible diagnoses include thrombotic thrombocytopenic purpura, and haemolytic uraemic syndrome. There is an uncommon association between these liver problems and fetal fatty acid oxidation defects (see next section).

Acute fatty liver of pregnancy

Acute fatty liver of pregnancy (AFLP) occurs between 1/6659 and 1/113,000 pregnancies, typically in late pregnancy. Symptoms include malaise, vomiting and abdominal pain. Jaundice and signs of hepatic encephalopathy may be evident. Coagulopathy, moderately elevated aminotransferases (500 U/L or below) and renal dysfunction are common. The uric acid is increased. Severe hepatic dysfunction is manifest by profound hypoglycaemia and high ammonia levels. DIC is almost universal, and the condition may progress to fulminant liver failure with death of the mother and the baby.

It can be difficult to differentiate AFLP and the HELLP syndrome, as a percentage of those with AFLP have pre-eclamptic features. The mechanism of the disease is different; AFLP is a severe metabolic disorder. The differentiation is more of an academic exercise, as the management is the same: expedient delivery. It is important to differentiate a severe pregnancy-related liver problem and fulminant viral hepatitis in the third trimester, as the clinical picture can be indistinguishable. Expedient delivery will not help the latter. Pre-eclamptic features favour a pregnancy-related problem, coexistent diabetes insipidus favours AFLP. Transaminases in the thousands favour viral hepatitis. Urgent viral serology is needed.

The pathogenesis of AFLP is unclear. The oxidative stress of pregnancy may cause defective mitochondrial fatty acid oxidation. Although liver biopsy is rarely done, this would show microvesicular steatosis. If a biopsy is needed to establish a diagnosis, a frozen section should be taken, with a histopathologist on standby to do special staining using Oil red O. Without this, the steatosis may not be appreciated.

After the delivery, the mother should make a full recovery without any long-term sequelae, although this may take up to a month. The condition was thought not to recur, but there are reports of an associated mitochondrial fatty acid oxidation enzyme deficiency in both mother and baby in some cases. These women are at risk of a recurrence during subsequent pregnancies (see below).

Fatty acid oxidation enzyme deficiency and severe maternal liver disease

About 20% of babies born to mothers with acute fatty liver of pregnancy have a homozygous deficiency of long-chain 3-hydroxyacyl-CoA dehydrogenase (LCHAD). This enzyme is needed for fatty acid oxidation at the mitochondria to produce glucose during periods of fasting. These babies are at risk of sudden death from hypoglycaemia, and develop severe microvesicular steatosis in the liver, heart and skeletal muscles, dying within months.

Mothers heterozygous for LCHAD do not have abnormal fatty acid metabolism. However, when the mother carries a fetus that cannot metabolise long chain fatty acids, these accumulate in the placenta, and spill over into the maternal circulation. Triglycerides (fatty acids) accumulate in the mother's hepatocyte mitochondria, leading to impaired function.

This problem does not explain most cases of AFLP. However, genetic counselling should be offered, and affected babies identified and given glucose at birth. Affected babies can be identified prenatally in subsequent pregnancies. There is also an association between LCHAD deficiency and the HELLP syndrome.

Hepatic haematoma and rupture

A rare but life-threatening problem occurring in the third trimester. It can occur with severe pre-eclampsia, the HELLP syndrome and AFLP. Other causes such as with cocaine use, liver neoplasm (e.g. enlarging adenomas) and liver abscess have been described. Hepatic haematomas generally occur in the right lobe, and can present with right upper quadrant pain, malaise and abnormal LFTs. A rupture will present, or progress into shock. This is a surgical emergency with high mortality. It is important to consider the diagnosis and image the liver. Women with less severe forms of HELLP, or AFLP earlier in pregnancy, being monitored in ICU should be imaged frequently.

LIVER DISEASES OCCURRING CONCOMITANTLY DURING PREGNANCY

Liver disorders that occur at the same time as the pregnancy are those most likely to be seen in the community.

Acute viral hepatitis

Acute viral hepatitis can occur any time during pregnancy. Most cases are due to hepatitis A virus (HAV) infection, but occasionally hepatitis B or C viruses will be the cause. Epstein–Barr virus and cytomegalovirus (CMV) can cause a mild hepatitis (but are associated with congenital defects). Rarely, hepatitis is seen with herpes simplex virus (HSV) and herpes zoster virus infections. Herpes simplex hepatitis can be severe in pregnancy; a rash will be seen and treatment with intravenous aciclovir is recommended. A history of intravenous drug use, recent travel or illnesses in other family members supports a diagnosis of viral hepatitis. Skin lesions (such as herpes) and stigmata of chronic liver disease may be apparent on examination. Depending on the clinical situation, the following tests might be ordered: HAV IgM, HbsAb (hepatitis B surface antigen), HCVAb (hepatitis C antibodies) as well as EBV IgM and CMV IgM, and perhaps HSV IgM.

Hepatitis E has a high association with fulminant hepatitis in the third trimester of pregnancy and should be considered in women returning from regions where it is seen, such as the Indian subcontinent.

Hepatic adenomas and focal nodular hyperplasia

Hepatic adenomas and focal nodular hyperplasia are both rare, occurring in 1/1,000,000 women. They are usually asymptomatic and may be picked up on a routine ultrasound. If diagnosed before conception, it is recommended that they be removed if they are greater than 6 cm in diameter, as they may increase in size during pregnancy and then spontaneously rupture. Some clinicians recommend symptomatic or larger lesions be removed during the second trimester.

Alcohol problems

Most young women with alcohol problems have insignificant liver problems and a normal fertility. Part of the alcohol counselling should include the risks of alcohol on a subsequent pregnancy and the potential of a baby developing fetal alcohol syndrome. Contraceptives need to be offered to women of child-bearing age with high-risk alcohol intakes.

A subset of this group will have more advanced liver disease or cirrhosis (see next section).

Budd-Chiari syndrome

Pregnancy heightens a procoagulant status. Pregnant women with a thrombophilic condition are at risk of hepatic vein thrombosis (Budd-Chiari syndrome), and will present with an enlarged tender liver and ascites. The condition is diagnosed by Doppler ultrasound. Budd-Chiari syndrome has a poor outcome and affected women need to be managed in a specialty unit. Fortunately, the condition is rare.

Cholelithiasis/cholecystitis and pancreatitis

The bile becomes more lithogenic during pregnancy, with gallstones being present in 12% of pregnancies. The risk of biliary and pancreatic problems increases during pregnancy and immediately postpartum. Cholelithiasis/cholecystitis and pancreatitis need to be excluded in any pregnant woman presenting with right upper quadrant or epigastric pain and/or abnormal liver function tests. Check the liver function tests, serum amylase and lipase, and perform an ultrasound. If imaging is required, nuclear magnetic resonance would be the next choice.

The management of acute cholelithiasis/ cholecystitis and pancreatitis is supportive, however about one-third do not settle and require intervention. Uncontrolled sepsis or acidosis is associated with a poor fetal outcome. Should the mother require endoscopic biliary treatment, aspiration techniques at biliary cannulation with very little screening is suggested. The woman should be imaged, rather than taking pictures, and images should not be magnified, to decrease radiation exposure to the fetus. More fetal X-ray protection is used. The patient should be intubated in later pregnancy, as pregnancy causes gastric stasis, which carries a risk of aspiration. Endoscopic sphincterotomy and/or biliary stenting usually manages the acute problem, so that cholecystectomy can be left until after delivery. Laparoscopic cholecystectomy can be safely performed in the second trimester, and there are cases reporting successful procedures performed safely during the third trimester. Fetal monitoring should be done intraoperatively, and quick-induction anaesthetic techniques used. The woman should be positioned with a 30-degree pelvic tilt on the theatre table during the third trimester. This is to prevent the gravid uterus blocking pelvic blood flow, which could cause placental insufficiency.

Gallstone pancreatitis is rare, but is associated with a poor fetal outcome if the woman becomes acidotic. There is a 70% recurrence rate of pancreatitis during the pregnancy, so endoscopic treatment is justified.

Preexisting chronic liver disease

Most women with chronic liver disease are not of childbearing age. In addition, women with chronic liver disease have a lower fertility rate due to the liver disease. The woman's history is very important, as it is difficult to diagnose chronic liver disease in late pregnancy based on clinical features alone.

Cirrhosis

Pregnant women with cirrhosis have an increased risk of hepatic decompensation and preterm delivery, and need to be closely monitored during pregnancy. If the mother has portal hypertension, a gastroscopy is recommended to screen for oesophageal varices. If there are oesophageal varices, prophylactic banding and/or non-selective beta-blockers may be recommended, depending on their size and risk of haemorrhage. However, there are reported cases of beta-blockers affecting the growth of the long bones. Women with non-cirrhotic portal hypertension have a normal fertility, but risk a complicated pregnancy, and should be counselled, preferably before conception.

Haemorrhage is the most likely adverse outcome. Ascites is rare during pregnancy, and should alert a search for a complication, such as a portal or hepatic vein block.

Chronic hepatitis B

Hepatitis B serology, HBsAg (hepatitis B virus [HBV] surface antigen) is part of routine antenatal screening in most countries. If the HBsAg is positive, check for markers of viral replication (HBV e antigen, HBV DNA). Liver function tests should be checked for evidence of more advanced liver disease and, if present, clotting factors and so forth should be undertaken as part of the work-up of chronic liver disease. Lamivudine has been used during the third trimester in women with a high viral load, to decrease the chance of vertical transmission. The mother should be followed up postpartum, to see if antiviral therapy is needed. As most cases of HBV infection are the result of congenital infection, other family members (e.g. siblings) need to be screened.

These women need to be identified antenatally, because of the high risk of HBV vertical transmission, with chronic hepatitis B developing in the offspring. The baby should receive vaccination and hyperimmune gamma globulin (hepatitis B immunoglobulin) at birth and follow-up vaccinations. The risk of vertical transmission drops to 5% in vaccinated babies.

Chronic hepatitis C virus

Women with chronic hepatitis C usually give a history of previous intravenous drug use, and routine antenatal screening generally includes hepatitis C serology (hepatitis C virus [HCV] antibody test).

The LFTs and HCV RNA status should be checked in women who are positive for HCV antibody (that is, anti-HCV positive). There is a 5% risk of vertical transmission in women who are HCV RNA positive. This rate is possibly influenced by the mode of delivery, but as yet there are no recommendations for preferred mode of delivery. Breastfeeding, however, appears to be safe.

The risk of vertical transmission relates to maternal viral load, and increases three-fold if the mother is coinfected with human immunodeficiency virus (HIV). This high rate decreases wth antiretroviral drug therapy.

The liver enzymes in patients with hepatitis C decrease during pregnancy, so these women need to be tested after delivery to get a more representative picture of the condition and its effect on the liver.

The usual treatment for hepatitis C, pegylated interferon and ribavirin, are contraindicated in pregnancy, and a hepatitis C vaccine has not yet been developed. These women should be followed up after finishing breastfeeding, and offered antiviral therapy, if appropriate.

Autoimmune chronic active hepatitis and Wilson's disease

Both autoimmune chronic active hepatitis and Wilson's disease (also called hepatolenticular degeneration) can occur in young women who want to have families. Pregnancy should be timed and the severity of liver disease assessed. Immunosuppressive drugs (corticosteroids and/or azathioprine) should be maintained in those with autoimmune chronic active hepatitis, and chelating agents (D-penicillamine) in those with Wilson's disease.

Non-alcoholic fatty liver disease and non-alcoholic steatohepatitis

Non-alcoholic fatty liver disease (NAFLD) and non-alcoholic steatohepatitis (NASH) are the most common causes of LFT abnormalities in the general community. As obesity rates rise, so does the incidence of associated liver problems. Liver histology in NAFLD and NASH shows macrovesicular fat, with or without an inflammatory reaction and increased fibrosis. These histological changes are similar to the histology seen with alcohol damage. Whereas the histological features with acute fatty liver of pregnancy are distinct (microvesicular steatosis), NAFLD and NASH remain stable throughout pregnancy and postpartum. The aminotransferases and gamma-glutamyl transpeptidase are minimally elevated. An ultrasound may show a hyperechoic liver consistent with fatty infiltration in the liver. Cirrhosis is unlikely to be seen in this age group. Affected women may give a family history of maturity onset diabetes, and have a higher body mass index. They are more likely to be older and have an increased risk of hypertension, diabetes and cholelithiasis.

The problem occurs in an overweight pregnant woman during the third trimester, where abnormal LFTs are identified on the first set of LFTs ordered. Check for echodensity changes in the liver on ultrasound, and if there is a personal or family history of insulin resistance. The woman needs to be monitored, as often it is difficult to differentiate this NASH from the beginning of a more serious pregnancy-related liver problem.

SUMMARY

The normal physiological changes in the LFTs during pregnancy are reviewed. LFTs are unchanged apart from a drop in the albumin and a rise in the alkaline phosphatase.

Liver diseases unique to pregnancy usually occur during the third trimester, the most common being cholestasis of pregnancy. This occurs in roughly 1% of pregnancies, and is characterised by the development of an itch in an otherwise asymptomatic woman. LFTs may be abnormal, and bile acids increased. Other disorders unique to pregnancy are life-threatening, and are associated with subtle constitutional symptoms and the development of pre-eclamptic features. The level of LFT abnormalities can underestimate the severity of the condition, and close monitoring in a high dependency setting and/or immediate delivery is/are required.

Other conditions occurring concurrently with the pregnancy, such as acute viral hepatitis, need to be excluded by appropriate serology. Likewise, cholelithiasis should be excluded by imaging.

Preexisting liver disorders, such as chronic hepatitis B or C, and autoimmune chronic active hepatitis, will be picked up by the history and appropriate serology. Those with unsuspected cirrhosis, alcoholic liver disease, or non alcoholic steatohepatitis can be a diagnostic problem, particularly if the first set of LFTs is done in the third trimester.

FURTHER READING

Benjaminov FS, Heathcote J. Liver disease in pregnancy. Am J Gastroenterol 2004; 99:2479–88.

Doshi S, Zucker SD. Liver emergencies during pregnancy. Gastroenterol Clin N Am 2003; 32:1213–27.

Glantz A, Marschall HU, Mattsson LA. Intrahepatic cholestasis of pregnancy: relationships between bile acid levels and fetal complication rates. Hepatology 2004; 40:467–74.

Guntupalli SR, Steingrub J. Hepatic disease and pregnancy: an overview of diagnosis and management. Crit Care Med 2005; 33:S332–9.

Kaaja RJ, Greer IA. Manifestations of chronic disease during pregnancy. JAMA 2005; 294:2751–7.

Tham TC, Vandervoort J, Wong RC, et al. Safety of ERCP during pregnancy. Am J Gastroenterol 2003; 98:308–11.

Chapter **49**

MEDICAL PROBLEMS AFTER LIVER TRANSPLANTATION

KEY POINTS

- Common medical problems after liver transplantation include acute rejection, infections, side effects of immunosuppressive medications, vascular and biliary complications and recurrence of primary disease.
- Acute rejection is characterised by specific histological features and usually responds to methylprednisolone.
- Clinicians should be aware that immunosuppressive treatment can attenuate responses to infections and conventional signs of sepsis may be absent.
- Drugs that alter cytochrome P450 activity may influence blood levels of immunosuppression.
- Long-term medical complications of immunosuppression include hypertension, diabetes mellitus, renal dysfunction and atherosclerosis.
- Recurrent hepatitis C virus infection is an important cause of morbidity and mortality after liver transplantation.

INTRODUCTION

Liver transplantation is a well established therapy for end-stage liver disease. Medical problems that occur in patients following liver transplantation include the following:
- Graft rejection
- Infections
- Side effects and drug interactions with immunosuppression
- Recurrence of the underlying disease
- Vascular and biliary complications.

REJECTION OF THE LIVER GRAFT

Hyperacute rejection

Hyperacute rejection occurs minutes after transplant and results in loss of the graft. Fortunately, this dramatic clinical picture is rare in liver transplantation.

Acute cellular rejection

Acute cellular rejection is the most common type of rejection following liver transplantation. Acute rejection may occur at any time after liver transplantation, but most frequently in the first month and may be provoked by adjustments in immunosuppression. Patients with acute rejection usually have no specific symptoms. Increases in serum alkaline phosphatase and gamma-glutamyltransferase with or without an increased serum bilirubin concentration is the usual pattern of biochemical disturbance. It is important to exclude biliary, vascular and infectious causes of abnormal liver function tests. Ultrasound examination and appropriate laboratory testing for infectious agents are usually performed to help exclude these other causes. However, the diagnosis of acute rejection is best established by liver biopsy, which shows endothelitis and biliary duct inflammation. Most cases of acute rejection respond to a pulse of methylprednisolone (1 g intravenously daily for 3 days).

Chronic rejection

Chronic rejection, despite the inference that it is a late event, can occur within 6 weeks of liver transplantation. It is characterised by an elevated serum bilirubin, alkaline phosphatase and gamma-glutamyltransferase. It is more insidious in progression than acute rejection and is characterised by histological features of paucity of bile ducts associated with arteriole obstruction by foamy macrophages. Chronic rejection does not respond to pulse methylprednisolone. Some patients who are on cyclosporine will benefit from conversion to tacrolimus, and patients already using tacrolimus may benefit from an increased dosage to achieve higher serum levels.

INFECTIONS IN THE LIVER TRANSPLANT RECIPIENT

Infections in the liver transplant recipient are common causes of morbidity and mortality. Physicians attending to liver transplant patients should be extremely vigilant as delays in diagnosis and therapeutic interventions can have very serious outcomes. Clinicians should also remember that immunosuppressive therapy can attenuate the usual systemic responses to infection, and conventional signs of underlying sepsis, such as fever and elevated white cell count, may be absent. Innocent symptoms such as mild fever, cough or vague abdominal pain may indicate serious underlying pathology and the threshold for investigation of such abnormalities should be very low.

It is useful to consider the type of infections in relationship to the time since liver transplantation. Bacterial infections are extremely common in the first month after liver transplantation and common sites of infection include the abdomen (peritonitis, cholangitis, hepatic abscess, wound infection), chest (pneumonia, empyema), urinary tract (a consequence of prolonged catheterisation) and intravenous access sites. A definitive focus of bacterial sepsis may not be found or may be unusually located (e.g. teeth or prostate gland). The viral infections that occur early after liver transplantation include herpes simplex virus (HSV) reactivation, which may be manifest by oral or genital lesions, and HHV-6, which may cause pancytopenia and interstitial pneumonia. Cytomegalovirus (CMV) is extremely common after liver transplant but tends to occur after the first month. The clinical manifestations may be protean and include cytopenia, hepatitis, upper and lower gastrointestinal tract ulceration, pulmonary involvement and an infectious mononucleosis syndrome. Diagnosis may be confirmed by the characteristic histological appearance of inclusion bodies in addition to the detection of a circulating structural protein (pp65) and direct identification of virus by polymerase chain reaction (PCR). However, it is recognised that diagnosis may be very difficult on occasions. Ganciclovir is the antiviral of choice and dose adjustments are required for patients with renal failure (see below for antimetabolite interactions). Similarly, reactivation of varicella tends to occur slightly later after liver transplant and can manifest as shingles, disseminated cutaneous disease or visceral involvement. Epstein-Barr virus infection tends to present as a post-transplant lymphoproliferative disorder that may respond to a reduction in the intensity of immunosuppression. The prevalence of opportunistic infections also relates to the intensity of the immunosuppressive regime. While the frequency of opportunistic infection is proportional to the intensity of the immunosuppression regime, patients are always at risk. Vigilance is required for infections with fungi (*Aspergillus*, *Cryptococcus*, *Candida*), protozoans (*Pneumocystis carinii*, *Toxoplasma gondii*) and bacteria (*Nocardia*, *Legionella*).

If the attending physician is suspicious of an underlying infection, a complete history and physical examination are required (including oral, dental and rectal examination). Laboratory tests including full blood count, blood cultures, urine examination (and culture) and chest X-ray should be performed. More specialised investigation will depend somewhat on the underlying symptoms. Abdominal ultrasound, computed tomography (CT) scan and cholangiogram may be performed to investigate the possibility of intra-abdominal sepsis, hepatic artery thrombosis or cholangitis. Fluid collections should be aspirated for laboratory evaluation and brain CT scan and lumbar puncture should be considered if there are any neurological symptoms or signs. Appropriate serology for various viral and opportunistic infections should be performed.

IMMUNOSUPPRESSION THERAPY

Advances in immunosuppression therapy have underpinned the dramatic developments in liver transplantation over recent decades. The most commonly used immunosuppressive agents used in transplantation are calcineurin antagonists (cyclosporine, tacrolimus), antimetabolites (azathioprine, mycophenolate) and corticosteroids (prednisone). Immunosuppressive regimens vary between different units but most patients who have had a liver transplant are maintained on a calcineurin antagonist with or without other added agents (e.g. azathioprine or prednisone).

Drug interactions

The terminal metabolism of cyclosporine and tacrolimus occurs via the cytochrome P450 system. Therefore, agents that alter cytochrome P450 activity—whether it be increased or decreased—have the potential to influence their blood levels resulting in drug toxicity or under-immunosuppression. Important inducers of cytochrome P450 metabolism include the following medications:

- Rifampicin
- Phenytoin
- Carbamazepine
- St John's wort.

Patients commenced on these medications will experience increased drug elimination necessitating dose adjustment. Close monitoring of drug levels should be performed when these medications are prescribed and often the dose of cyclosporine or tacrolimus may have to be doubled. There have been cases when ingestion of St John's wort has precipitated graft rejection. Similarly, cessation of these medications requires appropriate downward dose adjustments.

Agents known to decrease the elimination of cyclosporine and tacrolimus, and therefore increase blood levels, include:

- Ketoconazole
- Fluconazole
- Itraconazole
- Erythromycin
- Cimetidine
- Diltiazem.

The majority of these agents exert their effect by competing for cytochrome P450 metabolism and substantial dose adjustments are often required to avoid toxicity. Features of acute drug toxicity include a rapid decline in renal function as well as neurotoxicity manifesting as seizures, confusion or a fugue-like state.

Two other immunosuppressive drug interactions are worthy of note. An increased incidence of rhabdomyolysis has been reported in patients receiving concomitant cyclosporine and HMG-CoA reductase inhibitors ('statins') and rhabdomyolysis can occur at any time while patients are on these medications. Unfortunately, hyperlipidaemia is a well recognised side effect of cyclosporine and lipid lowering agents are frequently indicated in the post-transplant patient. Statins should be commenced at low dose and routine monitoring of creatinine phosphokinase is recommended. Grapefruit juice can markedly augment levels of immunosuppressive agents by selective post-translational down-regulation of intestinal wall cytochrome P450. There is significant interindividual variation in the susceptibility to this interaction, however patients should be warned about the potential for this interesting drug interaction.

There are two issues of note regarding drug interactions with azathioprine:

* Ganciclovir is usually prescribed in patients who develop CMV infection. A common side effect of both azathioprine and ganciclovir is leucopenia and it is therefore prudent to withhold azathioprine if ganciclovir is prescribed to avoid this potentially serious complication.
* Allopurinol is used to control gout. Allopurinol inhibits xanthine oxidase activity, which is an important step in the metabolism of azathioprine. Therefore, when these drugs are used in combination, the activity of azathioprine is potentiated and its dose must be reduced to approximately 25% of the usual dose.

Long-term medical complications

Many of the long-term medical complications seen in liver transplant patients are a result of side effects of cyclosporine, tacrolimus or other immunosuppressive agents. The major complications can be grouped according to body system.

Endocrine complications

Endocrine complications include diabetes mellitus and osteoporosis. The prevalence of diabetes appears to be higher in the early phase after liver transplantation and may relate to higher doses of corticosteroids and immunosuppression that are used during the early stage. Large studies have suggested that the prevalence of diabetes mellitus is higher in patients using tacrolimus compared with those using cyclosporine. Treatment is based on weight loss, oral hypoglycaemic agents and insulin. Osteoporosis is common in patients with end-stage liver disease who often have a number of different contributing factors. Bone loss is accelerated early in the early post-transplant period due to immobility and the effect of agents, including corticosteroids, used for immunosuppression. Preventive therapy is based on the use of calcium and vitamin D supplementation, as well as bisphosphonates, where indicated.

Renal complications

Renal dysfunction is common after liver transplantation and has multiple aetiologies. Hypertension, diabetes mellitus and drug-induced nephrotoxicity—either alone or in combination—

are responsible for the majority of cases of renal dysfunction. The renal effects of tacrolimus and cyclosporine can take several forms including renal vasoconstriction, thrombotic angiopathy and, in the chronic form, tubular atrophy and interstitial fibrosis with preservation of glomerular structure. A complete history and physical examination are important to exclude other potential contributing factors. The dose of cyclosporine or tacrolimus should be minimised, sometimes by using a small dose of another kidney sparing agent (e.g. azathioprine).

Cardiovascular complications

Prior to liver transplantation, most patients undergo an extensive cardiovascular evaluation. The majority of patients with significant coronary artery or valvular disease are identified in the pre-transplant work-up and appropriate therapy is undertaken or a decision is made not to proceed. Therefore, significant cardiovascular events are unusual in the early post-transplant period. However, accelerated atherosclerotic heart disease developing after all forms of solid organ transplantation is an important cause of morbidity and mortality. Metabolic complications such as diabetes mellitus, dyslipidaemia, obesity, arterial hypertension and renal disease form the basis of a very pro-atherogenic environment in the liver transplant patient. Clinicians involved in the care of liver transplant recipients should regularly screen for conditions that predispose to atherosclerosis. Yearly screening of patients with fasting lipid profiles, regular evaluation of fasting blood glucose, constant attention to weight gain and appropriate attention to blood pressure control are essential elements of care. Cigarette smoking is common in liver transplant patients and must be addressed and strongly and actively discouraged. Patients often have more than one risk factor for coronary artery disease and therefore stringent management of individual risk factors is indicated.

RECURRENCE OF THE UNDERLYING DISEASE

Chronic liver disease due to hepatitis C virus infection is the most common indication for liver transplantation worldwide. Unfortunately, the infection recurs in almost every patient following transplantation. An acute lobular hepatitis develops in 75% of patients within 6 months of liver transplantation, and this can be difficult to distinguish from acute rejection on liver biopsy. A small proportion of patients (approximately 5%) will develop a specific, accelerated course of liver injury termed fibrosing cholestatic hepatitis, which is usually fatal. Approximately 30% of patients will develop cirrhosis by 5 years after transplantation. Thus the course of liver disease in patients with recurrent HCV infection following liver transplantation is greatly compressed compared with non-transplant patients. A number of factors associated with aggressive recurrence have been identified (Table 49.1). Studies utilising pegylated interferon and ribavirin have reported sustained virological response of 25%–35% although dose reductions of both pegylated interferon and ribavirin are common (80%) and therapy has to be ceased in approximately 25% of patients.

Hepatitis B virus (HBV) infection was once regarded as a contraindication to transplantation because of an aggressive and usually fatal recurrence. Post-transplant prophylaxis with a regimen of hepatitis immunoglobulin and an oral nucleoside agent has greatly reduced the risk of recurrence and survival of patients transplanted with HBV is similar to that of patient groups. The frequency of lamivudine resistance due to YMDD and other mutations in viral DNA polymerase is much lower in transplant patients treated with this regimen compared with non-transplant patients treated with lamivudine monotherapy.

Recurrence of hepatocellular carcinoma is uncommon if patients are transplanted when there is a single tumour less than 5 cm in diameter, or no more than three lesions less than 3 cm (Milan criteria) and no evidence of portal vein invasion. Factors that predict increased likelihood of recurrence include vascular invasion and poorly differentiated tumours. Most units regard

---

TABLE 49.1: Risk factors associated with severe histological recurrence of hepatitis C virus

- Pulse methylprednisolone for acute cellular rejection
- Antithymocyte globulin use
- Recipient age
- Donor age
- Cytomegalovirus infection
- Pre-transplant viral load
- Post-transplant viral load

cholangiocarcinoma as a contraindication to transplantation as recurrence is almost universal. Extensive clinical research trials are being performed at some centres in an effort to identify patients with 'favourable' cholangiocarcinoma.

Autoimmune liver diseases such as primary biliary cirrhosis, primary sclerosing cholangitis and autoimmune hepatitis are all known to recur following transplantation, with several series showing recurrence rates of 10%–45%. Hereditary haemochromatosis does not appear to recur following liver transplantation whereas non-alcoholic steatohepatitis is an increasingly common finding after transplantation due to a combination of side effects of immunosuppression and excessive weight gain.

VASCULAR AND BILIARY COMPLICATIONS

Hepatic artery thrombosis

Hepatic artery thrombosis can produce a spectrum of outcomes ranging from an occult event (more likely when occurring as a late event some months post transplant) through multiple liver abscesses and biliary stricturing to acute hepatic failure. Confirmation of the presence of a hepatic artery thrombosis is usually obtained by duplex ultrasonography. Hepatic artery thrombosis requires urgent surgical review with consideration of revascularisation or re-transplantation. Hepatic artery thrombosis can occur months after transplantation and may be associated with a less catastrophic clinical presentation with biliary strictures or liver abscess formation. The most appropriate therapy in these latter situations varies depending on factors including graft function, patient condition and hepatic perfusion.

Mycotic aneurysm

Mycotic aneurysms usually occur at the hepatic arterial anastomosis and rupture of the aneurysm is usually fatal. Survival is dependent on early diagnosis and rapid surgical intervention.

Portal vein thrombosis

Portal vein thrombosis may occur early or some time after transplantation. Occlusion of the portal vein early after transplantation may be associated with a marked elevation of alanine aminotransferase and diagnosis is confirmed by duplex ultrasonography. Early surgical intervention or re-transplantation may be required. In the later postoperative course, portal vein occlusion may present with gastrointestinal bleeding associated with the development of collateral vessel formation or may be asymptomatic. The most appropriate management of a portal vein thrombosis in this situation is dependent on a number of different issues.

Bile leaks

Bile leaks occur early after transplantation and are often associated with abdominal pain, fever and an elevated white cell count. Bile leaks may be associated with hepatic artery thrombosis and a thorough evaluation of vascular patency is required. The site of the bile leak should be properly identified as this will determine appropriate management (e.g. anastomotic leaks often require surgical revision whereas leaks associated with T-tubes may be managed conservatively or by endoscopic stent placement).

Biliary strictures

Biliary strictures may occur at anastomotic or non-anastomotic sites and occur in the setting of bile duct ischaemia or recurrent primary sclerosing cholangitis. Clinical and laboratory features may include an episode of cholangitis or elevated liver function tests. Management of biliary strictures depends on the severity of symptoms, the location of the strictures and liver function. However, endoscopic or surgical management is often required.

SUMMARY

Liver transplantation is a widely available treatment for patients with liver disease. In the early years of transplantation, 1-year and 5-year survival were regarded as the core determinants of a successful transplant program. However, in recent years clinicians have recognised that medical complications related to immunosuppression are the most important determinant of long-term survival of liver transplant patients. As such, proper management of medical issues such as diabetes mellitus, hypertension and renal dysfunction are the central tenets of care of these patients. This chapter highlights the importance of these issues and provides basic instruction on the medical complications seen in the liver transplant patient (Figure 49.1).

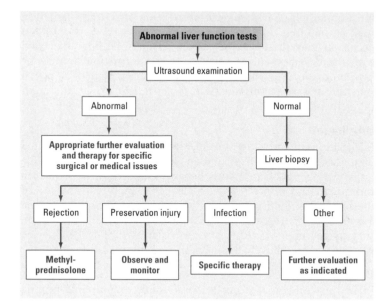

FIGURE 49.1: Approach to the liver transplant patient with abnormal liver function tests.

FURTHER READING

Fischer SA. Infections complicating solid organ transplantation. Surg Clin North Am 2006; 86:1127–45.

Killenberg PG, Clavien P-A, eds. Medical care of the liver transplant patient. 3rd edn. Malden MA: Blackwell Science; 2006.

Muñoz SJ, Elgenaidi H. Cardiovascular risk factors after liver transplantation. Liver Transpl 2005; 11(supp 1):S52–6.

Wilkinson A, Pham P. Kidney dysfunction in the recipients of liver transplants. Liver Transpl 2005; 11(supp 1):S47–51.

Index